T0195413

Global Oncology: Disparities, Outcomes and Innovations Around the Globe

Editors

MARY D. CHAMBERLIN
NARJUST FLOREZ

HEMATOLOGY/ONCOLOGY CLINICS OF NORTH AMERICA

www.hemonc.theclinics.com

Consulting Editors
GEORGE P. CANELLOS
EDWARD J. BENZ JR.

February 2024 • Volume 38 • Number 1

ELSEVIER

1600 John F. Kennedy Boulevard • Suite 1800 • Philadelphia, Pennsylvania, 19103-2899

http://www.theclinics.com

HEMATOLOGY/ONCOLOGY CLINICS OF NORTH AMERICA Volume 38, Number 1
February 2024 ISSN 0889-8588, ISBN 13: 978-0-443-18258-7

Editor: Stacy Eastman
Developmental Editor: Shivank Joshi

Hematology/Oncology Clinics (ISSN 0889-8588) is published bimonthly by Elsevier Inc., 360 Park Avenue South, New York, NY 10010-1710. Months of issue are February, April, June, August, October, and December. Business and Editorial Offices: 1600 John F. Kennedy Blvd., Ste. 1800, Philadelphia, PA 19103–2899. Customer Service Office: 3251 Riverport Lane, Maryland Heights, MO 63043. Periodicals postage paid at New York, NY and at additional mailing offices. Subscription prices are $498.00 per year (domestic individuals), $100.00 per year (domestic students/residents), $525.00 per year (Canadian individuals), $100.00 per year (Canadian students/residents), $597.00 per year (international individuals), and $255.00 per year (international students/residents). For institutional access pricing please contact Customer Service via the contact information below. International air speed delivery is included in all *Clinics* subscription prices. All prices are subject to change without notice. **POSTMASTER:** Send address changes to *Hematology/Oncology Clinics of North America*, Elsevier Health Sciences Division, Subscription Customer Service, 3251 Riverport Lane, Maryland Heights, MO 63043. Customer Service (orders, claims, online, change of address): Elsevier Health Sciences Division, Subscription **Customer Service, 3251 Riverport Lane, Maryland Heights, MO 63043. Tel: 1-800-654-2452 (U.S. and Canada); 314-447-8871 (outside U.S. and Canada). Fax: 314-447-8029. E-mail: journalscustomerservice-usa@elsevier.com (for print support); journalsonlinesupport-usa@elsevier.com (for online support).**

Reprints. For copies of 100 or more, of articles in this publication, please contact the Commercial Reprints Department, Elsevier Inc., 360 Park Avenue South, New York, New York 10010-1710; Tel.: 212-633-3874, Fax: 212-633-3820, E-mail: reprints@elsevier.com

Hematology/Oncology Clinics of North America is covered in *MEDLINE/PubMed (Index Medicus), EMBASE/ Excerpta Medica, and BIOSIS.*

Contributors

CONSULTING EDITORS

GEORGE P. CANELLOS, MD
William Rosenberg Professor of Medicine, Department of Medical Oncology, Dana-Farber Cancer Institute, Boston, Massachusetts, USA

EDWARD J. BENZ Jr, MD
Professor, Pediatrics, Harvard Medical School, Richard and Susan Smith Professor, Medicine, Harvard Medical School, Professor, Genetics, Harvard Medical School, President and CEO Emeritus, Office of the President, Dana-Farber Cancer Institute, Boston, Massachusetts, USA

EDITORS

MARY D. CHAMBERLIN, MD
Associate Professor of Medicine, Department of Medicine/Hematology-Oncology, Dartmouth Geisel School of Medicine, Dartmouth College of Medicine, Dartmouth Cancer Center at Dartmouth-Hitchcock Medical Center, Lebanon, New Hampshire, USA

NARJUST FLOREZ, MD
Associate Director of Cancer Care Equity, Medical Oncology, Dana-Farber Brigham Cancer Center, Boston, Massachusetts, USA

AUTHORS

OYEPEJU ABIOYE, MD
MSc Candidate, University of the Witwatersrand, School of Public Health, Johannesburg, South Africa

INAS ABUALI, MD
Division of Hematology and Oncology, Massachusetts General Hospital, Harvard Medical School, Boston, Massachusetts, USA

RIAZ AGAHI, PhD
Department of Diagnostic Health Sciences, Heimerer College, Evidence Synthesis Group, Prishtina, Kosovo

REGINA BARRAGAN-CARRILLO, MD
Department of Hemato-Oncology, Instituto Nacional de Ciencias Médicas y Nutrición Salvador Zubirán, Mexico City, Mexico

RICHARD J. BARTH JR, MD
Department of Surgery, Section of General Surgery, Dartmouth College of Medicine, Dartmouth Cancer Center at Dartmouth-Hitchcock Medical Center, Lebanon, New Hampshire, USA

SUYAPA BEJARANO, MD
Department of Radiation Oncology, Liga Contra el Cancer, San Pedro Sula, Honduras

STEVE P. BENSEN, MD
Dartmouth Geisel School of Medicine, Lebanon, New Hampshire, USA

PRARTHNA V. BHARDWAJ, MBBS, FACP
Division of Hematology-Oncology, University of Massachusetts Chan Medical School - Baystate, Springfield, Massachusetts, USA

CHRISTOPHER BOOTH, MD
Professor of Oncology and Public Health Sciences, Queen's University, Kingston, Canada

GABRIEL A. BROOKS, MD
Dartmouth Cancer Center, Lebanon, New Hampshire, USA

JETA BUNJAKU, MD, PhD
Evidence Synthesis Group, Prishtina, Kosovo

ANNE CHRISTINE BUTEAU, MD
Dartmouth-Hitchcock Medical Center, Lebanon, New Hampshire, USA

ALICIA CASTELO-LOUREIRO, MD
Medical Oncology Division, Hospital Universitario 12 de Octubre, Madrid, Spain

MARY D. CHAMBERLIN, MD
Associate Professor of Medicine, Department of Medicine/Hematology-Oncology, Dartmouth Geisel School of Medicine, Dartmouth College of Medicine, Dartmouth Cancer Center at Dartmouth-Hitchcock Medical Center, Lebanon, New Hampshire, USA

MARIE ANNE CHRISTINE BUTEAU, MD
Department of Hematology-Oncology, Dartmouth Geisel School of Medicine, Hanover, New Hampshire, USA

PAMELA CONTRERAS-CHAVEZ, MD
Division of Hematology and Oncology, Dana-Farber Cancer Institute, St. Elizabeth's Medical Center, Brighton, Massachusetts, USA

LUQMAN K. DAD, MD, MBA
Department of Radiation Oncology, Columbia University Irving Medical Center, New York, New York, USA

SHQIPTAR DEMACI, MD
Department of Thoracic Surgery, University Clinical Center of Kosovo, Prishtina, Kosovo

RENUKA DULALA, MD
Division of Hematology-Oncology, Holyoke Medical Center, Holyoke, Massachusetts, USA

VINCENT DUSABEJAMBO, MBBS
University of Rwanda College of Medicine and Health Sciences, Kigali, Rwanda

NARJUST FLOREZ, MD
Associate Director of Cancer Care Equity, Medical Oncology, Dana-Farber Brigham Cancer Center, Boston, Massachusetts, USA

VICTORIA FORBES, MD, MS
University of Connecticut Health Center, Carole and Ray Neag Comprehensive Cancer Center, Farmington, Connecticut, USA

RAMAPRIYA GANTI, MD, PhD
Department of Radiology and Medical Imaging, University of Virginia, Charlottesville, Virginia, USA

GOKSU GOÇ, MD
Department of Obstetrics and Gynecology, American Hospital, Prishtina, Kosovo

SYBIL R. GREEN, JD, RPh, MHA
American Society of Clinical Oncology, Alexandria, Virginia, USA

KRENARE GREZDA, MD
Evidence Synthesis Group, Prishtina, Kosovo

TEFTA ISUFAJ HALITI, MD, PhD Candidate
Clinic of Obstetrics and Gynecology, University Clinical Centre of Kosovo, Faculty of Medicine, University of Hasan Prishtina, Prishtina, Kosovo

NORRISA HAYNES, MD, MPH, MSHP
Yale University, New Haven, Connecticut, USA

KRESHNIKE DEDUSHI HOTI, MD, PhD
Faculty of Medicine, University of Hasan Prishtina, Clinic of Radiology, University Clinical Centre of Kosovo, Prishtina, Kosovo

ILIR HOXHA, MD, PhD, MPH
The Dartmouth Institute for Health Policy and Clinical Practice, Dartmouth Geisel School of Medicine, Lebanon, New Hampshire, USA; Evidence Synthesis Group, Research Unit, Heimerer College, Prishtina, Kosovo

LOT HOXHA, MD
Evidence Synthesis Group, Prishtina, Kosovo

ANDRIY HRYNKIV, MD
Chemotherapy Department, Lviv Regional Cancer Center of Ukraine, Lviv, Ukraine

DAFINA ADEMI ISLAMI, MD, PhD
Oncology Clinic, University Clinical Center of Kosovo, Prishtina, Kosovo

KATHYA JIMENEZ, MD
Universidad Evangelica de El Salvador, El Salvador

ANGANILE KALINGA, MD
Department of Radiology and Medical Imaging, Muhimbili University of Health and Allied Sciences Main campus, Dar Es Salaam, Tanzania

MEGAN KASSICK, MD, MPH
Department of Radiation Oncology, University of Pennsylvania, Philadelphia, Pennsylvania, USA

LINDA S. KENNEDY, MEd
Strategic Initiatives & Global Oncology at the Dartmouth Cancer Center, Dartmouth Health, Lebanon, New Hampshire, USA

OLGA KHAN, MD
World Bank Ukraine, Kyiv, Ukraine

LAUREN KIEL
Dana-Farber Cancer Institute, Harvard Medical School, Boston, Massachusetts, USA

ALBA J. KIHN-ALARCÓN, MD, MSc
Research Department, Liga Nacional Contra el Cáncer & Instituto de Cancerología, Guatemala City, Guatemala

ARBER LAMA, MD, PhD
Evidence Synthesis Group, Prishtina, Kosovo

ANDREW P. LOEHRER, MD, MPH
Dartmouth-Hitchcock Medical Center, Dartmouth Cancer Center, Lebanon, New Hampshire, USA

CHANDRAVATHI LOKE, MD
Division of Hematology-Oncology, University of Massachusetts Chan Medical School - Baystate, Springfield, Massachusetts, USA

FREDERICK L. MAKRAUER, MD
Assistant Professor of Medicine - Part Time, Harvard Medical School, Division of Gastroenterology, Hepatology and Endoscopy, Brigham and Women's Hospital, Boston, Massachusetts, USA

ROHINI MANDAL, BA
Dartmouth College, Hanover, New Hampshire, USA

ACHILLE MANIRAKIZA, MD
Oncology Unit, Department of Medicine, King Faisal Hospital, Rwanda

GUSTAVO NADER MARTA, MD, PhD
Department of Radiation Oncology, Hospital Sírio-Libanês, Sao Paulo, Brazil

KELLY MEZA, MD
Division of Internal Medicine, Baylor College of Medicine, Houston, Texas, USA

FRANK J. MINJA, MD
Department of Radiology and Imaging Sciences, Emory University School of Medicine, Atlanta, Georgia, USA

RUBENA MOJSIU, MD, PhD
Obstetric Gynecologic University Hospital "Koco Gliozheni," Tirana, Albania

FABIO YNOE MORAES, MD, MBA, PhD
Division of Radiation Oncology, Department of Oncology, Kingston General Hospital, Queen's University, Kingston, Ontario, Canada

MIDHET NASIM, MS
Evidence Synthesis Group, Prishtina, Kosovo; Japan International Cooperation Agency, Mother and Child Health Project, Lahore, Punjab, Pakistan

LETICIA NOGUEIRA, PhD, MPH
Scientific Director, Surveillance and Health Equity Sciences, American Cancer Society, Palm Harbor, Florida, USA

KATHRYN NUNES, BA
Sidney Kimmel Medical College, Philadelphia, Pennsylvania, USA

TOMA S. OMOFOYE, MD
Department of Breast Imaging, The University of Texas MD Anderson Cancer Center, Houston, Texas, USA

CINDY MEDINA PABON, MD
Division of Hematology and Oncology, The University of Texas MD Anderson Cancer Center, Houston, Texas, USA

JARED PASETSKY, MD
Department of Radiation Oncology, Columbia University Irving Medical Center, New York, New York, USA

CECÍLIA FÉLIX PENIDO MENDES DE SOUSA, MD
Department of Radiation Oncology, Hospital Sírio-Libanês, Sao Paulo, Brazil

TAWANDA PESANAYI, MS
Evidence Synthesis Group, Prishtina, Kosovo

DOUG PYLE, MBA
American Society of Clinical Oncology (ASCO), Alexandria, Virginia, USA

SENTHIL RAJAPPA, MD
Department of Medical Oncology, Basavatarakam Indo-American Cancer Hospital and Research Institute, Hyderabad, Telangana, India

IVY RIANO, MD
Division of Hematology and Oncology, Dartmouth Cancer Center, Dartmouth Geisel School of Medicine, Lebanon, New Hampshire, USA

TIMOTHY B. ROONEY, MD
Associate Professor and Division Chief of Breast Imaging, Department of Radiology and Medical Imaging, UVA Health, Charlottesville, Virginia, USA

FIDEL RUBAGUMYA, MD
Department of Oncology, Rwanda Military Hospital, Kigali, Rwanda

DEO RUHANGAZA, MD
Department of Pathology, Butaro Hospital, University of Global Health Equity, Rwanda

FITIM SADIKU, MS
Evidence Synthesis Group, Prishtina, Kosovo

VEAUTHYELAU SAINT-JOY, MD
Centre Hospitalier de la Basse-Terre, Basse-Terre, Guadeloupe, France

ERZA SELMANI, MSc
Research Unit, Heimerer College, Evidence Synthesis Group, Prishtina, Kosovo

JETON SHATRI, MD, PhD
Clinical of Radiology, University Clinical Center of Kosovo, Faculty of Medicine, Department of Anatomy, University of Prishtina, Prishtina, Kosovo

ENRIQUE SOTO-PEREZ-DE-CELIS, MD, PhD, FASCO
Department of Geriatrics, Instituto Nacional de Ciencias Médicas y Nutrición Salvador Zubirán, Mexico City, Mexico

CHARLES R. THOMAS JR, MD
Professor and Chief, Radiation Oncology, Dartmouth Cancer Center, Dartmouth Geisel School of Medicine, Hanover, New Hampshire, USA

OREST TRIL, MD
Regional Oncology Center for Treatment and Diagnostic, Lviv, Ukraine

GREGORY J. TSONGALIS, PhD
Pathology and Laboratory Medicine, Dartmouth Health, Dartmouth Cancer Center,
Lebanon, New Hampshire, USA; Dartmouth Geisel School of Medicine, Hanover, New
Hampshire, USA

VERNA VANDERPUYE, MD
Consultant Clinical Oncologist, National Center for Radiotherapy, Oncology and Nuclear
Medicine, Korlebu Teaching Hospital, Accra

ANA I. VELAZQUEZ, MD, MSc
Division of Hematology/Oncology, Department of Medicine, Helen Diller Family
Comprehensive Cancer Center, University of California, San Francisco, San Francisco,
California, USA

FAHREDIN VESELAJ, MD, PhD
Faculty of Medicine, Department of Surgery, University of Prishtina, Prishtina, Kosovo

LUCIA VIOLA, MD
Fundación Neumológica Colombiana, Centro de Tratamientoe Investigación Sobre
Cáncer Luis Carlos Sarmiento Angulo (CTIC), Bogotá, Colombia

TIM WALKER, MBBS, FRACP, MPHTM
Calvary Mater Newcastle, University of Newcastle, Newcastle, Australia

KAREN M. WINKFIELD, MD, PhD
Vanderbilt University Ingram Cancer Center, Meharry-Vanderbilt Alliance, Nashville,
Tennessee, USA

Contents

Part I: Global Oncology Around the Globe: Current Status by Region

> Inequity exists along the continuum of cancer and cancer care delivery in the United States. Marginalized populations have later stage cancer at diagnosis, decreased likelihood of receiving cancer-directed care, and worse outcomes from treatment. These inequities are driven by historical, structural, systemic, interpersonal, and internalized factors that influence cancer across the pathologic and clinical continuum. To ensure equity in cancer care, interventions are needed at the level of policy, care delivery, interpersonal communication, diversity within the clinical workforce, and clinical trial accessibility and design.

> Cervical cancer is a health crisis affecting women and their families across the world. It is known that developed countries have comprehensive protocols with recommendations regarding workforce, expertise, and medical resources to address this common cancer among women. In contrast, disparities in addressing cervical cancer remain present in Latin America and Caribbean countries. Here, we reviewed the current strategies of cervical cancer prevention and control in the region.

> Central America and the Caribbean is a highly heterogeneous region comprising more than 30 countries and territories with more than 200 million inhabitants. Although recent advances in the region have improved access to cancer care, there are still many disparities and barriers for obtaining high-quality cancer treatments, particularly for those from disadvantaged populations, immigrants, and rural areas. In this article, we provide an overview of cancer care in Central America and the Caribbean, with

selected examples of issues related to disparities in access to care and suggest solutions and strategies to move forward.

State of Cancer Control in South America: Challenges and Advancement Strategies

Ivy Riano, Ana I. Velazquez, Lucia Viola, Inas Abuali, Kathya Jimenez, Oyepeju Abioye, and Narjust Florez

Cancer is a major public health problem in South America. The cancer mortality burden is increasing in the region due to its presentation at later stages, which is related to limited access to cancer care. This results in a noticeable inequity in provisions of cancer care including specialized screening programs, as well as cancer-related treatments such as personalized medicine, radiation therapy, palliative care, and survivorship services. Consequently, South America faces many challenges for cancer control, most of them deriving from a lack of funding and unequal distribution of resources and cancer services, affecting mostly the underserved populations in the region.

Fighting Cancer in Ukraine at Times of War

Erza Selmani, Ilir Hoxha, Orest Tril, Olga Khan, Andriy Hrynkiv, Leticia Nogueira, Doug Pyle, and Mary D. Chamberlin

The resilience of the system in most specialized oncological institutions in Ukraine should be acknowledged, as well as the level of provision of high-quality special care quickly recovered in the center and areas close to a war zone. This situation has undoubtedly impacted global cancer research progress, as Ukraine is an important venue for many cancer trials.

Impact of Prostate Cancer in Eastern Europe and Approaches to Treatment and Policy

Riaz Agahi, Fahredin Veselaj, Dafina Ademi Islami, Erza Selmani, Olga Khan, and Ilir Hoxha

Prostate cancer is among the most prevalent cancer globally and within Eastern Europe, where there are also higher levels of mortality compared with Western Europe. Cancer control plans exist in most countries in the region. Attention should be given to devising and implementing optimal screening initiatives. Our review has identified that a lack of resources and health system dysfunctions hamper progress in ameliorating the burden of prostate cancer. Regional cooperation is needed as well as drawing on guidelines and findings from elsewhere. Health institutions must also know the latest developments and set up systems that allow swift adoption.

The Impact of Climate Change on Global Oncology

Leticia Nogueira and Narjust Florez

Climate change is the greatest threat to human health of our time, with significant implications for global cancer control efforts. The changing frequency and behavior of climate-driven extreme weather events results in more frequent and increasingly unanticipated disruptions in access to cancer care. Given the significant threat that climate change poses to cancer control efforts, oncology professionals should champion initiatives that help protect the health and safety of patients with cancer, such as enhancing emergency preparedness and response efforts and reducing emissions from our own professional activities, which has health cobenefits for the entire population.

Prarthna V. Bhardwaj, Renuka Dulala, Senthil Rajappa, and Chandravathi Loke

Breast cancer is the most common cancer in urban Indian women and the second most common cancer in all Indian women. The epidemiology as well as biology of this cancer seems to be different in the Indian subcontinent when compared with the West. The lack of population-based breast cancer screening programs and delay in seeking a medical consult due to financial and social reasons, including lack of awareness and fear related to a cancer diagnosis, results in delayed diagnosis.

Part II: Innovations to Improve Access and Outcomes

Ilir Hoxha, Fitim Sadiku, Lot Hoxha, Midhet Nasim, Marie Anne Christine Buteau, Krenare Grezda, and Mary D. Chamberlin

Lifestyle factors play a major role in the risk of breast cancer. This review aimed to examine the size of the effect of select lifestyle factors on risk for breast cancer and assess the quality of existing evidence. The authors performed an umbrella review of systematic reviews. The authors found an increased risk for breast cancer associated with obesity, alcohol intake, and smoking and a decreased risk due to physical activity. The evidence for sleep disruption and duration indicates risk for breast cancer, but it is limited in size, statistical significance, and quality of evidence.

Jeta Bunjaku, Arber Lama, Tawanda Pesanayi, Jeton Shatri, Mary D. Chamberlin, and Ilir Hoxha

This review explores the effect of common everyday factors, such as alcohol, tea and coffee consumption, on the risk for lung cancer. We performed an umbrella review of current systematic reviews. The risk for lung cancer was increased with alcohol or coffee intake and decreased with tea intake. While evidence for alcohol is of low quality, the effect of coffee may be confounded by the smoking effect. The protective effect of tea intake is present, but the evidence is also of low quality.

Victoria Forbes, Mary D. Chamberlin, Vincent Dusabejambo, Tim Walker, Steve P. Bensen, Norrisa Haynes, Kathryn Nunes, Veauthyelau Saint-Joy, and Frederick L. Makrauer

Our international partnerships have fostered longstanding collaborative relationships leading to the development of unique, locally-designed, and sustainable training programs that serve as models for global health education and cooperation.

> Due to the current limited capacity to provide digital mammography-based
> screening to all women, and the lack of modern surgical oncology meth-
> ods, mastectomy is still the predominant form of surgical treatment in
> many parts of the world. As such there is little incentive to detect breast
> cancer earlier and significant fear of treatment and outcomes continues
> to contribute to late presentations. Neoadjuvant chemotherapy, pre-oper-
> ative breast MRI and surgical mapping techniques can combine forces to
> allow for more women to be treated with breast conservation, decrease
> fear of treatment and improve outcomes.

> Diagnostic pathology services in low and middle-income countries are
> often hindered by lack of expertise, equipment, and reagents. However,
> there are also educational, cultural, and political decisions, which must
> be addressed in order to provide these services successfully. In this re-
> view, we describe some of the infrastructure barriers that must be over-
> come and provide 3 examples of implementing molecular testing in
> Rwanda and Honduras despite initial lack of resources.

> Radiation therapy is a critical modality for cancer treatment. Greater than
> 80% of the global population lack access to and expertise with the tech-
> nological advancements that allow for state-of-the-art treatments that
> are more accessible in the West. What follows is a review of a two-pronged
> solution to help address this global gap to technology and innovation: (1)
> trainee engagement and (2) industry partnerships. We hope to galvanize
> our readers to see the immense potential for success if we may synergize
> efforts in education and with our partners in private industry to help ad-
> dress critical unmet needs in emerging economies of the globe.

> Although current value frameworks and economic models have allowed us
> to better quantify the net benefit associated with cancer therapy, holistic
> cancer care must consider patient time, family and social values, and overall
> life expectancy. Training programs must include training in health services
> research, difficult conversations, and shared decision-making strategies
> that are developed in social and cultural frameworks for their settings.

We present subspecialty radiologist training for breast imaging at an Academic center in Dar Es Salaam, Tanzania. The training incorporates remote, in-person, asynchronous and synchronous teaching methods and multidisciplinary conferences. We use a team of US academic faculty under the auspices of the Radiological Society of North America Global Learning centers paradigm. Trainees are Tanzanian radiologists who are pursuing an additional specialization degree in Women's imaging, utilizing an approved 2-year curriculum. Challenges and opportunities in providing image-guided intervention and diagnosis training in the low- and middle-income settings are presented.

This study investigated whether combining International Ovarian Tumor Analysis (IOTA) Simple Rules with tumor biomarkers would improve the diagnostic accuracy for early detection of adnexal malignancies. Receiver operating characteristic curve analysis of suspected adnexal tumors was performed in 226 women admitted for surgery at the University Clinical Center of Kosovo. Primary outcome was the diagnostic accuracy of the combination of adnexal mass biomarkers and IOTA Simple Rules. IOTA Simple Rules combined with biomarker indications increased the diagnostic accuracy of classifying adnexal masses. Data analysis of individual measures showed that ferritin had the lowest rate of sensitivity.

HEMATOLOGY/ONCOLOGY
CLINICS OF NORTH AMERICA

SERIES OF RELATED INTEREST

Surgical Oncology Clinics
https://www.surgonc.theclinics.com
Advances in Oncology
https://www.advances-oncology.com

THE CLINICS ARE AVAILABLE ONLINE!
Access your subscription at:
www.theclinics.com

Erratum

In the December 2023 Hematology/Oncology Clinics (Volume 37, Issue 6) article, *"Chimeric Antigen Receptor T Cells in Hodgkin and T-Cell Lymphomas,"* support provided by Stand Up to Cancer Meg Vosburg T Cell Lymphoma Dream Team Grant should have been cited in the Acknowledgments on page 1121.

Hematol Oncol Clin N Am 38 (2024) xv
https://doi.org/10.1016/j.hoc.2023.11.001
0889-8588/24/© 2023 Elsevier Inc. All rights reserved.

Foreword

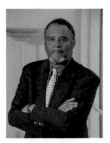

Charles R. Thomas Jr, MD,
Contributor

Global oncology is the highest priority for clinicians, policy-makers, and most importantly, patients, who seek to narrow the geographic disparities in access to care and outcomes from cancer diagnosis and treatment. A pair of the premier thought leaders in global oncology, Drs Mary Chamberlin and Narjust Florez, has assembled this two-issue focus on *Hematology/Oncology Clinics of North America*. The contributors not only have attempted to present the current state of cancer care around the world but also have made a superior effort to propose scalable solutions to the gaps in outcomes. I commend the contributors for centering the discussion on the unique challenges, including the social determinants of cancer outcomes that impact diverse societies, especially those from non-Western countries. These two issues of *Hematology/Oncology Clinics of North America* present a modern framework and will serve as a new baseline reference for approaching cancer care from a global perspective.

Charles R. Thomas Jr, MD
Dartmouth Cancer Center
Geisel School of Medicine at Dartmouth
1 Medical Center Drive
Lebanon, NH 03756, USA

E-mail address:
Charles.R.Thomas.Jr@Dartmouth.edu

Hematol Oncol Clin N Am 38 (2024) xvii
https://doi.org/10.1016/j.hoc.2023.06.006
0889-8588/24/© 2023 Published by Elsevier Inc.

hemonc.theclinics.com

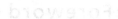

Preface

Conflict and Access to Health Care

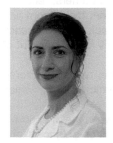
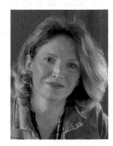
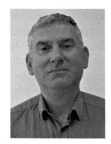

Victoria Forbes, MD, MS   Dafina Ademi Islami, MD, PhD   Ilir Hoxha, MD, PhD, MPH

Contributors

On a global scale, cancer is the second leading cause of death after cardiovascular disease, causing an estimated 10 million deaths per year. As such, it is estimated that 1 in 8 men and 1 in 11 women will die from cancer worldwide. Internationally, cancer causes more deaths than HIV/AIDS, tuberculosis, and malaria combined, and this number is increasing.

By the year 2030, the International Agency for Research on Cancer predicts there will be 17 million total deaths from cancer. Furthermore, it is estimated that globally, over 70% of the total number of deaths from cancer will occur in low- and middle-income countries (LMICs). Disparity gaps are highest in highly preventable cancers, such as cervical cancer, where an astounding 90% of new cases and deaths occur in LMICs. The survival rates of breast cancer in women in LMICs are also much lower compared with those in developed countries. With this in mind, there is a growing need to address the rising burden of cancer disparities in access to care, and we seek to do so through equitable partnerships and cultural humility, pillars maintained by the late Dr Paul Farmer, to whom this issue is dedicated.

A medical Anthropologist and Infectious Disease physician, Dr Farmer inspired many and set a profound example of viewing all citizens as equal partners whose responsibility was to care for one another. Clinically speaking, he believed that healthcare should be distributed based on need and founded Partners in Health (PIH), an organization offering medical services to the most disenfranchised among us. Last year PIH provided 3 million outpatient visits, 2.1 million women's health checkups, and over 2.2 million home visits by community health workers around the world. In this issue, as we delve into discussions of global healthcare approaches and programs, elucidate our passions, and share our stories, we remember Paul and aim to carry his memory and work forward.

Hematol Oncol Clin N Am 38 (2024) xix–xx
https://doi.org/10.1016/j.hoc.2023.07.006
0889-8588/24/© 2023 Published by Elsevier Inc.

hemonc.theclinics.com

It is known that conflicts of war severely compromise cancer care. For instance, the 1994 Genocide in Rwanda affected every aspect of society as healthcare providers fled the country and war ravaged. Rwanda rebuilt its medical infrastructure and made remarkable progress as the Rwandan government focused on community-based healthcare, invested in health information systems and technology, and collaborated with several organizations around the globe.

The penultimate war in Europe, more precisely in 1999 in Kosovo, seriously damaged health services, and due to political and socioeconomic barriers, recovery of such a damaged health system remains challenging. In Ukraine, the current war has compromised cancer care as Ukrainians fled areas under attack and emergency care took precedent, halting oncologic services and forcing many Ukrainians out of the country to seek cancer care.

Aside from conflicts, the joint battle for the fight against cancer has encountered other obstacles, such as the COVID-19 pandemic and economic inflation, which have widened disparities in cancer access and outcomes.

Based on such expansive challenges, global efforts should move in the direction of health education, prevention, implementing effective guidelines for diagnosis and treatment, enhancing health care systems, and include many partners involved in the field, policymakers, patient organizations, and civil society. We must further understand that without health digitization and data in LMICs, we cannot assess cancer incidence or mortality, employ prevention strategies or screening programs, or formulate proper treatment plans.

As health professionals, we are fortunate that our patients have chosen us as partners in their difficult journey for treatment and continue to trust us with their lives. We admire patients for the fight they have to move forward, for the inspiration and motivation they evoke, and for the role they play in raising awareness about cancer and advancing treatment for future patients with cancer.

Globally, we will fight against cancer together!

Victoria Forbes, MD, MS
University of Connecticut Health Center
Carole and Ray Neag Comprehensive Cancer Center
263 Farmington Avenue
Farmington, CT 06030, USA

Dafina Ademi Islami, MD, PhD
Oncology Clinic
University Clinical Center of Kosovo
Prishtina 10000, Kosovo

Ilir Hoxha, MD, PhD, MPH
The Dartmouth Institute for
Health Policy and Clinical Practice
Geisel School of Medicine at Dartmouth
Lebanon, NH 03766, USA

E-mail addresses:
vforbes@uchc.edu (V. Forbes)
dafinaademi@hotmail.com (D. Ademi Islami)
ilir.s.hoxha@dartmouth.edu (I. Hoxha)

Part I: Global Oncology Around the Globe: Current Status by Region

Inequity in Cancer and Cancer Care Delivery in the United States

Andrew P. Loehrer, MD, MPH[a,b,]*, Sybil R. Green, JD, RPh, MHA[c],
Karen M. Winkfield, MD, PhD[d,e]

KEYWORDS

- Disparities • Cancer care delivery • United States equity
- Social determinants of health • Political determinants of health

CLINICS CARE POINTS (KEY POINTS)

- Inequities in cancer exist along clinical continuum from incidence/epidemiology through survivorship.
- Cancer inequities are driven by multilevel and intersecting drivers of health and health care.
- Solutions to inequities require multipronged approaches including addressing the political determinants of health, engaging community-driven initiative, increasing diversity of medical workforce, increasing enrollment in clinical trials, and transdisciplinary research.

INTRODUCTION

While overall outcomes for cancer care have improved considerably in the United States over the past century, as evidenced by decreases in incidence and mortality of certain cancers, inequities in access, affordability, outcomes and the overall burden of cancer persist for many populations. At the individual and community levels, socioeconomic status, race and ethnicity, language, gender identity and sexual orientation, disability status, and rural place of residence, to name but a few, contribute to inequities for those faced with the disease. Such gaps in care are present across the globe, but there is a specific historical context that shapes the inequity of health status,

[a] Dartmouth-Hitchcock Medical Center, One Medical Center Drive, Lebanon, NH 03756, USA;
[b] Dartmouth Cancer Center, Lebanon, NH, USA; [c] American Society of Clinical Oncology, 2318 Mill Road, Suite 800, Alexandria, VA 22314, USA; [d] Vanderbilt University Ingram Cancer Center, 2220 Pierce Avenue, Nashville, TN 37232, USA; [e] Meharry-Vanderbilt Alliance, 1005 Dr DB Todd Jr Boulevard, Nashville, TN 37208, USA
* Corresponding author. Dartmouth-Hitchcock Medical Center, One Medical Center Drive, Lebanon, NH 03756.
E-mail address: andrew.p.loehrer@hitchcock.org

Hematol Oncol Clin N Am 38 (2024) 1–12
https://doi.org/10.1016/j.hoc.2023.08.001
0889-8588/24/© 2023 Elsevier Inc. All rights reserved.

incidence of cancer, type of care received, and patient experience and outcomes in the United States.

Here, we will provide an overview of important historical factors that have shaped the current health and health care inequities in the United States. We will outline examples of inequities in incidence and mortality as well as gaps along the continuum of cancer care, spanning screening and timely diagnosis through treatment outcomes, survivorship, and end of life care. We will then provide a conceptual framework with which we can begin to understand the drivers of these inequities, while keeping an eye toward solutions for addressing cancer inequities. Finally, we will discuss community-grounded and action-oriented approaches to addressing cancer inequities, including public policy, care delivery transformation, diversification and empowerment of the cancer care workforce, and an expansion of transdisciplinary research that targets inequity.

HISTORY

Of all the forms of inequality, injustice in health is the most shocking and the most inhuman.
        The Rev. Martin Luther King, Jr. at the Second National Convention of the Medical Committee for Human Rights. Chicago, IL, March 25, 1966.

Inequality in health and health care, especially for Black and poor communities, has been present since the inception of the United States of America. Systematic and structural disparities in the incidence and treatment of disease were manifest during the genocidal displacement of native populations and the nearly 250 years of chattel slavery. Inequities in health and health care have been especially well-documented since the turn of the 20th century when W.E.B. Du Bois systematically documented the social and political drivers of health outcomes. In his seminal works, *The Philadelphia Negro* and *The Health and Physique of the Negro American*, Du Bois refuted claims of the physiologic inferiority of Black persons as the cause of disparities. To the contrary, he documented a multitude of social drivers of unequal health and health care outcomes, notably (1) discrimination in life insurance coverage, (2) community education, (3) public health infrastructure, (4) socioeconomic stresses, (5) poor diet and access to quality food, (6) lack of access to high-quality hospitals, and (7) lack of diversity in the health care workforce or the medical school pipeline.[1–3] In the decades before the Civil Rights Era, efforts aimed at health inequality, such as the creation of Black medical schools and hospitals, as well as the National Negro Health Week movement, indeed improved the overall wellbeing and health care for Black communities, but it did so without addressing the underlying structural inequality that drove ongoing gaps in care. While the Civil Rights Act, Voting Rights Act, and creation of Medicare and Medicaid technically eliminated de jure segregation in the United States, long-standing systems remained in place, including in health care delivery, which allow de facto inequities to persist to this day.

In addition to the legacy of slavery, Jim Crow, and segregation, America is also unique in terms of our lack of universal health care coverage. Even after implementation of the 2010 Affordable Care Act (ACA), there are currently an estimated 27.5 million people, under the age of 65 living in the United States without health insurance coverage.[4] The influence of policy decisions on these gaps in coverage is immediately evident when most uninsured Americans reside in states that opted against expanding coverage to the country's most vulnerable populations via Medicaid under the ACA. Furthermore, insurance coverage for the other nearly 300 million Americans is spread out across multiple different payors, comprised of private insurance companies

(54.6%) and government insurance for low-income Americans (Medicaid, 21.1%) and the military (1.3%).[5] Less than 1% of Americans over the age of 65 are uninsured, since Medicare provides coverage for most of that population.[5] Moreover, payors have a large degree of discretion in terms of what services are covered by insurance, and where patients can receive this care. The variation in payors, covered services, participation by health systems, and costs to patients results in a system that is fragmented, difficult to navigate, and fraught with inefficiencies, often resulting in underinsurance for patients, variation in health care utilization, and discrepant spending.[6] These challenges are compounded for patients who face the uncertainty and complexity of multidisciplinary cancer care, with consequences ranging from financial toxicity and increased stress to increased mortality for marginalized populations across the country.[7]

DISCUSSION

Inequities exist along the continuum of cancer care, and contribute to the disparate incidence of select cancer, more advanced disease at time of diagnosis, decreased receipt of and responsiveness to treatment, and impaired survivorship experience (**Fig. 1**). Historically marginalized (hereinafter "marginalized") populations include, but is certainly not limited to, marginalized racial and ethnic identities, communities of lower socioeconomic status, low English proficiency, and limited ability status, as well as populations living in rural areas of the country, older adults, and sexual and gender minorities. Significant gaps in care exist for a multitude of populations of marginalized and intersectional identities. Applying the appropriate lens, definitions, and frameworks are essential in understanding the drivers of cancer inequities and formulating targeted interventions to specifically improve inequities in cancer care.

Framing Inequities

Drawing on the World Health Organization definition, disparities in cancer care can be understood as systematic differences in cancer incidence, treatment, or outcomes for different populations or groups. However, such disparities are better described with the more normative term of "inequity" when these differences are rooted in deeper social, historical, and structural inequities and injustice.[8] The more disparities in health are evaluated over time, the more we can appreciate the extent to which differences in outcomes between populations are driven by these deeper systemic and structural

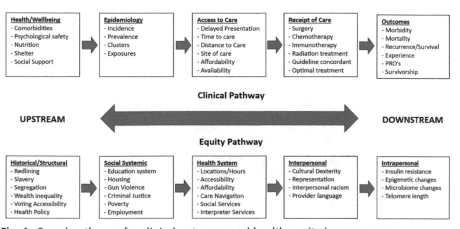

Fig. 1. Causal pathways for clinical outcomes and health equity in cancer care.

factors rather than some fixed, immutable, or innately biologic process. As such, the systematic differences in cancer care are best conceptualized as inequities, and the drivers of these inequities include different levels of racism, social or economic marginalization or oppression, or structural exclusion.[4,9–11] Across many demographics, reflecting income, race, ethnicity, language, gender identity, sexual orientation, age, and geography, there are many forms of health inequities such as gaps in access to, receipt of, and outcomes from cancer care.

Drivers of Inequities

Health and cancer inequities are not fixed, immutable realties, but rather are shaped by specific policies, systems and structures, personal choices, interpersonal relationships and dynamics, and internalized racism (**Fig. 2**). The political determinants of health (PDOH) framework recognizes that specific policies, regulations, legislation, and legal decisions shape the social environment in which we all live.[12] These determinants in turn shape the more frequently considered social determinants of health (SDOH). SDOH considers the intersection between factors like education, housing, employment, neighborhood environment, food availability, transportation, etc., and their remarkable impact on access to care through primary care and specialty providers, overall health, development of chronic medical conditions, outcomes, and life expectancy. These broader social conditions undoubtedly also influence the individual met and unmet social needs of individual patients. While the concepts are interrelated, understanding the multiple different levels that influence community and patient health is fundamental to developing specific strategies to address inequities at the level of the individual patient, community, and larger social systems in which they live.

The interpersonal drivers of inequity are very well described, especially in the context of how interpersonal racism influences care in the United States, and are deeply rooted in mistrust based on historical treatment.[13] Marginalized patients have delayed access to care but also are less likely to receive indicated care even when they present at the same stage as others. For example, Black patients are significantly less likely to receive cancer-directed surgery compared to non-Hispanic White patients.[14–16] Furthermore, patient experience of bias or racism in the clinical setting has been associated with decreased completion of recommended services.[17] Educational initiatives and trainings addressing cultural competence, cultural dexterity, and trauma-informed care target these interpersonal drivers of inequity.[18–20]

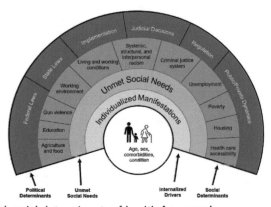

Fig. 2. Political and social determinants of health framework.

Finally, the intrapersonal, or internalized, drivers of inequity have also been most well described in the context of Black health in the United States. Perceived racism has been shown to be associated with multiple physiologic and even intergenerational changes on the human body with deleterious ramifications. Racism is associated with increased cortisol levels, increased insulin insensitivity, and decreased telomere length.[21–24] The rise of epigenetic, multi-omic, and microbiome sciences are further elucidating the ways in which social and moral drivers, like racism, have fundamental physiologic manifestations within the human body.[25–28] As such, transdisciplinary research that incorporates the span of social and medical sciences should play a central role in unpacking the mechanisms and solutions for inequities in cancer care in the years to come.[29,30]

Current Evidence

Incidence of Cancer

Overall incidence of cancer remains relatively stable for males at around 449.4 new cases per 100,000 in the United States, although it continues to rise slightly for female patients up to approximately 423.3 new diagnoses per 100,000 people.[31] The most common diagnosis for males and females are cancers of the prostate (29%) and breast (31%) for males and females, respectively. This is followed by cancer of the lung and bronchus cancers, and colorectal cancer for both men and women.

Overall, non-Hispanic Black communities have a higher rate of nearly all cancers.[32] There remain persistent disparities in the incidence of select cancers, especially in the rate of prostate, colorectal, liver, gastric, and lung cancer for Black men.[8,9] While the overall rates of prostate, lung, and colorectal cancers have been declining for men overall, there has been a very significant shift in the incidence of young-onset (<50 years of age at diagnosis) colorectal cancer within younger men, especially White patients where there has been nearly a 50% increase from the mid-1990s to the early 2010s.[33] This is driven largely by the disproportionate increase in colon cancer for White patients while rates have stabilized for non-Hispanic Black patients. There remains considerable uncertainty regarding the overall increase in young-onset colorectal cancer as well as the disproportionate increase in White patients with colon cancer.

Access to Timely Diagnosis and Care

One of the leading causes of inequitable outcomes of cancer in the United States stems from decreased access to cancer screening and increased probability of presenting with advanced-stage disease. Lower socioeconomic status and lack of insurance in the United States are consistently shown to be associated with later stage cancer at the time of diagnosis.[9] Additionally, multiple studies have shown insurance expansion to be associated with earlier and less-emergent diagnosis with colon cancer along with an increase in the proportion of patients presenting with stage I breast, colon, and lung cancer.[34,35]

Prevention of cancer development and early diagnosis are contingent upon both preventive services and screening of appropriate cancer. From a preventative standpoint, multiple studies have shown marginalized communities as having decreased awareness of specific cancer risks and behavioral contributors to cancer development.[36–39] Gaps in cancer screening rates have been well documented, especially for cervical, breast, and colorectal cancers.[40] National programs, including through the ACA, have been developed and implemented to improve early detection and policies implemented to increase screening services.[41] Despite this concerted effort, there are still significant gaps in cancer screening for marginalized populations, including populations with low–English-speaking proficiency, low health literacy, and limited transportation.[42–46]

Receipt of Care Cancer Treatment

While later stage at the time of presentation may be a leading mechanism of inequities, additional aspects of care delivery also contribute to inequitable outcomes. Uninsured and low-income patients and communities have significantly less likelihood of receiving guideline-concordant care, even when accounting for later stage at the time of presentation.[47–49] Uninsured patients are significantly less likely to receive cancer-directed surgery for solid organ malignancy including cancer of the breast, colon and rectum, and lung.[50,51] Furthermore, patients with residence in communities of lower socioeconomic status or rural geography (for example, areas with fewer than 50,000 residents) are significantly less likely to receive cancer-directed surgery, suggesting that the gaps in receiving care are not solely based on insurance coverage alone.[52] Multiple studies have shown interpersonal racism, communication and cultural barriers, and patient-provider race/ethnicity discordance play a major role in the failure of patients receiving cancer-directed surgery. Additionally, the referral patterns and site of care delivery also play important roles in gaps in cancer-directed surgery, with uninsured, low-income, and marginalized patients having lower likelihood of being evaluated by a surgical specialist or at a high surgical volume facility.

The increasingly multidisciplinary approach to cancer also requires critical coordination of therapeutic modalities, including surgery, chemotherapy, and radiation. As was the case in surgical care, low-income and marginalized communities are significantly less likely to receive guideline-recommended chemotherapy (for example, in stage III colon cancer), radiation (for example, in rectal cancer), and appropriate sequencing or use of multiple treatment modalities.[37,47,49,53] As the complexity of cancer care continues to increase, the advances also create new opportunities for gaps in care to occur that ultimately influence outcomes. Care coordination with the use of clinical pathways or nurse navigators has shown promise at not only improving overall care delivery but also decreasing disparities in care across communities. However, many of the mission-driven clinics and institutions providing care for low-income and marginalized communities are themselves under-resourced due to unfavorable payor-mix and lack of inadequate supplemental funding. When compared to other countries, this is a component of the US health care structure that may fail patients and perpetuate inequities.

Beyond guideline-concordant cancer-directed therapies, it is also important to consider inequities in access to clinical trials and use of palliative and hospice care for patients with more advanced disease as additional treatments. Structural racism in how clinical trials are conducted has been recognized for decades and there are now important investments and strategies to increase access to trials across North America. These efforts are critical not only to ensure all patients are able to benefit from potentially cutting-edge therapeutics, but also to ensure that the science behind our clinical guidelines is truly representative of all communities. Finally, end-of-life and survivorship care often represents the tailing aspects of cancer care delivery. While the cancer community attempts to better understand how to expand and integrate palliative care, hospice, and survivorship programs, there are data to suggest that communities are presently not having equal access to, or use of, these services most effectively and equitably. For example, rural place of residence has been shown to be associated with decreased use of palliative care for advanced pancreatic cancer.[54] Low-income and marginalized communities have also been shown to have decreased receipt of hospice care and an increased use of inpatient hospitalization at the end of life.[55–57]

Outcomes of Cancer Care

In addition to disparities in the access to and receipt of cancer-directed treatment, there are significant inequities in outcomes from care. While overall survival from cancers is improving in the United States, there are multiple gaps in care that persist. The increase in insurance coverage associated with the Patient Protection and Affordable Care Act has been associated with earlier stage at diagnosis, which in turn is associated with increased survival. However, even when possessing the same insurance coverage in the United States, patients residing in communities of greater socioeconomic disadvantage have significantly worse survival with cancer.[58] Similarly, cancer deaths for non-Hispanic Black patients have decreased significantly over the past decade, but there remain considerable gaps in survival between non-Hispanic Black and White patients.[59] Similarly, the introduction of newer screening or treatment options may have overall benefit, especially for better-insured and White populations, but their asymmetric introduction, uptake, or use has the potential to simultaneously introduce new racial or socioeconomic disparities.[60] Among cancer survivors, socioeconomic and racial inequities in quality of life and financial toxicity remain a challenge. Looking at 301 survivors of colorectal cancer, low-income patients had significantly worse quality of life, including higher pain interference, lower physical function, and higher depression scores as compared to higher-income patients.[61]

Approaches to Addressing Inequities

There are multiple levels at which cancer care inequities are being addressed in the United States.[62] These range from the upstream public policy and regulations at the federal and state levels to downstream care redesign and diversification of clinical trials (**Table 1**). On the health policy front, these inequities may be addressed by further increasing health insurance coverage through expanded Medicaid eligibility in states that have not done so already, increased Medicaid payment parity, and ensuring Medicaid payment for certain services, including care in clinical trials which are an

Table 1 Approaches to addressing inequity in cancer research, care delivery, and outcomes	
Domains	**Example**
Health policy	• Affordable Care Act[63,64] • State-based insurance expansions and other policies[34,65] • Funding for systems addressing social determinants of health[66] • Cancer Moonshot[67]
Care redesign	• Alternative payment models[68] • Equity-oriented interventions to close racial disparities[69] • Increased navigation services at cancer centers[70]
Health care workforce	• Increasing pipeline of future oncologists through community engagement, scholarships, and addressing institutional discrimination[71,72]
Cancer care research	• Community trials network expanding access to and diversity in clinical trials[73] • Pragmatic trial design[74,75] • Transdisciplinary research bridging upstream and downstream drivers and outcomes[27,28] • Clinical Treatment Act[76]

important point of access to drugs and other cutting-edge approaches to treatment. Additionally, national policy guidelines targeting equity could help establish health equity outcome measures and toolkits to empower practices. Federal legislation can also help expand patient navigation and promote reimbursement for such services. Finally, as the Oncology Care Model and other bundled care payments are rolled out, we must identify mechanisms to ensure access to and receipt of quality cancer care for marginalized populations.

Beyond policy, efforts to address equity in cancer care should both engage and empower community partners, yielding priorities, funding, and deliverables to the community rather than keeping influence and products within the health system. The research community can help develop toolkits to collect SDOH data and operationalize data to specifically target equity as a quality improvement goal. Finally, there can be considerable improvements in increasing diversity and representation within the clinical trial process. Expansion of trial eligibility and participation has been recognized as a top priority of the National Cancer Institutes, the American Society of Clinical Oncology, and the Centers for Medicare and Medicaid Services.

SUMMARY

Cancer inequity in the United States spans the clinical continuum and is influenced by historical, structural, systemic, interpersonal, and intrapersonal racism and oppression. These gaps in cancer outcomes exist for marginalized populations from increased incidence of select cancer, later stage at diagnosis, decreased receipt of cancer-directed therapy, and worse survival. Understanding PDOH and SDOH and causal framework is important for strategically ensuring equity in cancer care in the United States.

DISCLOSURE

A.P. Loehrer has no financial conflicts of interest to report. Time spent on this work was supported in part by a grant from the National Institutes of Health, United States (NCI K08CA263546). S.R. Green and K.M. Winkfield have no financial conflicts or disclosures to report.

REFERENCES

1. Du Bois WEB. The Philadelphia Negro: a social study. New York: Schocken Books; 1899.
2. Du Bois WEB. The health and Physique of the Negro American. Atlanta: The Atlanta University Press; 1906.
3. Loehrer AP, Chang DC, Hutter MM, et al. Surgical quality and equity: Revisiting the class of 1895. Ann Surg 2016;264(2):235–6.
4. Cohen, RA, Cha, AE. Health insurance coverage: early release of estimates from the national health interview survey, january-june 2022, Centers for disease control, https://www.cdc.gov/nchs/data/nhis/earlyrelease/insur202212.pdf.
5. Health Insurance Coverage of the Total Population. Kaiser Family Foundation; 2021. https://www.kff.org/other/state-indicator/total-population/?dataView=0&currentTimeframe=0&selectedDistributions=employer–non-group–medicaid–medicare–military–uninsured–total&sortModel=%7B%22colId%22:%22Location%22,%22sort%22:%22asc%22%7D.
6. Cooper Z, Stiegman O, Ndumele CD, et al. Geographical Variation in Health Spending Across the US Among Privately Insured Individuals and Enrollees in

Medicaid and Medicare. JAMA Netw Open 2022;5(7):e2222138. Erratum in: JAMA Netw Open. 2022 Aug 1;5(8):e2230459.

7. Parikh-Patel A, Morris CR, Kizer KW. Disparities in quality of cancer care: The role of health insurance and population demographics. Medicine (Baltim) 2017 Dec; 96(50):e9125.

8. Braveman PA, Kumanyika S, Fielding J, et al. Health disparities and health equity: The issue is justice. Am J Public Health 2011;101(Suppl 1):S149–55.

9. Boyd RW, Lindo EG, Weeks LD, et al. On racism: A new standard for publishing on racial health inequities. Health Affairs Blog 2020. https://doi.org/10.1377/hblog20200630.9399347.

10. Jones CP. Levels of racism: a theoretic framework and a gardener's tale. Am J Public Health 2000;90:1212–5.

11. Loehrer AP, Cevallos PC, Jiménez RJ, et al. Reporting on race and racial disparities in breast cancer: The neglect of racism as a driver of inequitable care. Ann Surg 2023;277:329–34.

12. Dawes DE, Williams DR. The political determinants of health. 1st Edition. Baltimore, MD: Johns Hopkins University Press; 2020.

13. Gordon HS, Street RL Jr, Sharf BF, et al. Racial differences in trust and lung cancer patients' perceptions of physician communication. J Clin Oncol 2006;24(6): 904–9.

14. Gordon HS, Street RL Jr, Sharf BF, et al. Racial differences in doctors' information-giving and patients' participation. Cancer 2006;107(6):1313–20.

15. McCann J, Artinian V, Duhaime L, et al. Evaluation of the causes for racial disparitiy in surgical treatment of early stage lung cancer. Chest 2005;128(5):3440–6.

16. Nocon CC< Ajmani GS, Bhayani MK. A contemporary analysis of racial disparities in recommended and received treatment for head and neck cancer. Cancer 2020;126(2):381–9.

17. Penner LA, Dovidio JF, Gonzalez R, et al. The effects of oncologist implicit racial bias in racially discordant oncology interactions. J Clin Oncol 2016;34(24): 2874–80.

18. Changoor N, Udyavar N, Morris MA, et al. Surgeons perceptions toward providing care for diverse patients: The need for cultural dexterity training. Ann Surg 2019;269(2):275–82.

19. Butler SS, Winkfield KM, Ahn C, et al. Racial disparities in patient-reported measures of physician cultural competency among cancer survivors in the United States. JAMA Oncol 2020;6(1):152–4.

20. Griggs J, Maingi S, Blinder V, et al. American Society of Clinical Oncology Position Statement: Strategies for reducing cancer health disparities among sexual and gender minority populations. Obstet Gynecol Surv 2017;35:2203–8.

21. Brody GH, Yu T, Chen E, et al. Racial discrimination, body mass index, and insulin resistance: A longitudinal analysis. Health Psychol 2018;37(12):1107.

22. Fuller-Rowell TE, Homandberg LK, Curtis DS, et al. Disparities in insulin resistance between black and white adults in the United States: The role of lifespan stress exposure. Psychoneuroendocrinology 2019;107:1–8.

23. Chae DH, Nuru-Jeter AM, Adler NE, et al. Discrimination, racial bias, and telomere length in African-American men. Am J Prev Med 2014;46(2):103–11.

24. Duru OK, Harawa NT, Kermah D, et al. Allostatic load burden and racial disparities in mortality. J Natl Med Assoc 2012;104(1–2):89–95.

25. Thayer ZM, Kuzawa CW. Biological memories of past environments: epigenetic pathways to health disparities. Epigenetics 2011;6(7):798–803.

26. Martin CL, Ghastine L, Lodge EK, et al. Understanding health inequalities through the lens of social epigenetics. Annu Rev Publ Health 2022;43:235–54.

27. Martini R, Gebregzabher E, Newman L, et al. Enhancing the trajectories of cancer health disparities research: improving clinical applications of diversity, equity, inclusion, and accessibility. Cancer Discov 2022;12(6):1428–34.

28. Royston KJ, Adedokun B, Olopade OI. Race, the microbiome and colorectal cancer. World J Gastrointest Oncol 2019;11(10):773.

29. Findley K, Williams DR, Grice EA, et al. Health disparities and the microbiome. Trends Microbiol 2016;24(11):847–50.

30. Salas LA, Peres LC, Thayer ZM, et al. A transdisciplinary approach to understanding the epigenetic basis of race/ethnicity health disparities. Epigenomics 2021;13(21):1761–70.

31. Siegel RL, Miller KD, Wagle NS, et al. Cancer statistics, 2023. CA Cancer J Clin 2023;73:17–48.

32. Islami F, Guerra CE, Minihan A, et al. American Cancer Society's repor on the status of cancer disparities in the United States, 2021. CA Cancer J Clin 2022;72:112–43.

33. Murphy CC, Wallace K, Sandler RS, et al. Racial disparities in incidence of young-onset colorectal cancer and patient survival. Gastroenterology 2019;156:958–65.

34. Loehrer AP, Song Z, Haynes AB, et al. The impact of insurance expansion on the treatment of colorectal cancer. J Clin Oncol 2016;34(34):4110–5.

35. Takvorian SU, Oganisian A, Mamtani R, et al. Association of Medicaid expansion under the Affordable Care Act with insurance status, cancer stage, and timely treatment among patients with breast, colon, and lung cancer. JAMA Netw Open 2020;3(2):e1921653.

36. Oh A, Shaikh A, Waters E, et al. Health disparities in awareness of physical activity and cancer prevention: findings from the National Cancer Institute's 2007 Health Information National Trends Survey (HINTS). J Health Commun 2010;15(sup3):60–77.

37. Goding Sauer A, Siegel RL, Jemal A, et al. Current prevalence of major cancer risk factors and screening test use in the United States: disparities by education and race/ethnicity. Cancer Epidemiol Biomarkers Prev 2019;28(4):629–42.

38. Jacobsen AA, Galvan A, Lachapelle CC, et al. Defining the need for skin cancer prevention education in uninsured, minority, and immigrant communities. JAMA dermatology 2016;152(12):1342–7.

39. Fyffe DC, Hudson SV, Fagan JK, et al. Knowledge and barriers related to prostate and colorectal cancer prevention in underserved black men. J Natl Med Assoc 2008;100(10):1161–7.

40. Benavidez GA, Zgodic A, Zahnd WE, et al. Disparities in Meeting USPSTF Breast, Cervical, and Colorectal Cancer Screening Guidelines Among Women in the United States. Prev Chronic Dis 2021;18:E37.

41. Miller JW, Plescia M, Ekwueme DU. Public health national approach to reducing breast and cervical cancer disparities. Cancer 2014;120(S16):2537–9.

42. Cataneo JL, Kim TD, Park JJ, et al. Disparities in Screening for Colorectal Cancer Based on Limited Language Proficiency. Am Surg 2022;88(11):2737–44.

43. Jerant AF, Fenton JJ, Franks P. Determinants of Racial/Ethnic Colorectal Cancer Screening Disparities. Arch Intern Med 2008;168(12):1317–24.

44. Cooper GS, Kou TD Dor A< Koroukian SM, Schluchter MD. Cancer preventive services, socioeconomic status, and the Affordable Care Act. Cancer 2017;123:1585–9.

45. Sosa E, D'Souza G, Akhtar A, et al. Racial and socioeconomic disparities in lung cancer screening in the United States: A systematic review. CA: a cancer journal for clinicians 2021;71(4):299–314.

46. May FP, Yang L, Corona E, et al. Disparities in colorectal cancer screening in the United States before and after implementation of the Affordable Care Act. Clin Gastroenterol Hepatol 2020;18(8):1796–804.

47. Hamad A, DePuccio M, Reames BN, et al. Disparities in stage-specific guideline-concordant cancer-directed treatment for patients with pancreatic adenocarcinoma. J Gastrointest Surg 2021;25:2889–901.

48. Fang P, He W, Gomez D, et al. Racial disparities in guideline-concordant cancer care and mortality in the United States. Adv Rad Oncol 2018;3(3):221–9.

49. Ju MR, Wang SC, Mansour JC, et al. Disparities in guideline-concordant treatment and survival among border county residents with gastric cancer. JCO Oncology Practice 2022;18(5):e748–58.

50. Markey C, Weiss JE, Loehrer AP. Influence of race, insurance, and rurality on equity of breast cancer care. J Surg Res 2022;271:117–24.

51. Leech MM, Weiss JE, Markey C, et al. Influence of race, insurance, rurality, and socioeconomic status on equity of lung and colorectal cancer care. Ann Surg Oncol 2022;29(6):3630–9.

52. Loehrer AP, Chen L, Wang Q, et al. Rural disparities in lung cancer-directed surgery: A Medicare cohort study. Ann Surg 2023;277(3):e657–63.

53. de Oca MK, Wilson LE, Previs RA, et al. Healthcare access dimensions and guideline-concordant ovarian cancer treatment: SEER-Medicare analysis of the ORCHiD study. J Natl Compr Cancer Netw 2022;20(11):1255–66.

54. Ramkumar N, Wang Q, Brooks GA, et al. Association of rurality with utilization of palliative care and hospice among patients who died from pancreatic cancer. J Rural Health 2023. https://doi.org/10.1111/jrh.12739. Online ahead of print.

55. Perry LM, Walsh LE, Horswell R, et al. Racial disparities in end-of-life care between black and white adults with metastatic cancer. J Pain Symptom Manag 2021;61(2):342–9.

56. Coltin H, Rapoport A, Baxter NN, et al. Locus-of-care disparities in end-of-life care intensity among adolescents and young adults with cancer: a population-based study using the IMPACT cohort. Cancer 2022;128(2):326–34.

57. Shen MJ, Prigerson HG, Paulk E, et al. Impact of end-of-life discussions on the reduction of Latino/non-Latino disparities in do-not-resuscitate order completion. Cancer 2016;122(11):1749–56.

58. Abdelsattar AM, Hendren S, Wong SL. The impact of health insurance on cancer care in disadvantaged communities. Cancer 2016;123(7):1219–27.

59. Lawrence WR, McGee-Avila JK, Vo JB, et al. Trends in cancer mortality among black individuals in the US from 1999 to 2019. JAMA Oncol 2022;8(8):1184–9.

60. Jatoi I, Sung H, Jemal A. The emergence of the racial disparity in U.S. breast-cancer mortality. N Engl J Med 2022;386:2349–52.

61. McDougall JA, Blair CK, Wiggins CL, et al. Socioeconomic disparities in health-related quality of life among colorectal cancer survivors. J Cancer Survivorship 2019;13:459–67.

62. Winkfield KM, Regnante JM, Miller-Sonet E, et al. Development of an actionable framework to address cancer care disparities in medically underserved populations in the United States: expert roundtable recommendations. JCO Oncology Practice 2021;17(3):e278–93.

63. Han X, Jemal A, Zheng Z, et al. Changes in noninsurance and care unaffordability among cancer survivors following the Affordable Care Act. JNCI: J Natl Cancer Inst 2020;112(7):688–97.
64. Takvorian SU, Oganisian A, Mamtani R, et al. Association of medicaid expansion under the affordable care act with insurance status, cancer stage, and timely treatment among patients with breast, colon, and lung cancer. JAMA Netw Open 2020;3(2):e1921653.
65. Loehrer AP, Chang DC, Hutter MM, et al. Health insurance expansion and treatment of pancreatic cancer. J Am Coll Surg 2015;221:1015–22.
66. Alcaraz KI, Wiedt TL, Daniels EC, et al. Understanding and addressing social determinants to advance cancer health equity in the United States: A blueprint for practice, research, and policy. CA A Cancer J Clin 2020;70:31–46.
67. The White House, Fact Sheet: President Biden Reignites Cancer Moonshot to End Cancer as We Know February 1, 2022, www.whitehouse.gov/cancermoonshot/, Accessed July 19, 2023.
68. Liao JM, Lavizzo-Mourey RJ, Navathe AS. A National Goal to Advance Health Equity Through Value-Based Payment. JAMA 2021;325(24):2439–40.
69. Cykert S, Eng E, Walker P, et al. A system-based intervention to reduce Black-White disparities in the treatment of early stage lung cancer: A pragmatic trial at five cancer centers. Cancer Med 2019;8(3):1095–102.
70. Rodday AM, Parsons SK, Snyder F, et al. Impact of patient navigation in eliminating economic disparities in cancer care. Cancer 2015;121(22):4025–34.
71. Patel MI, Lopez AM, Blackstock W, et al. Cancer Disparities and Health Equity: A Policy Statement from the American Society of Clinical Oncology. J Clin Oncol 2020;38(29):3439–48.
72. Winkfield KM, Flowers CR, Patel JD, et al. The American Society of Clinical Oncology strategic plan for increasing racial and ethnic diversity in the oncology workforce. J Clin Oncol, chrome-extension://efaidnbmnnnibpcajpcglclefindmkaj/https://old-prod.asco.org/sites/new-www.asco.org/files/content-files/practice-and-guidelines/documents/2017-diversity-strategy.pdf, Accessed July 19, 2023.
73. Guerra C, Pressman A, Hurley P, et al. Increasing racial and ethnic equity, diversity, and inclusion in cancer treatment trials: Evaluation of an ASCO-Association Of Community Cancer Centers site self-assessment. JCO Oncology Practice 2023;19(4):e581–8.
74. Cykert S, Eng E, Walker P, et al. A system-based intervention to reduce Black-White disparities in the treatment of early stage lung cancer: A pragmatic trial at five cancer centers. Cancer Med 2019;8(3):1095–102.
75. Cykert S, Eng E, Manning MA, et al. A multi-faceted intervention aimed at Black-White disparities in the treatment of early stage cancers: the ACCURE pragmatic quality improvement trial. J Natl Med Assoc 2020;112(5):468–77.
76. H.R.133 - 116th Congress (2019-2020): Consolidated Appropriations Act, 2021. (2020, December 27). https://www.congress.gov/bill/116th-congress/house-bill/133, Accessed July 19, 2023.

An Overview of Cervical Cancer Prevention and Control in Latin America and the Caribbean Countries

Ivy Riano, MD[a,1,*], Pamela Contreras-Chavez, MD[b,1],
Cindy Medina Pabon, MD[c], Kelly Meza, MD[d], Lauren Kiel[e],
Suyapa Bejarano, MD[f,2], Narjust Florez, MD[e]

KEYWORDS

- Cervical cancer • Human papillomavirus • Papanicolaou stain • Cervical cytology
- Latin America • HPV Vaccine

KEY POINTS

- Cervical cancer remains a major health problem in Latin America and the Caribbean despite declining trends in incidence and mortality during the past decade.
- Several Latin America and the Caribbean countries have implemented screening programs, yet the impact of those programs is limited due to suboptimal coverage, unequal access to health care, loss of follow-up, and low adherence.

Continued

[a] Division of Hematology and Oncology, Dartmouth Cancer Center, Geisel School of Medicine Dartmouth, One Medical Drive, Lebanon, NH 03766, USA; [b] Division of Hematology and Oncology, Dana Farber Cancer Institute, St. Elizabeth's Medical Center, 736 Cambridge Street, Brighton, MA 02135, USA; [c] Division of Hematology and Oncology, The University of Texas MD Anderson Cancer Center, Unit 0463, 1515 Holcombe Boulevard, FC11.3055, Houston, TX 77030, USA; [d] Division of Internal Medicine, Baylor College of Medicine, One Baylor Plaza, Houston, TX 77030, USA; [e] Dana Farber Cancer Institute, Harvard School of Medicine, 450 Brookline Avenue - DA1230, Boston, MA 02215, USA; [f] Department of Radiation Oncology, Liga Contra el Cancer, San Pedro Sula, Honduras
[1] Shared first authorship.
[2] Present address: Barrio el Benque 8 calle 10 y, 11 Avenida Southeast, San Pedro Sula 21104, Honduras.
* Corresponding author.
E-mail address: Ivy.Riano@dartmouth.edu
Twitter: @IvyLorena_Md (I.R.); @PamChMD (P.C.-C.); @cmpabon (C.M.P.); @KellyMezaMD (K.M.); @NarjustFlorezMD (N.F.)

Hematol Oncol Clin N Am 38 (2024) 13–33
https://doi.org/10.1016/j.hoc.2023.05.012
0889-8588/24/© 2023 Elsevier Inc. All rights reserved.

Continued

- Even though human papillomavirus (HPV) testing is commercially available, only a few countries have integrated the technology into their national screening programs, leaving cytology as the primary screening test.
- To ensure consistent quality of care, each country in the region should strengthen its health-care system and use the data collected, implement population-based cancer registries, and use the data collection more effectively for treatment and care decisions.
- The coronavirus disease 2019 pandemic posed new challenges for cervical cancer screening and HPV vaccination but its full impact has yet to be determined, given limited accurate official reports.

INTRODUCTION

Globally, cervical cancer is the fourth most frequent cancer in women with 604,000 new cases reported during 2020.[1] Of the estimated 342,000 deaths from cervical cancer in 2020, about 90% occurred in low and middle-income countries (LMICs).[1] Latin America and the Caribbean has the second highest cervical cancer mortality worldwide, with the highest rates in the Caribbean (8.2 per 100,000), followed by South America (7.8 per 100,000) and Central America (6.8 per 100,000).[2] Almost all cervical cancer cases (99%) are linked to infection with high-risk human papillomaviruses (HPVs), a common virus transmitted through sexual contact.[3] Cervical cancer can be prevented by effective HPV vaccination (primary prevention) and/or screening and treatment of precancerous lesions (secondary prevention).[1,3] Individuals at greatest risk for cervical cancer are often women from marginalized or underserved groups who do not participate in regular screening for a variety of reasons that will be addressed in this article.[4]

Cervical cancer is one of the most prominent diseases reflecting global inequities. LMICs face the greatest burden of cervical cancer due to the lack of access to public health services, therapies, and timely screening. As a result, in May 2018 the World Health Organization (WHO) designated cervical cancer as a public health problem, thereby adopting the Global Strategy for Cervical Cancer Elimination in August 2020.[5] To understand the main challenges of this global initiative, we review the epidemiology, cancer control strategies, and treatment barriers of cervical cancer in countries in Latin American and the Caribbean. The elimination of cervical cancer in this region still requires substantial political and economic commitments. For instance, there is a need to address key factors such as lack of widely implemented screening, difficulties interacting with the health-care system (eg, limited knowledge and health literacy, lack of provider recommendation/contact), financial burden (eg, lack of insurance), and logistical barriers (eg, competing demands, scheduling issues), which ultimately will influence the cervical cancer rates across all underserved groups.

WHO's Global Strategy to Accelerate Cervical Cancer Elimination

To eliminate cervical cancer as a public health complication, in 2020, the WHO launched a global strategy plan that called for all nations to work toward a cervical cancer incidence of less than 4/100,000 women, using platforms sensitive to women's needs and the health service access barriers that they may face.[5] Particularly, the WHO developed the following 90-70-90 milestones for all nations to implement by 2030.[5]

- Ninety percent of girls must be fully vaccinated with HPV vaccine by 15 years of age (primary prevention).
- Seventy percent of women screened using a high-performance test by 35 years of age and again by 45 years of age (secondary prevention).
- Ninety percent of women identified with cervical disease are treated (tertiary prevention; 90% of women with precancer are treated; 90% of women with invasive cancer are managed).[1]

To accomplish such milestones, the WHO recommended strategies for primary prevention such as creating vaccine delivery platforms (including school immunization programs), advocacy and social mobilization efforts to overcome vaccine hesitancy, and age-appropriate information regarding safe sexual behaviors.[5] For secondary prevention, the WHO recommended testing for HPV as the primary screening method, with the option of self-sampling. An increase in cervical cancer screening must be accompanied by a matching increase in capacity for lesion treatment, and market-shaping initiatives to secure affordable, high-quality diagnostic supplied should also be prioritized.[5] According to the WHO, for invasive cervical cancer to be treated effectively, surgical capacity should be expanded, radiotherapy and chemotherapy must be improved, as well as palliative care involving psychosocial and spiritual support for women and their families to be integrated into cancer treatment plans.[5]

Finally, the WHO called for investment in the primary care workforce, to remain the preferred entry point for cervical cancer prevention interventions but for service structures to accommodate women presenting at any given time.[5] Partnerships with global institutions, resource entities, and multisectoral collaborations should also be established. Advocacy groups such as nongovernmental organizations, civil society organizations, and women's groups should aid communities in reducing barriers to care, and communication should promote relevant interventions and counter misinformation.[5] National and regional surveillance and monitoring systems, including cancer registries and vital registration, will help to understand the impact of implemented policies and interventions, as well as help identify next steps to improve cervical cancer outcomes.[5]

Moreover, the Pan American Health Organization (PAHO) adopted the Regional Strategy and Plan of Action for Comprehensive Cervical Cancer Prevention and Control to work with countries in the Americas in different ways including alternative approaches in several countries in Latin America and the Caribbean, technical assistance provided to the region to strengthen their cervical cancer programs, and HPV vaccine funding enabling bulk purchase at one unique price for all countries of the Americas. For instance, a cost-effectiveness model was developed by PAHO's ProVac Initiative to support decision-making about HPV vaccines introduction.[6] By 2030, PAHO aims to eliminate cervical cancer as a public health problem in the Americas by reducing incidence and mortality rates by one-third.[7]

Epidemiology of Cervical Cancer in Latin America and the Caribbean Region

Cervical cancer has been identified in the top 5 of most common cancer among women worldwide.[1] Its incidence and mortality rates vary widely among high and LMICs (**Fig. 1**).[2] The most updated epidemiologic data revealed that in 2020, there were an estimated of 59,439 new cervical cancer cases (rank No. 7 of all cancers) and 31,582 deaths (rank No. 8) in countries from Latin America and the Caribbean, although the age-standardized incidence and mortality rates was of 14.9 and 7.6 per 100,000 representing the third most common cancer in women from the region.[8] These trends revealed great variations between countries/territories despite similar

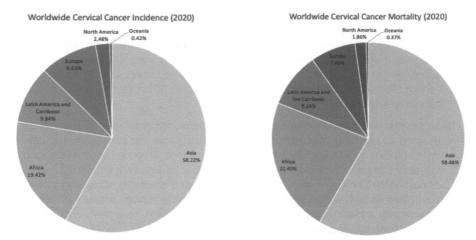

Fig. 1. Patterns of incidence and mortality of cervical cancer worldwide (2020) from the global cancer observatory. (*Reprinted from* Cancer Cancer IAfRo. Global Cancer Observatory. Accessed March 20, 2023, https://gco.iarc.fr/. Copyright 2023.)

income levels across the region. Precisely, incidence rates have been reported lower in Central America (13.0 per 100,000) than in South America (15.2) and the Caribbean (15.5) while mortality rates were higher in the Caribbean (8.5) than in South America (7.1) and Central America (7.0).[9] In terms of country, Martinique exhibited the lowest incidence and mortality rates in 2018 (7.6 and 1.9, respectively), whereas Bolivia had the highest estimated incidence rate (38.5) and Jamaica the highest mortality rate (20.1). Moreover, although cervical cancer is the leading cause of cancer-related mortality in El Salvador, it represents the sixth cause in Chile and fourth in Costa Rica and Cuba.[10] Such differences in cervical cancer incidence and mortality rates per region raise questions about what other aspects may be contributory. One of the key factors is the robustness of the nation's health-care system, which is essential to implementing comprehensive cancer care services.[11,12] This is mostly affected by the several inequities of the region, with state-run hospitals and clinics over-stressed by continuous demand for treatment of high rates of noncommunicable diseases.

Overall, trends in cervical cancer mortality and morbidity have decreased during the past 10 years.[13] For instance, mortality rates have decreased in Chile (−2%), Colombia (−2%), Ecuador (−3%), Cuba (−1%), El Salvador (−4%), Mexico (−2%), and Paraguay (−2%) and stayed stable in the remaining countries. Specifically, a decline in mortality rates among women aged 0 to 29 years was observed across all countries/territories, except for Brazil, where rates have significantly increased (+4%). Most countries/territories also exhibited decreasing mortality rates at ages 30 years and older.[9] Several factors may contribute to this decrease, including reduced fertility rates, lower parity, and an overall improvement in socioeconomic and educational levels in the region including structured screening, vaccination, and treatment programs.[9,14,15]

Cervical cancer is associated with infection by high-risk HPV strains.[2] Efforts to mitigate this have led to the development of HPV vaccines targeting children and teenagers. In the Latin America and Caribbean region, 29 of the 47 countries/territories have implemented HPV vaccination programs for girls.[16] Although controversy in some Latin American countries remains due to the association of HPV infections with sexual activity, several countries have developed vaccination programs to strategically educate and offer the vaccine to individuals. However, these programs are difficult to implement across these countries because of economic, political, and logistical obstacles.[16] This continues to be an evolving initiative by many public health services, with the acknowledgement that cervical cancer screening will continue to be especially important for future generations, until HPV vaccination is more widely accepted.

The approach for cervical cancer screening begins with a cytology-based test or Papanicolaou (Pap) smear and/or preferably with a DNA-based testing for HPV. When abnormal results are obtained, patients undergo colposcopy and potentially further testing procedures. The colposcopy itself requires a colposcope, acetic acid, and expertise in distinguishing clinically normal and abnormal results. Furthermore, if results on colposcopy are abnormal, additional procedures may include ablative cryotherapy, cold knife cone biopsy, or loop electrosurgical excision procedure (LEEP).[17] Although this is a well-established algorithm, the level of instruments, techniques, expertise, and workforce involved in such procedures are often not available in LMICs. Thus, many individuals with abnormal screening results need to travel to main referral facilities that are usually located in urban areas to receive the recommended diagnostic and treatment procedures. Even when patients can attend the first consultation, follow-up visits may pose challenges due in part to distance, costs, and unfamiliarity with the health-care system. Consequently, many women in Latin American countries may present with late-stage cervical cancer due to a lack of screening and treatment opportunities.[18] It is also important to note that access to cervical cancer screening and care is often based on insurance status and existing health systems infrastructure. For instance, Argentina and Mexico offer HPV screening within their public health system, whereas in other countries, it is mainly available through the private sector.[11] Thus, expenses for routine screening further reduce patient interest and compliance with cervical cancer prevention.

In efforts to bridge such gaps in access to care in more rural areas of Latin America and the Caribbean, partnerships between institutions with resources and experience with screening and their counterparts have been developed. With these collaborations, countries with more resources aim to strengthen the infrastructure, improve population outcomes in the long term and provide training on effective specialty cancer care to lower resource settings.[18] Successful partnerships have existed in pediatric oncology between Nicaragua and Italy, the United States and El Salvador, Honduras, and Guatemala, as well as with St. Jude Children's Research Hospital in the United States and the Amazon region of Brazil.[2] Additionally, teleconference technology has allowed for the development of mentorship programs that may improve the capacity and access to care in underserved communities.[19] Examples of such initiatives include Project ECHO (Extension for Community Healthcare Outcomes), developed at the University of New Mexico, which was adapted by the MD Anderson Cancer Center to educate and support local providers in the management of cervical dysplasia and invasive cervical cancer in the Texas-Mexico Border and low-resources regions of Latin America.[19] Other efforts of visiting underserved sites to train local providers have been directed by the Central America Gynecologic Oncology Education Program, providing training in preventive and therapeutic gynecologic cancers treatment and prevention with 6 Central American countries.[20]

Finally, it is important to note the impact that the coronavirus disease 2019 (COVID-19) pandemic has had on delivering comprehensive cervical cancer care. Recently, an infodemiology study analyzed the Google search trends from 2018 to 2021 in the following topics "cervical cancer," "Pap smear," "HPV vaccine," or "colposcopy," among others, and they found a sharp decline in global online search interest in cervical cancer during the course of the pandemic, indicating potential reduced efforts to cervical cancer screening. This study highlighted the need for maintained awareness initiatives in the community so as not to diminish the progress made in cervical cancer care thus far.[21]

Cervical Cancer Control

Challenges in cancer control

Despite the initiatives to address cancer disparities in the Latin American region, gaps in cancer care persist.[12,22] Main identified challenges of cervical cancer control in the region are.

- Limited trained personnel: Compared with the number of patients with cancer in Latin American countries, there are few oncologists, radiotherapists, cancer surgeons, and palliative care professionals.[12] For example, only a few countries in the South American region, including Ecuador, Venezuela, Uruguay, and Brazil, have implemented palliative care in primary health-care facilities[11] (Table 1).
- Fragmented health-care system: This system modality results in delayed diagnosis and more cases of advanced cervical cancer, which frequently necessitates costly diagnostic testing and treatments.[23] The most significant impediment of a fragmented health-care system tends to be various administrative delays as communication between hospitals is lacking, particularly between level 1 to 2 and level 3 facilities.[24] Health maintenance organizations have complete authority over deciding authorizations and require a lengthy administrative regulatory process before individuals can receive care.[24]
- Limited number of centers and geographical barriers: According to government hospital service regulations, patients must be sent to facilities in ascending order, which leads to treatment delays. Some level 1 and 2 facilities have more technology than others; some also have computerized medical records, whereas others use handwritten records.[24] Additionally, most cancer specialists in Latin American countries work in large metropolitan tertiary cancer centers. Due to their inequitable geographic distribution, patients residing outside of urban areas must travel long distances for specialized care, on top of first needing to attend level 1 or 2 facilities.[24] In Brazil, for example, it has been reported that riverside women in the Amazon face notable delays and hurdles to accessing cervical cancer screening tests.[25] Therefore, populations in rural or remote areas, indigenous women, the poor, and uninsured are disproportionately affected by screening barriers.[26]
- Socioeconomic barriers: The lower socioeconomic status of Latin Americans makes health-care problems worse and more likely to occur.[27] In South America, development and access to health-care facilities vary widely from one region to the next.[9] Additionally, there are misunderstandings, societal stigmas, and a general lack of information, including the assumption that cancer is communicable, causes discomfort with physical touch, and necessitates sexual abstinence.[28] Furthermore, socioeconomic constraints can have a negative impact on those seeking medical care as other expenses, such as housing and food, may overwhelm a family's income, leaving little or no financial means for medical needs such as transportation. Finally, in many cases, patients are obliged to deliver biopsy samples to the pathology laboratory themselves, leading to issues related to sample preservation and specimen loss in the absence of quality control.[24]

Initiatives to improve cervical cancer control

Cancer control requires not only the integration of preventive, screening, and high-quality diagnosis, and treatment systems but also a comprehensive range of social

Table 1
Current landscape of cervical cancer policies in Latin America and the Caribbean region

	Argentina	Ecuador	Bolivia	Colombia	Peru	Venezuela	Chile	Uruguay	Paraguay	Brazil
Incidence of cervical cancer per 100,000 women	19.8	17.4	34.1	18.3	25.7	25.7	15.5	15.2	33.5	16.4
Cervical cancer deaths	2500	840	1100	2300	1900	2000	780	170	520	9500
Relationship between mortality and incidence of cervical cancer	0.56	0.53	0.53	0.53	0.54	0.57	0.53	0.58	0.55	0.52
Cancer policies, strategies, and action plans										
(1) Population cancer registry	Yes	Yes	Yes	Yes	Yes	No	Yes	Yes	Yes	Yes
(2) HPV included in the national vaccination program	Yes	Yes	Yes	Yes	Yes	No	Yes	Yes	Yes	Yes
(3) National cervical cancer screening program	Yes	Yes	Yes	Yes	Yes	Yes	Yes	Yes	Yes	Yes
Screening test used	HPV test	Cytology/ HPV test	Cytology	Cytology	Cytology	Cytology	Cytology	Cytology	Cytology	Cytology
(4) Program/guidelines to strengthen early detection of early symptoms in primary care	Yes	Yes	Yes	Yes	Yes	No	Yes	Yes	No	Yes
(5) National cervical cancer treatment guidelines	Yes	No	Yes	Yes	Yes	Yes	Yes	Yes	Yes	Yes
Palliative care in primary health-care services	No	Yes	NS	No	No	Yes	No	Yes	No	Yes
Number of radiotherapy units per 10,000 oncological patients	10	9	5	8	8	8	8	9	7	6
Number of brachytherapy units per 10,000 oncological patients	3	2	3	3	3	2	2	9	2	2

services, such as rehabilitation, survivorship, and palliative care. In recent years, several initiatives have started in Latin America and the Caribbean region, such as the inclusion of HPV vaccination on national immunization schedules, the implementation of cervical cancer screening programs and cancer programs and registries, as well as the training of specialized health-care professionals.[16]

Human papillomavirus vaccine included in the national immunization schedule. According to the PAHO, 80% of adolescent women in Latin America and the Caribbean should now have access to the HPV vaccine, as Argentina, Ecuador, Bolivia, Mexico, Honduras, Panama, Guatemala, Dominican Republic, Colombia, Peru, Chile, Uruguay, Paraguay, and Brazil are among the nations that have implemented the HPV vaccination and include it in their national guidelines.[6,29] Notably, Venezuela has not included HPV immunization in its national vaccination program in South America[11] (see **Table 1**). Only a handful of countries, although, have reported the proportion of girls who have received the full dose of the 3-dose or 2-dose HPV vaccine. In the 2 years following the addition of the HPV vaccine in Argentina's national immunization schedule, more than 80% of girls in the target age range received the first dose of the vaccine, whereas only 60% and 50%, respectively, received second and third doses.[6,29] In Panama, 89% of 10-year-old girls received one dose of the vaccine, whereas 46% received all 3 doses. In Mexico, 1-dose coverage was 85% and full 2-dose coverage was 67%.[29] Monitoring HPV vaccine uptake and effects can assist governments in better evaluating national trends and implementing more efficient policies based on local circumstances.[6]

Decentralization of cancer services. Improving primary care in rural areas is crucial to enhancing cancer control. In 2014, as part of the Xingu Project in Brazil, local health workers were trained to collect samples for cytology tests from the Xingu region's indigenous population.[25,30] These medical professionals administered cytology tests to 76% of the local indigenous women and answered their questions regarding cervical cancer.[30] Such an example of the relocation of specialist facilities in key locations that can serve rural people is a tactic to encourage the decentralization of resources. The National Cancer Control Plan (NCCP), known as Plan Esperanza, in Peru also included the decentralization of cancer services as a component.[31,32] Additionally, telemedicine networks have been implemented in Peru, Ecuador, and Colombia to enhance health care in remote and rural areas.[33]

National cancer plans and cancer registries. In 2021, WHO stated that a large number of South American nations had a program or standards in place to improve the early detection of symptoms in primary care.[11] A successful NCCP established in Latin America is Plan Esperanza in Peru, where a multidisciplinary team, including authorities, collaborated to gather and develop cancer control policies such as cross-sectional public health promotion, system performance and budget management, health-care professional care, competence, and quality services.[34]

Cancer control plans should be rich in high-quality epidemiological data and thorough cancer registries should be a crucial prerequisite for NCCP implementation success. In 2011, just 21% of Latin American nations reported having a population-based cancer registry; by 2014, that number had increased to 67%.[11] By 2021, 90% of South American countries now have cancer registries. Although 45% are population-based, 36% are subnational, and more than 60% are national.[11]

The Cali Cancer Registry in Colombia, which began as an academic project in 1962, is one of the most effective examples of a high-quality epidemiological registry because it has been one of Latin America's most trustworthy and reputable sources of epidemiological cancer data.[24] The data is gathered by actively searching hospital and other medical facility files on a regular basis. This registry has prompted health officials in the region to develop specialized public health policies and allowed the identification of cofactors that act together with HPV to increase the risk of progression from HPV-persistent infection to cervical cancer: tobacco, high parity, long-term use of oral contraceptives and past infections with herpes simplex type 2 and *Chlamydia trachomatis*. It also contributed to establish the important role of male sexual behavior in the risk of developing cervical cancer.[35]

Multicentric initiatives. The implementation of localized training and specialized support, encouragement of research, support for advocacy efforts, and the creation of networks are important actions in each region that enable nations to create national cancer registries through collaborative learning. Project ECHO is an example of a low-cost, high-impact initiative that connects experienced interdisciplinary specialized teams with community primary care practitioners via monthly TeleECHO sessions, thereby increasing the capacity and accessibility of specialist treatment of rural and underserved communities.[19,36] The ECHO telementorship program is supplemented by hands-on training for diagnostic and therapeutic surgical procedures in locations with limited resources, such as colposcopy and LEEP courses.[36]

Implementation of palliative care. There are critical components in the care of patients with cervical cancer including the expansion of palliative care programs, the incorporation of educational courses for specialization in palliative care, the increased use of opioids for pain control, and increased awareness of the importance of palliative care. The publication of the Atlas of Palliative Care in Latin America signaled a significant advancement in recent palliative care progress, as measured by an increase in palliative care services, palliative physicians *per capita*, palliative care education and training programs, and the availability of powerful analgesics.[26] Moreover, in a survey held by the Lancet Commission only 10 of 19 Latin American countries included have formal training in palliative care, and roughly 70% of certified professionals practice in Argentina, Chile, and Mexico. These countries, in addition to Costa Rica, were classified as having the highest palliative care development in Latin America.[26]

Cervical Cancer Screening

Cancer screening and human papillomavirus testing

Almost all Latin American and Caribbean countries use cytology-based cervical cancer screening (Pap smear) as gold standard.[29] The American Cancer Society (2020) recommends cervical cancer screening with an HPV test alone every 5 years for everyone with a cervix from age 25 until age 65 years. If HPV testing alone is not available, women can get screened with an HPV/Pap cotest every 5 years or a Pap test every 3 years.[37] Despite these recommendations, many women in Latin America do not get screened timely. Insufficient screening programs, limitations in techniques, poor quality of histopathological assessment, low-population coverage, insufficient monitoring, and follow-up for women with abnormal cytology results, among other difficulties, have limited cervical cancer screening success.[38,39] Moreover, there is a lack of awareness or access to cervical cancer screening among women from lower socioeconomic backgrounds, often with less education than their counterparts and less access to screening tests.[26,39] Venezuela and Brazil, specifically, have screened around 40% of 30 to 49-year-old women for cervical cancer during the last 5 years, whereas Bolivia and Ecuador have screened 50%[40] (**Fig. 2**). Screening barriers vary by

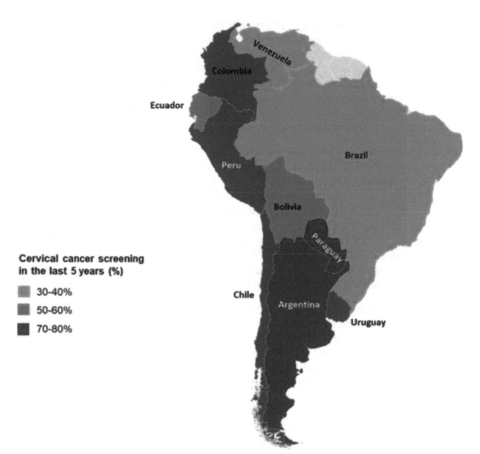

Fig. 2. Cervical cancer screening in the last 5 years in South America. *Reprinted with permission from* Elsevier. The Lancet Global Health. Aug 2022;10(8):e1115-e1127.

geographical region and demographic but disproportionately affect vulnerable populations.[27]

Another critical component is the quality of the screening. If this is poor, or follow-up and treatment of premalignant lesions found by cytology test are insufficient, the proportion of persons with cervical cancer will remain high, even with accessible screening.[33] This may be the case in Boa Vista, Brazil; even though 86% of eligible women participate in screening, the incidence of cervical cancer remains high.[33] Poor-quality cytology tests have also been documented in Latin America and the Caribbean countries. High-quality Pap smears, and a pathologist or cytotechnologist to interpret them, make high-level cytology-based screening programs challenging to implement in resource-constrained areas. For screening programs to be effective, it is crucial to define target populations, screen tests, and screen intervals properly.[41,42] Experts agree that cervical cancer screening should be changed.[30] Currently, there are 3 different screening tests that may be used, depending on the capacity and conditions in a region. If available, the recommended primary screening test is an HPV nucleic acid amplification test (HPV NAAT). The other 2 types of screening tests are cytology and visual inspection with acetic acid (VIA).[43] Given constraints, see-and-treat screening with VIA or DNA-based HPV testing may be more effective than cytology-based screening in the region. Latin American governments presently use VIA in 15 nations including Costa Rica, El Salvador, Guatemala, Nicaragua, Argentina, Colombia, Venezuela, Antigua and Barbuda, Bahamas, Barbados, Guyana, Saint Kitts and Nevis, Saint Lucia, Suriname, Trinidad and Tobago.[29]

Finally, because HPV DNA testing requires less training and quality assurance than cytology-based and VIA screening programs, it offers a unique way to avoid resource limitations.[44] It also enables women to self-sample, which is favored by Latin American women over a clinical pelvic examination.[31,45] Self-sampling with HPV DNA screening has also been assessed in a study in Argentina, where 86% of participants had screening (HPV DNA self-sampling) compared with only 20% in the control group; this difference was independent of socioeconomic variables.[46] As a result of these results, the Ministry of Health in Argentina plans to introduce HPV self-sample screening at the national level in the near future. International Agency for Research on Cancer (IARC) is leading an international research project name the ESTAMPA study in Latin America to evaluate approaches to coordinated cervical screening based on HPV testing and to minimize cervical cancer mortality in the region.[47] In South America, the governments of Argentina and Ecuador have included HPV testing as a screening test in their policies, whereas in other South American nations, such as Bolivia, Colombia, Peru, Venezuela, among others, where resources remain limited, cytology is recommended for screening[11] (see **Table 1**).

In addition, the PAHO recommends 2 screening approaches: (1) in a "screen-and-treat" approach, the decision to proceed with treatment is made without triage testing (no second screening test and no histopathological diagnosis). HPV NAATs are the recommended screening test in this approach but VIA can also be used while transitioning to the use of HPV NAATs. (2) In a "screen, triage, and treat" approach, when the primary screening test is positive, the decision to proceed with treatment is based on the result of a second/triage test. HPV NAATs are the recommended primary screening test in this approach but cytology can also be used while transitioning to the use of HPV NAATs.[43]

Human papillomavirus vaccination

Given how cervical cancer is a preventable disease, vaccination of teenagers and screening of adult women with HPV tests have generated a realistic expectation for cervical cancer elimination in the present and near future. HPV vaccine availability and accessibility has increased substantially since its initial market launch in the late-2000s in Latin America and the Caribbean countries. Still, improving uptake at the population-level, specifically among teenagers, girls and other vulnerable populations, will be crucial to achieving the regional and global targets for cervical cancer control.[48]

Currently, a bivalent vaccine containing high-risk HPV types 16 and 18 and a quadrivalent vaccine containing low-risk HPV types 6, 11, 16, and 18 antigens are in use in vaccination programs around the world. After the Food and Drug Administration approved the quadrivalent HPV vaccine in 2006, the United States was the first country to adopt it. Panama was the first nation in the region to introduce the vaccine in 2008 followed by Mexico. Between 2011 and 2015, 14 countries in Latin America and the Caribbean introduced HPV vaccines into their national immunization programs, and since 2016, the other remaining 27 HPV vaccine introductions have occurred in the region.[48] Currently, 42 countries use the quadrivalent HPV vaccine.[49] By the end of 2021, 44 countries/territories in Latin America and the Caribbean had implemented HPV vaccines in their national immunization programs (**Table 2**), thereby providing access to teenager girls in 89% of PAHO Member States.[29]

The targeted age for vaccination ranges from 9 to 13 years old, although Colombia and Mexico define the target cohort by school grade, rather than age. In general, the

Table 2
Coverage status of human papillomavirus vaccination in Latin America and the Caribbean region

Country	Year of HPV Vaccine Implementation	Target Sex	Schedule
Argentina	2011	F/M	2 doses
Bolivia	2017	F	2 doses
Brazil	2014	F/M	2 doses
Chile	2014	F/M	2 doses
Colombia	2012	F	3 doses
Costa Rica	2019	F	2 doses
Dominican Republic	2014	F	2 doses
Ecuador	2014	F	2 doses
El Salvador	2020	F	N/A
Guatemala	2018	F	N/A
Honduras	2016	F	2 doses
Mexico	2008	F	2 doses
Panama	2008	F/M	2 doses
Paraguay	2013	F	3 doses
Peru	2011	F	2 doses
Uruguay	2013	F/M	3 doses

Adapted from: https://ais.paho.org/imm/IM_JRF_COVERAGE.asp.[61]

vaccination schedule corresponds to that indicated by the vaccine manufacturer, although Colombia and Brazil use an extended schedule with 3 doses at 0, 6, and 60 months; Mexico, Chile, and other countries use 2 doses (0–6 months).[50] The delivery strategy in Uruguay is focused on health centers, while the remaining countries use a school-based strategy (Peru, Paraguay, and Colombia) or a combination of schools and health-care centers (Argentina, Brazil, Mexico, and Panama).[10]

In 2020, all HPV vaccination coverage indicators in the region, including program performance measures and assumed levels of protection afforded by historical HPV vaccination, were affected by the unprecedented impacts of the COVID-19 pandemic on immunization service delivery.[48] Additionally, among teenage girls initiating their HPV vaccination series in 2020, the proportion of girls who did not complete their vaccination series was substantial across countries, ranging from a 4% dropout rate in Chile to as high as a reported 63% of girls in Peru.[51] Since the COVID-19 vaccine has been prioritized, adding an additional vaccine to the immunization schedule and increasing health budgets, it will be critical to redouble efforts to ensure HPV vaccine implementation remains a priority, as part of national immunization programs with regular monitoring and reporting.[48]

Challenges remain in optimizing national immunization programs in the Latin America and the Caribbean region, particularly in terms of engaging government members with advocacy groups, scientists, clinicians, key influencers in the community, and policy makers to lead tailored campaigns focused on cancer prevention and adolescent health.

Overview of Current Therapeutic Options

As is tradition in oncology, therapeutic choices are based on staging and resources available. Although targeted therapy has become a large topic of discussion in novel cancer therapeutics, there are not yet any first-line therapies in cervical cancer directed at specific molecular/genetic mutations. For specifics on staging, refer to **Table 3**, adapted from the 2022 United States' National Comprehensive Cancer Network and the 2018 International Federation of Gynecology and Obstetrics (FIGO) Surgical Staging of Cancer of the Cervix Uteri.[52]

Early stage (stage IA2–IIA)

Early-stage cervical cancer has excellent cure rates when treated aggressively upfront with a radical hysterectomy and pelvic lymphadenectomy.[53] However, this is not without consequences because such therapy can lower quality of life, resulting in early menopause and eliminating fertility. Significant amounts of counseling and shared

Table 3
Staging of cervical cancer adapted from the 2022 United States' National Comprehensive Cancer Network and 2018 International Federation of Gynecology and Obstetrics Surgical Staging of Cancer of the Cervix Uteri[52]

Early	*Stage I*	The carcinoma is strictly confined to the cervix
	IA	Invasive carcinoma that can be diagnosed only by microscopy with maximum depth of invasion ≤5 mm *IA1* Measured stromal invasion ≤3 mm in depth *IA2* Measured stromal invasion >3 mm and ≤5 mm in depth
	IB	Invasive carcinoma with measured deepest invasion >5 mm (greater than stage IA); lesion limited to the cervix uteri with size measured by maximum tumor diameter *IB1* Invasive carcinoma >5 mm depth of stromal invasion and ≤2 cm in greatest dimension *IB2* Invasive carcinoma >2 cm and ≤4 cm in greatest dimension *IB3* Invasive carcinoma >4 cm in greatest dimension
	Stage II	The cervical carcinoma invades beyond the uterus but has not extended onto the lower third of the vagina or to the pelvic wall
	IIA	Involvement limited to the upper two-thirds of the vagina without parametrial invasion *IIA1* Invasive carcinoma ≤4 cm in greatest dimension *IIA2* Invasive carcinoma >4 cm in greatest dimension
	IIB	With parametrial invasion but not up to the pelvic wall
Locally advanced	*Stage III*	The carcinoma involves the lower third of the vagina and/or extends to the pelvic wall and/or causes hydronephrosis or nonfunctioning kidney and/or involves pelvic and/or para-aortic lymph nodes
	IIIA	Carcinoma involves lower third of the vagina, with no extension to the pelvic wall
	IIIB	Extension to the pelvic wall and/or hydronephrosis or nonfunctioning kidney (unless known to be due to another cause)
	IIIC	Involvement of pelvic and/or paraaortic lymph nodes (including micrometastases), irrespective of tumor size and extent *IIIC1* Pelvic lymph node metastasis only *IIIC2* Paraaortic lymph node metastasis
Metastatic	*Stage IV*	The carcinoma has extended beyond the true pelvis or has involved (biopsy proven) the mucosa of the bladder or rectum. A bullous edema, as such, does not permit a case to be allotted to stage IV
	IVA	Spread of the growth to adjacent organs
	IVB	Spread to distant organs

decision-making between providers and patients should take place before proceeding forward.

For those who do decide to proceed with definitive surgery, there are limited centers with such expertise in Latin America. As an approach to foster less-invasive procedures that can be more readily provided by local gynecologists, MD Anderson Cancer Center has partnered with institutions in Mexico, Colombia, Brazil, Peru, and Argentina in a prospective study to evaluate the feasibility, safety, and effectiveness of performing more conservative surgeries in women with early-stage cervical cancer (ConCerv trial); results are not yet available.[54]

In 2019, an expert panel composed of specialists from more than 38 countries from Africa, Asia, Europe, and Latin America congregated to develop treatment recommendations for early-stage cervical cancer.[55] Acknowledging that resources may be limited in certain settings, and considering varied patient priorities and preferences in their care, they came up with the following recommendations.

- For patients with stage IA2 cervical cancer wishing to preserve fertility, trachelectomy is advised.
- For patients with a clinically visible tumor (stage IB3–IIA), chemoradiation alone is recommended in areas where gynecologic surgery services are not available.
- For patients with a clinically visible tumor (stage IB3–IIA) where radiation therapy is unavailable, neoadjuvant chemotherapy (generally with a platinum-based regimen) is advised, followed by surgery. If gynecologic oncology services were unavailable, simple hysterectomy would suffice.
- For patients with early-stage cervical cancer undergoing surgery with at least one high-risk feature (positive surgical margins, pathologically involved pelvic nodes, or positive involvement of the parametria), adjuvant radiotherapy and chemotherapy should be provided, if available.
- In areas where brachytherapy is unavailable, both primary and adjuvant external radiotherapy can be administered to women with early-stage cervical cancer.[55]

The Chilean Society of Radiation Oncology (SOCHIRA) also convened to provide graded recommendations on radiation therapy.[56] The grades were in an A to C scale, with A being recommended, B being suggested cautiously, and C not being advised. SOCHIRA gave a grade B recommendation to definitive radiation therapy (external beam radiation therapy, [EBRT], plus brachytherapy) in patients with early stage (IB1–IIA1) cervical cancer, in the case where surgery was unavailable or contraindicated.[56] The advised dosing for radiation by SOCHIRA was 45 Gy in 25 fractions, although they acknowledged that other appropriate schedules may exist. They further stressed that referral for radiation must be urgent, at most within 50 or lesser to 56 days from the initiation of treatment.[56]

Locally advanced (stages IIB–IVA)

Standard therapy for locally advanced cervical cancer is chemoradiation. This includes EBRT to the pelvis with potential attention to para-aortic lymph nodes, if involved. Treatment is generally given on weekdays for a total of 5 to 6 weeks and is then followed by 2 to 5 sessions of brachytherapy. The concurrent chemotherapy is generally cisplatin or carboplatin if cisplatin-ineligible; SOCHIRA gave a grade A recommendation to this approach for patients with an advanced stage (IB2–IVA).[56]

Unfortunately, many regions in Latin America lack the appropriate radiation therapy specialists and units required for treatment. This combined shortage results in delays in treatment and requires patients to travel from afar if no local providers/equipment for radiotherapy is available. Additionally, this oftentimes can lead to incomplete treatment of locally advanced cervical cancer because patients only end up receiving partial radiation or chemotherapy.[57]

Many organizations have investigated alternative standards of care for locally advanced cervical cancer in low-resource settings. Presently, the National Institute of Neoplastic Diseases in Peru is assessing neoadjuvant chemotherapy followed by surgery in place of chemoradiation, with results pending at this time.[57]

The International Gynecological Cancer Society consensus meeting in 2019 led to the following recommendations in the setting of locally advanced cervical cancer.[55]

- If available, concomitant chemoradiation is the recommended approach for stages IIB to IVA cervical cancer.
- Chemoradiation alone is recommended for patients with locally advanced disease in areas where gynecologic oncology surgical services are not available, and for immunocompromised patients.
- A 2-dimensional conventional brachytherapy technique is recommended for eligible patients with stages IB3 through IVA disease after external radiation.
- For patients with known para-aortic node involvement, chemoradiation with extended-field radiotherapy is recommended.
- Weekly cisplatin is the preferred chemotherapy for the general patient population receiving concurrent chemoradiation (generally 40 mg/m^2 every week).[55]

Finally, SOCHIRA gave a grade A recommendation to adjuvant EBRT in individuals who did not receive concurrent chemotherapy while meeting Sedlis criteria and adjuvant EBRT for those who did receive concurrent chemotherapy and met Peters criteria.[56]

Distant metastases or recurrent disease (stage IV)

Patients with localized recurrence may still be candidates for radical treatments including radiation, chemotherapy, and surgical approaches. If there is recurrence in an area that recently underwent chemoradiation, other systemic agents such as carboplatin, paclitaxel, or gemcitabine may be considered. With respect to surgical options, those who have central pelvic recurrence may be considered for pelvic exenteration that removes the vagina, cervix, uterus, ovaries, and tumor deposits, as well as the bladder, anus, and a portion of the intestine. This is an aggressive approach in preventing recurrence and could result in many side effects and lifelong medical needs that may pose challenges for individuals in low-resource settings.[55]

The standard of care for distant metastatic cervical cancer is quality supportive care with the intent of life prolongation and a reasonable quality of life because these cases are generally not curable. As such, care of these patients may include a coordinated approach with pain specialists, emotional and spiritual resources, and palliative therapies (radiation, systemic, surgical options). In this setting, combination chemotherapies may be pursued, including first-line regimen cisplatin, paclitaxel, and bevacizumab. If molecular profiling is available, those who are programmed cell death ligand 1 (PD-L1) positive or with microsatellite instability-high (MSI-H)/a mismatch repair deficient (dMMR) cervical tumors may be eligible for second-line pembrolizumab immunotherapy. Alternative second-line therapies include nab-paclitaxel, docetaxel, fluorouracil, gemcitabine, ifosfamide, irinotecan, mitomycin, pemetrexed, topotecan, and/or vinorelbine, depending on the availability in each region. Currently, there is no study or available data to provide insights on the access to molecular profiling or turn-around-time for such tests in Latin America countries.[55]

The International Gynecological Cancer Society consensus meeting in 2019 led to the following recommendations in the setting of (distant) metastatic or recurrent cervical cancer.[55]

- For patients not amenable to salvage locoregional treatment and not eligible to receive cisplatin, carboplatin plus paclitaxel should be the regimen of choice.
- The best intervention to treat fecal incontinence due to rectovaginal fistula is surgical management by a diverting colostomy.
- Either paclitaxel or gemcitabine can be considered as appropriate treatment options for women with metastatic cervical cancer at any point, according to its availability and lower price.[55]

Pregnancy

Oftentimes with pregnant patients, neoadjuvant systemic therapies are used to quell the disease while the baby finishes developing and is delivered, then after allowing for more definitive surgical and radiation therapies. A multicenter retrospective review was conducted among 12 institutions, including 6 in Latin America, to observe outcomes of patients diagnosed with stage IB1–IVA cervical cancer during pregnancy who received neoadjuvant chemotherapy.[58] Centers involved in the study included Instituto Nacional de Enfermedades Neoplásicas, Peru; Instituto Regional de Enfermedades Neoplásicas, Arequipa, Peru; Hospital Cayetano Heredia, Peru; Instituto Nacional de Cancerología, Colombia; Hospital Militar Central, Colombia; Instituto de Cancerología Las Américas-AUNA, Colombia; Unidad de Terapia Antineoplásica Centro Médico Guerra Méndez Valencia, Venezuela; Hospital Oncológico de Buenos Aires Marie Curie, Argentina; Hospital de Cáncer de Barretos, Brazil; Hospital Pereira Rossell, Uruguay; Clínica Médica Uruguaya, Uruguay; and Servicio Oncológico Hospitalario de Caracas, Venezuela.[58] Following this review, the group summarized the following for pregnant patients wishing to preserve their pregnancy while diagnosed with cervical cancer.

- Chemotherapy during first trimester is contraindicated.
- Cisplatin can be administered safely during the second or third trimester of pregnancy.
- Potential toxicity from platinum-based chemo the second and third trimester mainly negatively influences growth and birth weight. In a review of 88 neonates, however, 71 had no anomalies, suggesting low rates of chemotherapy-related sequelae for the baby.[59]

Accessibility to clinical trials

Clinical trials are often advised for patients with late-stage disease; however, access is mainly attainable through large academic centers and usually requires frequent travel and associated health-care expenses that may not be feasible for the general Latin American population.[60]

Several groups including the Gynecologic Cancer InterGroup and the Cervical Cancer Research Network (CCRN) have been developing methods of expand access to clinical trials through low-resource settings including Latin America, Africa, and the Indian subcontinent.[44,60] CCRN has representation from surgical, medical, and radiation oncologists and has been involved in bringing regional symposia to these areas for more direct teaching and sharing of resources.[60] Although clinical trials are not yet widely accessed in Latin America and the Caribbean region, there is hope that this will continue to improve in the decades to come with such efforts.

Patient Education

The task of demystifying cervical malignancies is difficult. Yet, by educating patients and developing long-lasting educational programs, numerous myths and stigmas have diminished. Integrating patient navigators and/or community health professionals to engage vulnerable populations in HPV vaccination and cervical cancer screening programs bridges the patient-health-care system gap and informational barriers, aiding in demystification.[24]

A successful example in Latin America is Partners for Cancer Care and Prevention (PFCCAP) and its sister organization in Colombia, Fundación para la Prevención y Tratamiento del Cáncer, nonprofit organizations established in 2012.[24] As an addition to the navigation program, PFCCAP created a mobile application, Amate Cuida tu Salud, a smartphone application intended to deliver basic cervical cancer education, identify people at risk, and help patients navigate their disease more effectively.[16] Notably, it is also a low-cost and accessible tool for identifying women at risk for cervical cancer and detecting impediments to early cancer diagnosis.[24] This novel strategy has the potential to reach rural communities and can be duplicated in other underdeveloped countries. To date, more than 1500 women and their families have benefited from group conferences, individual education, support groups, and outreach activities from these 2 organizations. Similar projects should be implemented in other Latin American nations.[24]

SUMMARY

Cervical cancer is one of the most common cancers among women worldwide and its incidence and mortality rates varies between developed and developing countries. Interventions in Latin America and the Caribbean countries continue to be needed to address gaps in care such as limited trained personal, fragmented health-care systems, and difficulties to accessing medical centers due to geographical and socioeconomic barriers. Screening with cervical cytology and HPV vaccinations programs continue to be key in decreasing the burden of cervical cancer in Latin America and the Caribbean region. Although availability and accessibility of HPV vaccines have increased in recent years, optimizing immunization programs, and delivering high-quality oncological care remain an essential paradigm for engaging government members with clinicians, advocacy groups, and community members. Collaboration with higher level cancer centers from the United States and around the world is currently taking place to train clinicians and develop viable treatment systems and surgical approaches; such efforts remain key in addressing cervical cancer management. Virtually, by combining HPV vaccine programs with HPV-based testing via screening programs, the cervical cancer burden could be eliminated in every country of the Latin America and the Caribbean region. Further political and economic commitments and efforts are needed.

CLINICS CARE POINTS

- Cervical cancer represents the third most common cancer in women from the region.
- The WHO's Global Strategy to Accelerate Cervical Cancer Elimination aims to decrease the rate of cervical to less than 4 cases per 100,000 women.
- To eliminate cervical cancer by 2030, the goals are to vaccinate 90% of girls against HPV by age 15, achieve more than 70% screening coverage using a high-performance test for women aged 35 to 45 years, and treat 90% of cases.

- The PAHO recommends the introduction of new technologies in "screen and treat" or "screen, triage, and treat" approaches to reduce cervical cancer inequalities, overcoming loss of follow-up, and improving detection and treatment rates.
- HPV vaccination programs potentially can reduce the long-term future burden of cervical cancer; currently the WHO recommends effective and cost-effective interventions such as vaccinations against HPV (2 doses) of girls aged 9 to 13 years, and high-quality screening programs to prevent cervical cancer among unvaccinated older women.
- Obtaining reliable cancer incidence data is critical for cervical cancer elimination monitoring.
- Collaborations to increase expertise of professionals in oncology treatments will ensure quality of care of women with cervical cancer in all stages of disease.

DISCLOSURE

I. Riano, P. Contreras-Chavez, C. Pabon, K. Meza, and S. Bejarano have nothing to declare. N. Florez: Consulting/Advisory to Merck, Astrazeneca, Pfizer, DSI, BMS, Novartis, Neogenomics, and Janssen.

REFERENCES

1. WHO. Cervical Cancer. Available at: https://www.who.int/news-room/fact-sheets/detail/cervical-cancer. Accessed March 20, 2022.
2. Cancer IAfRo. Global Cancer Observatory. Available at: https://gco.iarc.fr/. Accessed March 20, 2023.
3. WHO. Cervical Cancer: Health Topic. 2023. Available at: https://www.who.int/health-topics/cervical-cancer#tab=tab_1.
4. Bongaerts THG, Ridder M, Vermeer-Mens JCJ, et al. Cervical cancer screening among marginalized women: a cross-sectional intervention study. Int J Womens Health 2021;13:549–56.
5. WHO. Cervical Cancer Elimination Initiative. Available at: https://www.who.int/initiatives/cervical-cancer-elimination-initiative. Accessed March 20, 2023.
6. PAHO. Cervical Cancer. Available at: https://www.paho.org/en/topics/cervical-cancer. Accessed March 20, 2023.
7. PAHO. Plan of Action for Cervical Cancer Prevention and Control 2018-2030. Available at: https://iris.paho.org/handle/10665.2/38574. Accessed March 20, 2023.
8. IARC. Latin America and the Caribbean. Available at: https://gco.iarc.fr/today/data/factsheets/populations/904-latin-america-and-the-caribbean-fact-sheets.pdf. Accessed March 20, 2023.
9. Pilleron S, Cabasag CJ, Ferlay J, et al. Cervical cancer burden in Latin America and the caribbean: where are we? Int J Cancer 2020;147(6):1638–48.
10. Murillo R, Herrero R, Sierra MS, et al. Cervical cancer in Central and South America: Burden of disease and status of disease control. Cancer Epidemiol 2016;44(Suppl 1):S121–30.
11. WHO. Cervical cancer country profiles. Available at: https://www.who.int/teams/noncommunicable-diseases/surveillance/data/cervical-cancer-profiles. Accessed March 20, 2023.
12. Goss PE, Lee BL, Badovinac-Crnjevic T, et al. Planning cancer control in Latin America and the Caribbean. Lancet Oncol 2013;14(5):391–436.

13. Bray F, Ferlay J, Soerjomataram I, et al. Global cancer statistics 2018: GLOBO-CAN estimates of incidence and mortality worldwide for 36 cancers in 185 countries. CA Cancer J Clin 2018;68(6):394–424.

14. Simms KT, Steinberg J, Caruana M, et al. Impact of scaled up human papillomavirus vaccination and cervical screening and the potential for global elimination of cervical cancer in 181 countries, 2020-99: a modelling study. Lancet Oncol 2019; 20(3):394–407.

15. Vaccarella S, Laversanne M, Ferlay J, et al. Cervical cancer in Africa, Latin America and the Caribbean and Asia: Regional inequalities and changing trends. Int J Cancer 2017;141(10):1997–2001.

16. Nogueira-Rodrigues A. HPV Vaccination in Latin America: Global Challenges and Feasible Solutions. Am Soc Clin Oncol Educ Book 2019;39:e45–52.

17. WHO. WHO guideline for screening and treatment of cervical pre-cancer lesions for cervical cancer prevention. Available at: https://www.who.int/publications/i/item/9789240030824. Accessed March 20, 2023.

18. Lopez MS, Baker ES, Maza M, et al. Cervical cancer prevention and treatment in Latin America. J Surg Oncol 2017;115(5):615–8.

19. Lopez MS, Baker ES, Milbourne AM, et al. Project ECHO: A Telementoring Program for Cervical Cancer Prevention and Treatment in Low-Resource Settings. Journal of Global Oncology 2017;3(5):658–65.

20. Schmeler KM, Ramirez PT, Reyes-Martinez CA, et al. The Central America Gynecologic Oncology Education Program (CONEP): improving gynecologic oncology education and training on a global scale. Gynecol Oncol 2013; 129(3):445–7.

21. Eala MAB, Tantengco OAG. Global online interest in cervical cancer care in the time of COVID-19: An infodemiology study. Gynecol Oncol Rep 2022;41:100998.

22. Nuche-Berenguer B, Sakellariou D. Socioeconomic determinants of cancer screening utilisation in Latin America: a systematic review. PLoS One 2019; 14(11):e0225667.

23. Nnaji CA, Kuodi P, Walter FM, et al. Effectiveness of interventions for improving timely diagnosis of breast and cervical cancers in low-income and middle-income countries: a systematic review. BMJ Open 2022;12(4):e054501.

24. Sardi A, Orozco-Urdaneta M, Velez-Mejia C, et al. Overcoming Barriers in the Implementation of Programs for Breast and Cervical Cancers in Cali, Colombia: A Pilot Model. J Glob Oncol 2019;5:1–9.

25. da Silva DCB, Garnelo L, Herkrath FJ. Barriers to access the pap smear test for cervical cancer screening in rural riverside populations covered by a fluvial primary healthcare team in the amazon. Int J Environ Res Public Health 2022; 19(7). https://doi.org/10.3390/ijerph19074193.

26. Strasser-Weippl K, Chavarri-Guerra Y, Villarreal-Garza C, et al. Progress and remaining challenges for cancer control in Latin America and the Caribbean. Lancet Oncol 2015;16(14):1405–38.

27. Soneji S, Fukui N. Socioeconomic determinants of cervical cancer screening in Latin America. Rev Panam Salud Publica 2013;33(3):174–82.

28. Nnebue CC. The epidemiological transition: policy and planning implications for developing countries. Niger J Med Jul-Sep 2010;19(3):250–6.

29. PAHO. PAHO. Cancer in the Americas. Basic Indicators, 2013. Available at: https://www.paho.org/en/documents/paho-cancer-americas-basic-indicators-2013. Accessed March 20, 2023.

30. Cendales R, Wiesner C, Murillo RH, et al. [Quality of vaginal smear for cervical cancer screening: a concordance study]. Biomedica 2010;30(1):107–15. La

calidad de las citologías para tamización de cáncer de cuello uterino en cuatro departamentos de Colombia: un estudio de concordancia.

31. Abuelo CE, Levinson KL, Salmeron J, et al. The Peru Cervical Cancer Screening Study (PERCAPS): the design and implementation of a mother/daughter screen, treat, and vaccinate program in the Peruvian jungle. J Community Health 2014; 39(3):409–15.

32. Kirkwood MK, Bruinooge SS, Goldstein MA, et al. Enhancing the American Society of Clinical Oncology workforce information system with geographic distribution of oncologists and comparison of data sources for the number of practicing oncologists. J Oncol Pract 2014;10(1):32–8.

33. Navarro C, Fonseca AJ, Sibajev A, et al. Cervical cancer screening coverage in a high-incidence region. Rev Saude Publica 2015;49:17.

34. Vallejos C. National plan for prevention, early detection, and cancer control in Peru. Am Soc Clin Oncol Educ Book 2013. https://doi.org/10.1200/EdBook_AM. 2013.33.e245.

35. Muñoz N, Bravo LE. Epidemiology of cervical cancer in Colombia. Colomb Méd 2012;43(4):298–304.

36. Komaromy M, Duhigg D, Metcalf A, et al. Project ECHO (Extension for Community Healthcare Outcomes): a new model for educating primary care providers about treatment of substance use disorders. Subst Abus 2016;37(1):20–4.

37. NCI. ACS's Updated Cervical Cancer Screening Guidelines Explained. Available at: https://www.cancer.gov/news-events/cancer-currents-blog/2020/cervical-cancer-screening-hpv-test-guideline#:~:text=ACS%20recommends%20cervical%20cancer%20screening,Pap%20test%20every%203%20years Accessed March 20, 2023.

38. Parkin DM, Almonte M, Bruni L, et al. Burden and trends of type-specific human papillomavirus infections and related diseases in the latin america and Caribbean region. Vaccine 2008;26(Suppl 11):L1–15.

39. Villa LL. Cervical cancer in Latin America and the caribbean: the problem and the way to solutions. Cancer Epidemiol Biomarkers Prev 2012;21(9):1409–13.

40. Bruni L, Serrano B, Roura E, et al. Cervical cancer screening programmes and age-specific coverage estimates for 202 countries and territories worldwide: a review and synthetic analysis. Lancet Global Health 2022;10(8):e1115–27.

41. de Sanjose S, Holme F. What is needed now for successful scale-up of screening? Papillomavirus Res 2019;7:173–5.

42. Fernández-Deaza G, Caicedo-Martínez M, Serrano B, et al. Cervical cancer screening programs in Latin America: current recommendations for facing elimination challenges. Salud Publica Mex 2022;64(4, jul-ago):415–23.

43. WHO. World Health Organization Department of Sexual and Reproductive Health and Research (WHO/SRH) and Johns Hopkins Bloomberg School of Public Health/Center for Communication Programs (CCP), Knowledge SUCCESS. Family Planning: A Global Handbook for Providers.Available at: https://fphandbook. org/sites/default/files/WHO-JHU-FPHandbook-2022Ed-v221114b.pdf. Accessed March 20, 2023.

44. Sankaranarayanan R, Nene BM, Shastri SS, et al. HPV screening for cervical cancer in rural India. N Engl J Med 2009;360(14):1385–94.

45. Levinson KL, Abuelo C, Salmeron J, et al. The peru cervical cancer prevention study (PERCAPS): the technology to make screening accessible. Gynecol Oncol 2013;129(2):318–23.

46. Arrossi S, Thouyaret L, Herrero R, et al. Effect of self-collection of HPV DNA offered by community health workers at home visits on uptake of screening for

cervical cancer (the EMA study): a population-based cluster-randomised trial. Lancet Global Health 2015;3(2):e85–94.

47. Almonte M, Murillo R, Sánchez GI, et al. Multicentric study of cervical cancer screening with human papillomavirus testing and assessment of triage methods in Latin America: the ESTAMPA screening study protocol. BMJ Open 2020;10(5): e035796.

48. De Oliveira LH, Janusz CB, Da Costa MT, et al. HPV vaccine introduction in the Americas: a decade of progress and lessons learned. Expert Rev Vaccines 2022;21(11):1569–80.

49. PAHO. 2021 : DTP3 District Coverage - Region of the Americas. Available at: https://ais.paho.org/imm/IM_ADM2_COVERAGE-MAPS-Americas.asp.   Accessed March 20, 2023.

50. Herrero R, González P, Markowitz LE. Present status of human papillomavirus vaccine development and implementation. Lancet Oncol 2015;16(5):e206–16.

51. Toh ZQ, Russell FM, Garland SM, et al. Human papillomavirus vaccination after COVID-19. JNCI Cancer Spectr 2021;5(2):pkab011.

52. Berek JS, Matsuo K, Grubbs BH, et al. Multidisciplinary perspectives on newly revised 2018 FIGO staging of cancer of the cervix uteri. J Gynecol Oncol 2019; 30(2):e40.

53. Guimarães YM, Godoy LR, Longatto-Filho A, et al. Management of early-stage cervical cancer: a literature review. Cancers 2022;14(3). https://doi.org/10. 3390/cancers14030575.

54. Schmeler KM, Pareja R, Lopez Blanco A, et al. ConCerv: a prospective trial of conservative surgery for low-risk early-stage cervical cancer. Int J Gynecol Cancer 2021;31(10):1317–25.

55. Maluf FC, Dal Molin GZ, de Melo AC, et al. Recommendations for the prevention, screening, diagnosis, staging, and management of cervical cancer in areas with limited resources: Report from the International Gynecological Cancer Society consensus meeting. Front Oncol 2022;12:928560.

56. Carvajal F, Carvajal C, Merino T, et al. Radiotherapy for cervical cancer: chilean consensus of the Society of Radiation Oncology. Rep Practical Oncol Radiother 2021;26(2):291–302.

57. Aguilar A, Pinto JA, Araujo J, et al. Control of cervical cancer in Peru: current barriers and challenges for the future. Mol Clin Oncol 2016;5(2):241–5.

58. Lopez A, Rodriguez J, Estrada E, et al. Neoadjuvant chemotherapy in pregnant patients with cervical cancer: a Latin-American multicenter study. Int J Gynecol Cancer 2021;31(3):468–74.

59. Song Y, Liu Y, Lin M, et al. Efficacy of neoadjuvant platinum-based chemotherapy during the second and third trimester of pregnancy in women with cervical cancer: an updated systematic review and meta-analysis. Drug Des Dev Ther 2019; 13:79–102.

60. McCormack M, Gaffney D, Tan D, et al. The cervical cancer research network (gynecologic cancer intergroup) roadmap to expand research in low- and middle-income countries. Int J Gynecol Cancer 2021;31(5):775–8.

61. PAHO. Country reports and PAHO/WHO-UNICEF Joint Reporting Forms (JRF). Available at: https://ais.paho.org/imm/IM_JRF_COVERAGE.asp. Accessed March 20, 2023.

Disparities in Cancer Control in Central America and the Caribbean

Anne Christine Buteau, MD[a], Alicia Castelo-Loureiro, MD[b],
Regina Barragan-Carrillo, MD[c], Suyapa Bejarano, MD[d],
Alba J. Kihn-Alarcón, MD, MSc[e],
Enrique Soto-Perez-de-Celis, MD, PhD[f],*

KEYWORDS

- Central America • Caribbean region • Cancer care facilities
- Health services accessibility • Health-care disparities • Cancer

KEY POINTS

- Central America and the Caribbean is a highly heterogeneous region with an increasing burden of cancer facing many challenges for providing equitable access to high-quality cancer care.
- Barriers for obtaining cancer care across the region include socioeconomic barriers, health-care system fragmentation, immigration, rural–urban disparities, and low availability of human and technological resources.
- Although recent initiatives have improved access and outcomes for patients with cancer in Central America and the Caribbean, regional and global initiatives are needed to further increase the capacity of health-care systems to provide care for a growing population of patients.

INTRODUCTION

The Central American and Caribbean region are home to more than 180 million people in Central America and about 44 million people in the Caribbean Island nations.[1,2] These populations are spanned over 7 mainland countries in Central America

[a] Dartmouth-Hitchcock Medical Center, 1 Medical Center Drive, Lebanon, NH 03766, USA; [b] Medical Oncology Division, Hospital Universitario 12 de Octubre, Av. de Córdoba, s/n, 28041, Madrid, Spain; [c] Department of Hemato-Oncology, Instituto Nacional de Ciencias Médicas y Nutrición Salvador Vasco de Quiroga 15, Sección XVI, Tlalpan, Mexico City, Mexico; [d] Excelmedica, Liga Contra el Cancer Honduras, Condominios Médicos del Valle I Apt 318, San Pedro Sula, Honduras; [e] Research Department, Liga Nacional Contra el Cáncer & Instituto de Cancerología, 6a Avenida 6-58, Cdad. de Guatemala 01011, Guatemala; [f] Department of Geriatrics, Instituto Nacional de Ciencias Médicas y Nutrición Salvador Zubirán, Vasco de Quiroga 15, Sección XVI, Tlalpan, Mexico City, Mexico
* Corresponding author.
E-mail address: enrique.sotop@incmnsz.mx

Hematol Oncol Clin N Am 38 (2024) 35–53
https://doi.org/10.1016/j.hoc.2023.07.007
0889-8588/24/© 2023 Elsevier Inc. All rights reserved.

(Panama, Costa Rica, Nicaragua, Honduras, El Salvador, Guatemala, and Belize) and 31 countries and territories in the Caribbean including 13 independent states (Antigua and Barbuda, The Bahamas, Barbados, Cuba, Dominica, Dominican Republic, Grenada, Haiti, Jamaica, St Kitts and Nevis, St Lucia, St Vincent and the Grenadines, Trinidad and Tobago) (**Fig. 1**).[3,4] Although these countries have a shared heritage of European colonialism and American influence, climate change vulnerability, and inequality, there is diversity in their culture, population, language, economic and health-care systems. In this article, we provide an overview of existing cancer care disparities in this very diverse, and often overlooked, region of the world, including a summary of existing projects for reducing those disparities.

In this article, we provide an overview of issues related to disparities in access to cancer care faced in selected countries in the Central American and Caribbean region, highlighting relevant problems and offering solutions regarding strategies to overcome them.

Central America

For the Central American region, we have focused on crucial cancer control issues in 4 territories: (1) Southeastern Mexico, which bears a large proportion of the burden of cancer in Mexico, faces visible disparities compared with the wealthier north of the country, and has a large rural population; (2) Guatemala, which showcases a country in the region transitioning from a low-income to a middle-income economy; (3) Honduras, a country still suffering from low human development index; and (4) Costa Rica, which is one of the few countries in the region, which has achieved universal health coverage.

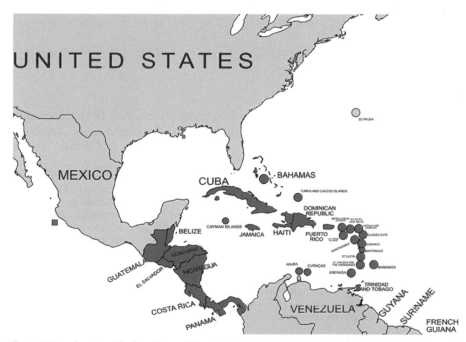

Fig. 1. Map showing the location of the Central American and Caribbean region (in purple) within the Americas.

Southeastern Mexico

Mexico is a diverse country where access to specialized cancer care can widely vary among regions. Cancer is the third cause of death in Mexico, with an incidence and mortality of 25.1 and 11.7 cases per 100,000 inhabitants, respectively.[5,6] Mexico's south-eastern region comprises 5 states (Campeche, Quintana Roo, Tabasco, Yucatan, and Chiapas) and a population is approximately 7,509,844 inhabitants, accounting for 10% of the country's population.[7] This region shares a common border with Guatemala and Belize, is characterized by slow economic growth, geographical barriers limiting transportation, higher alcohol consumption, lower educational levels, and exposure to carcinogens from wood burning and contaminated water.[8]

Mexico's indigenous populations are concentrated in the south. These populations are culturally and ethnically heterogeneous, with Mayan, Olmec, Mixtec, and Zapotec heritage, traditions, and languages.[9] South-eastern Mexico has the highest percentage of speakers of Mesoamerican languages, with Maya spoken by 30% to 40% of Yucatan's population.[10] The lack of cultural and linguistic inclusivity within the Mexican health-care system hinders access to care and generates mistrust in the system, leading to an increased reliance on local healers or shamans.[8]

People in south-eastern Mexico have increased cancer mortality compared with those from northern and central regions.[11] Among the 5 states comprising this area, 3 have a high or very high cancer mortality-to-incidence ratios of 0.68, 0.61, 0.60 to 0.58 deaths per cancer diagnosis, respectively.[12] Furthermore, 60% of the country's cancer workforce is based in cities in the central and northern regions,[13] with only 76 oncology specialists registered in the southeastern region (unpublished data obtained from the Mexican Society of Oncology, 2022). Access to chemotherapy and novel treatments such as targeted therapies and immunotherapies is also limited outside of large metropolitan areas and is only available for some patients with private insurance coverage or as an out-of-pocket expense.[14,15]

Simialrly, radiation therapy, imaging, and high-quality pathology are only available in some southeastern states' capital cities, making access difficult for poor patients from rural areas with limited access to transportation, many of which are indigenous.[16] Early detection is also limited with scarce availability of mammography equipment (from 0.41 to 2.61 per 100.000 inhabitants) and limited uptake of cervical cytology among indigenous populations, which might be an explanation for the increasing incidence of breast and cervical cancer in the region.[17–19]

Guatemala

Guatemala is an upper-middle income country of 17 million inhabitants. Of the 80,000 yearly deaths in the country, 59% are related to noncommunicable diseases (NCDs), with cancer being the second cause after cardiovascular disease.[20–22] Guatemala does not have a national cancer registry, and only one hospital-based registry is available but existing data show that the most common cancers are liver, gastric, breast, and cervical.[23,24]

Since 2013, general practitioners and specialists are required to report new cancer cases every 3 months. The National Commission for the Prevention of Noncommunicable Diseases and Cancer, which is a governmental task force created by the federal government to guide national policies on cancer and other chronic diseases, is tasked with analyzing those reports to develop policies and actions aimed at decreasing the incidence, prevalence, mortality, and disability associated with NCDs. This National Commission has managed to draft a cervical cancer guideline and a cervical cancer designated program, which has shown the positive impact of screening on the reduction of premature deaths. However, efforts are still needed to create awareness regarding breast cancer and improving access to early diagnosis and treatment.[25,26] Moreover, further understanding of the risk factors causing other malignancies highly present in the population, such as liver and gastric cancer, might help to create other prevention and early detection programs.

Currently, 2 public systems cover the cost of oncological surgeries and systemic therapy but there are only 2 comprehensive cancer centers in the country (both nongovernmental organizations): *Unidad Nacional de Oncología Pediátrica* for pediatric patients and *Liga Nacional Contra el Cáncer-INCAN*, which provides services at reduced cost for the general population and radiotherapy to adult patients referred by the National Health System. In addition, several private practices and hospitals offer cancer care for patients who can afford it. According to the most recent data by the International Atomic Energy Agency, there are only 8 radiotherapy units in the country, all located in Guatemala city. Considering that approximately 49% of the population lives in rural areas, radiotherapy is out of reach or requires traveling long distances for a significant number of Guatemalans.[27,28]

Cancer care in Guatemala is also hampered by a limited clinical workforce. The main reason for this is that in the past there were no opportunities for oncology training in the country both in medical school and in fellowship, making it necessary to obtain training abroad. Although oncology fellowships are now available in Guatemala, there are few professionals dedicated to cancer, including 62 cancer specialists (medical oncologists, hematologists, pediatric hemato-oncologists, surgical oncologists, gynecological oncologists, and radiation oncologists) and 11 palliative care physicians.[29,30]

Honduras

Honduras has a population of 9,656,299 inhabitants.[31] In 2019, Honduras was placed as the 132nd country in the world by Human Development Index, reflecting poor sanitary, educational, environmental, and social conditions. Sixty-one percent of Honduran households live in poverty, which was worsened by the coronavirus disease 2019 (COVID-19) pandemic and, out of a gross domestic product (GDP) of US$22.98 billion, public health-care represents around 2.7%.[32] Health care in Honduras has mixed coverage with the public sector (SESAL) providing care for 60% of the population, the Honduran Institute of Social Security for 12% and the profit/nonprofit private sector to another 10%. The Ministry of Health of Honduras governs and leads the main health strategies, and although attempts to create a cancer control plan have occurred since 2009, to date Honduras lacks a national policy for cancer control.[32] Disparities in Honduras are further deepened among diverse racial and ethnic groups. There are 8 native ethnic groups in Honduras, 2 of which preserve their own language.[31]

Strategies for gynecologic cancer care are embedded in the reproductive health policy. Screening for cervical cancer with cytology has a coverage of 42% for women aged 26 years or older.[33] In 2016, the quadrivalent vaccine against human papillomavirus for 11-year-old schoolgirls was introduced in the national vaccination program, although coverage dropped to 48% during the COVID-19 pandemic.[34]

Although Honduras does not have a national population-based cancer registry, 3 nonexhaustive regional efforts have been started to provide an initial picture of the cancer burden in Honduras (**Table 1**).

Educational campaigns, such as those sponsored by the *Fundación Hondureña para el Niño con Cáncer* on warning symptoms for the early detection of childhood cancer and on early referrals for patients with a diagnosis have given results, including a reduction in treatment abandonment from 36% to 9%, and a 10% reduction in the number of newly diagnosed advanced stages.[35] However, there is still a lack of awareness regarding cancer control among health personnel at the first level of care.

Table 1 Population-based cancer registries in Honduras			
Location	Tegucigalpa Metro Area (Ministry of Health) (2020)[a]	San Pedro Sula Metro Area (LCC) (2019–2020)[b]	Copán Department WHGCPI (2013–2017)[66]
Registered tumors	Breast Prostate Gastric Cervix uteri Leukemia Liver	Breast Cervix uteri Gastric Corpus uteri Prostate Leukemia	Cervix uteri Gastric Colorectal Prostate

Abbreviation: WHGCPI, Western Honduras gastric cancer prevention initiative.
[a] Source IARC 2020.
[b] LCC. Liga Contra el Cáncer, Honduras.
Source. Bejarano S. Institutional unpublished data 2021.

There is availability of cancer care in the country (**Table 2**) but resource distribution is highly unequal. The interval between symptom onset to cancer treatment is considerable, and there is a gap in the continuum of care due to the limited capacity of diagnostic and therapeutic centers, many of which are underequipped and understaffed to provide high-quality precision diagnosis.

Although the scenario seems unfavorable, there are many opportunities for promoting cancer policies in Honduras to improve access to equitable cancer care and early diagnosis, increase coverage of cancer prevention and screening for the main cancers, as well as improve communications between organizations of the public/private sector and civil society and academia to guide cancer control strategies.

Costa Rica
Costa Rica has an area of 51,100 km², a population of 5,180,000 people and a population density of 101 inhabitants per square kilometer.[36] It is a middle-income country with a strongly unequal income distribution, as in most Latin American countries.

Table 2 Existing cancer care units in Honduras by health-care system provider					
	Type of Provider/Service Available				
Institution	Medical Oncology	Surgical Oncology	Radiation Therapy	Number of Essential Oncology Drugs Included in Health-Care Plan	Number of Opioid Medications Available
Secretaría de Salud (SESAL)	3	3	1	30	5
Instituto Hondureño de Seguridad Social	2	2	2[a]	45	7
Nongovernmental organizations	2	1	2	NA	NA
Private	NA	NA	2	NA	NA

[a] Through private provider.

However, Costa Rica has one of the highest life expectancies in the region of approximately 81 years in 2021.[36] This effect is probably due to the decision to cease investment in national defense, which freed funds to invest in water purification, education, and health care, developing a strong universal health-care system (*Caja Costarricense de Seguro Social*). This explains why Costa Rica does not have negative social gradients in health as described in developed countries.[37] In fact, most Costa Ricans and legal residents are treated in public hospitals, especially for the most serious conditions, including cancer.

In Costa Rica, cancer is the second leading cause of death after cardiovascular diseases (relegated to third place by the COVID-19 pandemic in 2020). Each year, 13,139 new cases are diagnosed, with a prevalence of 35,534 in 2020. In order of incidence and excluding nonmelanoma skin cancer, the most frequent tumors are prostate (14.5%), breast (12.4%), colorectal (9.6%), gastric (7.2%), and thyroid (5.3%).[38] As for the distribution by sex, prostate (29.3%), colorectal (9.4%), and stomach (8.4%) are the most frequent in men, whereas breast (24.5%), colorectal (9.8%), and thyroid (9.1%) are the most frequent in women.[38] In terms of mortality, stomach cancer (12.9%) is the deadliest, followed by colorectal (9.3%), breast (7.2%), prostate (6.8%), and lung cancers (6.2%).[38] As for geographic distribution, an increased incidence of lung, colorectal, breast, uterine, ovarian, prostate, testicular, kidney, and bladder cancers is found in urban areas, whereas a higher incidence of gastric, cervical, penile, and skin cancers is found in rural areas. In addition, the incidence of cervical cancer is higher in coastal areas, where populations tend to be of lower socioeconomical levels.[39,40]

In Costa Rica, obstacles and issues related to cancer care prevail, including insufficient human and financial resources. There are significant shortages of oncology equipment (such as linear accelerators for radiotherapy) that lead to long waiting or transport times, which affect treatment outcomes, particularly for patients living in rural communities.[41] In terms of human resources, there is a shortage of oncology specialists, which is widespread in much of the region and affects suburban and rural areas even more. This deficit of human and material resources is expected to worsen in the coming years due to the aging process of the population. Currently, the older population is close to 409,000 people (8.2% of the total) and, by 2050, this number could increase to 1.3 million people (20.7% of the total).[36,42] Population aging produces a change in the health profile, which shows a higher prevalence of NCDs, such as neoplasms, which would increase health spending in 2030 by 86%, in comparison to 2016.[42]

To address these problems, Costa Rica developed the National Cancer Control Plan (PNCC) in 1998, with a last update in 2012. The objectives were to reduce cancer incidence and mortality, increase coverage in comprehensive care, improve the quality of care, and thus improve the quality of life of people with cancer.[43] An important clinical initiative aimed at improving access to care is the project for the Strengthening of Comprehensive Cancer Care, which includes the training of professionals, the articulation of a structured network of services, the strengthening of infrastructure, and the generation of information and knowledge.[44]

Efforts have also been made to increase research outputs. The Directorate of Scientific and Technological Development of the Ministry of Health carried out the Analysis of the Situation in Health Research and Technological Development report. This revealed that out of 100% of institutional spending, only 4.4% was dedicated to health research, which demonstrates the need to allocate larger budgets to research, especially in priority areas such as cancer because one of the main obstacles to research is the lack of financial resources.[45]

Another set of initiatives aimed at decreasing disparities in cancer outcomes in Costa Rica have focused on educational projects aimed at the public. Dietary guidelines have been developed and healthy lifestyles have been incorporated into school curricula. In addition, the Ministry of Health coordinates the Costa Rican Network of Physical Activity for Health (RECAFIS).[46] The Costa Rican Social Security Fund includes projects to promote healthy lifestyles, such as healthy sexuality, breastfeeding clinics, smoking cessation clinics, and detection of risk factors for cervical cancer.[47]

The Caribbean

The Caribbean is home to more than 44 million people of different ethnic, cultural, historical, and economic background.[2] It comprises 13 independent countries and 12 dependencies and about 7000 islands. Belize, Guyana, and Suriname are often considered to be part of the Caribbean and are included in **Table 3**.[3]

The Caribbean has been plagued by an increasing burden of NCDs, including cancer. Per the Global Cancer Observatory (GLOBOCAN), the Caribbean region accounted for 113,280 new cancer cases in 2020 with 65,954 deaths (**Fig. 2**).[38] Prostate, lung, and colorectal malignancies are the leading new cancer cases in men in the region with breast, colorectal, and lung cancers affecting women.[48] Cancer now comes right after cardiovascular disease as the leading cause of death in these islands.[49] Cancer mortality rates there are higher compared with the United States for example especially for prostate and breast cancers with many of patients diagnosed at advanced stages of their disease.[50]

There are significant disparities between major Caribbean countries in terms of available resources and strategies to combat the growing cancer burden and mortality (**Table 4**). Eight territories (Belize, Cuba, Jamaica, Guadeloupe, Martinique, Puerto Rico, Suriname, and Trinidad and Tobago) among which only 5 are independent states, have national cancer-control plans.[51,52] Most countries in the region do not have robust cancer-screening programs. Breast, colorectal, and cervical cancers are mostly screened opportunistically by different health actors and not through national screening programs except in Puerto Rico, Martinique, St Lucia (cervical and breast), Guadeloupe (breast and colorectal), Aruba (breast), and Jamaica (cervical).[52] There are also significant contrasts in available diagnostic tools and human resources when comparing countries. For example, Puerto Rico had 111 medical oncologists in 2018 compared with 4 in Haiti for populations of 4 million and 11 million, respectively.[52] Most countries do not have radiotherapy centers and most machines (around two-thirds) are concentrated in the Dominican Republic and Puerto Rico.[52] Despite the increasing disease burden and mortality, palliative care is not an integral part of health services and cancer programs. With public expenditure on health representing less than 4% of GDP for most of the Caribbean countries, the majority of the patients have to pay out of pocket for these scarce services and have to travel, when feasible, to neighboring or North-American or European countries for necessary care.[53] It is often the case that even when resources are available, there are significant economic, geographic, and cultural barriers that keep the most vulnerable populations in the region from accessing cancer care.

There are relevant health-related migrations between certain Caribbean countries. For example, many Haitian patients seek care in the Dominican Republic or Cuba. Some patients from Turks and Caicos have oncologic treatments including radiation in Jamaica, the Bahamas, and the Cayman Islands.[52] These are usually not the result of state-sponsored care but rather organized and paid for by the patients and their families. There are international partners that fund certain health-related projects in the region including the European Union, the American and Canadian governments,

Table 3
Caribbean countries and territories at a glimpse

Country/Territory	Population 2022 (Thousands)[3]	Income Classification[21]	Independence/Political Affiliation
Anguilla	15.9	High income	UK territory
Antigua and Barbuda	93.8	High income	Independent
Aruba	106.4	High income	Netherlands territory
Bahamas	410.0	High income	Independent
Barbados	281.6	High income	Independent
Belize	400.0 (World bank 2021)	Upper middle income	Independent
Bermuda	63.87 (World bank 2021)	High income	UK territory
Bonaire	22.5 (www.statista.com)	High income	Municipality of the Netherlands
British Virgin Islands	31.12 (World bank 2021)	High income	UK territory
Cayman Islands	68.7	High income	UK territory
Cuba	11,212.2	Upper middle income	Independent
Curacao	191.2	High income	Country of the Netherlands
Dominica	72.7	Upper middle income	Independent
Dominican Republic	11,228.8	Upper middle income	Independent
Grenada	125.4	Upper middle income	Independent
Guadeloupe	395.8	High income	Department of France
Guyana	808.7	Upper middle income	Independent
Haiti	11,585.0	Lower middle income	Independent
Jamaica	2827.4	Upper middle income	Independent
Martinique	367.5	High income	Department of France
Montserrat	4.4	High income	UK territory
Puerto-Rico	3252.4	High income	US territory
Saba	1.9 (www.statista.com)	High income	Municipality of the Netherlands
St Kitts and Nevis	47.7	High income	Independent

St Lucia	179.9	Upper middle income	Independent
St Vincent and the Grenadines	103.9	Upper middle income	Independent
Sint Eustatius	3.2	High income	Municipality of the Netherlands
Sint Maarten	44.2	High income	Country of the Netherlands
Suriname	618.0	Upper middle income	Independent
Trinidad and Tobago	1531.0	High income	Independent
Turks and Caicos Islands	45.7	High income	UK territory
Virgin Islands	99.5	High income	US territory

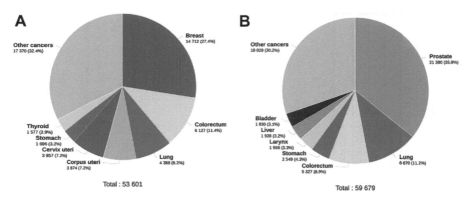

Fig. 2. Cancer incidence in the Caribbean region for the year 2020 according to GLOBOCAN for men (*A*) and women (*B*).

the Inter-American Development Bank, the World Health Organization, and the Pan American Health Organization. Regionally, some institutions such as the CARICOM (Caribbean Community and Common Market) and the Caribbean Public Health Agency attempt to shape collective action and health policy. Although the work and funding from these regional and international organizations help fill a gap in certain national health systems and cancer care, their actions is not always harmonized. Yet, there are effective collaborations strategies that have been developed recently among which the International Agency for Research on Cancer (IARC) Caribbean Regional Cancer Registry Hub, which provides personnel training and government counsel to help establish effective national cancer registries.[50] The National Comprehensive Cancer Network has collaborated with the Caribbean Association for Oncology and Hematology in 2018 to create treatment guidelines for the Caribbean. Pediatric oncologists in the region have established a network with their counterparts in the United States (St. Jude Children's Research Hospital) and Europe (University of Milan-Bicocca in Italy) to exchange knowledge and identify funding sources with goals to provide optimal and cohesive care. The SickKids Capacity Building in the Caribbean Initiative (SCI) is a similar joint project between the Hospital for Sick Children in Toronto and certain English speaking Caribbean Institutions including the University of the West Indies.[50] Partners in Health (International Nonprofit organization) provides cancer care and palliative services essentially free of cost to a large rural population in Haiti while emphasizing on training local providers and strengthening communities.

In the following sections we highlight 2 countries in the Caribbean region with unique challenges for providing cancer care in an equitable manner: (1) Cuba, which has an aging population and faces the limitations placed on the local industry by the United States-led blockade and (2) the Dominican Republic, which faces the challenges of a growing refugee population from neighboring Haiti.

Cuba

Cuba is a country of 11,326,616 inhabitants, with a life expectancy of 78.89 years in 2020.[2] The constitution of Cuba obliges to provide universal health services, based on equity, prevention, scientific and technical evidence, community participation, public institutions, and government participation in medicine. There are no private hospitals in Cuba and the production of medicines is in the hands of the state. The Cuban pharmaceutical industry works in coordination with the National Health System (SNS), produces, and distributes medicines according to the epidemiological profile of the country.[38,54,55]

Table 4
Available cancer care resources in the 5 most populous Caribbean countries

Country	Total Population 2022 (in Millions).[67]	Number of New Cancer Cases in 2020.[48]	National Cancer Control Plan (Yes/No)[68]	Number of Pathologists. (2018)[55,69]	Palliative Care Availability.[68-70]	Cancer Management Guidelines. (2019)[68]	Population-Based Cancer Registry (PBCR)[68]
Cuba	11.3	46,794	Yes	No precise information available	Yes	Yes (2019)	PBCR
Dominican Republic	11.1	19,816	No	No precise information available	Yes	Yes	Registration activity
Haiti	11.7	12,404	No	14	Available in one center (per source in the country)	Yes	No information
Puerto Rico	2.8	13,080	Yes	93	Yes	Yes	High-quality PBCR
Jamaica	3	7197	Yes	21	Yes	Yes	High-quality PBCR

Cancer is the second leading cause of death in Cuba (after cardiovascular events) but it is estimated that in a few years it will become the leading cause (this is already the case in 8 of the 14 provinces). A total of 46,794 new cases of cancer are diagnosed every year, with a prevalence of 121,131 cases in 2020. In order of incidence and excluding nonmelanoma skin cancer, the most frequent tumors are lung (14.3%), prostate (13.6%) and colorectal cancers (10.4%). As for the distribution by sex, prostate (25.5%), lung (16.3%), and colorectal cancers (8%) are the most frequent in men, whereas breast (21.4%), colorectal (13.2%), and lung cancers (12%) are the most frequent in women. Cancers in order of mortality: lung (22.4%), prostate (12.5%), and colorectal cancers (9.5%). Finally, in terms of prevalence, the most frequent are prostate, breast, colorectal, and lung cancers.[38]

The challenges facing Cuba are compounded by its rapidly aging population (17.6% of the population is older than 60 years of age), smoking rates greater than 35% in adults, and obesity affecting 20% of adults. Specifically, the smoking rate places lung cancer as the leading cause of death from cancer. Cuba has the highest physician per person ratio in the world, with 6.7 physicians and 8.2 nurses for every 1000 people (compared with 2.8 physicians per 1000 people in the United States).[56] Although the rate of medical oncologists far exceeds the Latin American average, there is a deficit of palliative care specialists (traditionally handled by anesthesiologists and oncologists), surgical, and radiation oncologists. There is also a deficit in terms of technological resources. In Cuba, more than 20,000 cases requiring radiotherapy are diagnosed each year but there are only 9 services with 18 external radiotherapy teams in the country, which can only treat 9000 patients (500 patients a year each), leaving the rest without coverage.[57] Because of the US economic, commercial, and financial blockade against Cuba, the country is unable to acquire many technologies, raw materials, reagents, diagnostic means, medicines, devices, equipment, and spare parts, which must be obtained in geographically distant markets or through a third country, with an increase in costs that directly affects the SNS and the population in general.[55,58]

In Cuba, the first cancer control program was implemented in 1968 and was aimed at the early detection of cervical cancer. In subsequent years, other neoplasms have been included, until the current Comprehensive Program for Cancer Control (2017). Its purposes are to reduce cancer mortality by 2% per year, increase survival, and improve quality of life. To this end, human, technological, and training resources are implemented in all health areas. The Cancer Control Knowledge Network has also been set up, which is intended to function as a channel for sharing knowledge. In addition, the Cuban Ministry of Public Health created the Independent Cancer Control Section as an expression of the government's political will to achieve the expected impact on a population scale to reduce the incidence and mortality from this cause.[59]

Dominican Republic
The Dominican Republic shares the island of Hispaniola with Haiti. It has 48,442 km^2 and a population of 10,847,904 inhabitants. It has a life expectancy of 74.4 years (lower than the average for the Region of the Americas); however, it has increased by 7.2 years compared with what was reported in 2000.[60]

The Dominican health system is highly fragmented and has unequal coverage. There is strong socioeconomic inequality, especially among the Haitian migrant population, which accounts for about 5% of the population (excluding Haitian descendants).[61] This population is heavily relegated to rural areas, suffering from poverty and food insecurity, and is more vulnerable to poor health outcomes. In addition, this population suffers higher levels of perceived discrimination, which results in detrimental mental and social health outcomes.[62]

Cancer is the second leading cause of death; 19,816 new cases are diagnosed annually with a prevalence of 50,037 in 2020. In order of incidence and excluding non-melanoma skin cancer, the most frequent tumors are prostate (24.3%), breast (17.2%), and lung cancers (8.1%). As for the distribution by sex, prostate (46.5%), lung (8.9%), and colorectal cancers (7.1%) are the most frequent in men, whereas breast (36%), cervix (11.3%), and colorectal cancers (8.2%) are the most frequent in women. Cancers in order of mortality: prostate (18.4%), breast (13.0%), and colo-rectal cancers (12.2%). Finally, in terms of prevalence, the most frequent are prostate, breast, colorectal and cervical cancers.[38]

The Dominican Republic lacks a high-quality PNCC, although it is briefly included in the National Plan for the Prevention and Control of Non-Communicable Diseases 2019 to 2024 and in the Institutional Strategic Plan 2021 to 2024.[63,64] There are significant gaps in technical equipment and human resources are highly insufficient, with marked inequality (almost a complete absence) in rural or periurban areas. To improve access to high-cost cancer treatments, the Ministry of Health created the Office for Access to High-Cost Medications (DAMAC), which provides support for the purchase of expen-sive medications, including cancer drugs, for more than 16,000 Dominicans per year.[65]

In 2008, the subregional plan for cancer prevention and control in Central America and the Dominican Republic was developed with the aim of promoting the

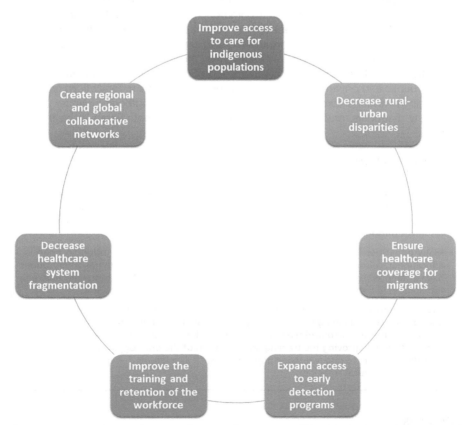

Fig. 3. Recommendations for the reduction of cancer care disparities in Central America and the Caribbean.

development of national plans, establishing cancer prevention and control networks, establishing strategies for the acquisition of medicines, and promoting training and information programs on cancer. However, its objectives have not been achieved in the Dominican Republic and so far, no updates have been made.[63]

Summary and Opportunities to Move Forward

Although this article does not pretend to be an exhaustive description of the state of disparities in cancer care in Central American and the Caribbean, clearly there are many challenges to achieve optimal cancer control in the region and that, despite some advances, a lot remains to be done to improve cancer care. Strategies aimed at reducing disparities and increasing access to high-quality cancer care should include all relevant stakeholders and leverage implementation science, novel technologies, and artificial intelligence to address limited resources, improve data gathering, and increase access to management. Governments across the regions should be encouraged to make efforts to reduce health-care system fragmentation, increase national spending in health, and prioritize universal health coverage for their citizens. As countries move from low-income to middle-income economies, plans should be put in place to face the impending demographic change and to strengthen the infrastructure needed to provide care for chronic diseases, including cancer, as recommended by the United Nations Sustainable Development Goals. This should include the establishment of cancer registries, national cancer policies, and cancer control programs aimed at the most common malignancies within each territory. Intraregional collaborations represent an excellent platform to share and expand resources, while collaboration with organizations in high-income nations may allow for a more unified front to advocate more effectively on the international scene. Our recommendations for future actions are summarized in **Fig. 3**. Concerted actions between national public and private sectors, regional and international organizations as well as academic institutions across the region with a goal of strengthening cancer prevention, early diagnosis, and effective and affordable treatments seem to be the path forward.

CLINICS CARE POINTS

- Patients with cancer living in Central America and the Caribbean face many disparities when attempting to access high quality care due to healthcare system fragmentation and limited resources throughout the region.

- Many disparities limiting access to care exist throughout the region, including financial, educational, cultural, racial and urban-rural. Governments and international organizations have attempted to decrease disparities by creating programs aimed at improving coverage for vulnerable populations, and progress is occurring, albeit at a slow pace.

- Future initiatives for the improvement of cancer control in Central America and the Caribbean include building regional and global collaborative networks, creating comprehensive cancer control plans aimed at expanding access and decreasing system fragmentation, improving the training and retention of the oncology workforce, and providing support to disadvantaged populations such as migrants, indigenous groups and people living in rural areas.

DISCLOSURE

The authors have no conflicts of interest to disclose.

REFERENCES

1. Central America Population 2023. Available at: https://worldpopulationreview. com/continents/central-america-population. Accessed June 16, 2023.
2. Caribbean Population 2023. Available at: https://worldpopulationreview.com/ continents/caribbean-population. Accessed June 16, 2023.
3. World Resources Institute. The Caribbean Region. Available at: https://www.wri. org/data/caribbean-region. Accessed June 4, 2023.
4. Bushnell, David and Woodward, Ralph Lee. "Central America". Encyclopedia Britannica, 13 Jun. 2023. Available at: https://www.britannica.com/place/Central-America. Accessed June 18, 2023.
5. INEGI. Estadística de defunciones registradas de Enero a Junio de 2022. Available at: https://www.inegi.org.mx/contenidos/saladeprensa/boletines/2023/DR/ DR-Ene-jun2022.pdf. Accessed April 4, 2023.
6. Ferlay J, Ervik M, Lam F, et al. Global cancer observatory: cancer today. Lyon, France: International Agency for Research on Cancer; 2018. Available at: https://gco.iarc.fr/today. Accessed June 4, 2023.
7. INEGI. Censo de Población y Vivienda 2020. Available at: https://www.inegi.org. mx/programas/ccpv/2020/#:~:text=Con%20el%20Censo%202020%2C% 20el,cuales%20se%20realizan%20desde%201895. Accessed January 4, 2023.
8. Aguilera R. Can AMLO rescue Mexico's poorest southern states, like Oaxaca, Chiapas, and Guerrero? London School of Economics and Political Science. Available at: https://blogs.lse.ac.uk/latamcaribbean/2019/03/08/can-amlo-rescue-mexicos-poorest-southern-states-like-oaxaca-chiapas-and-guerrero/. Accessed March 9, 20123.
9. Fideicomiso para el Desarrollo Regional del Sur Sureste. The South Southeast, a rich but lagging region. FIDESUR Trust for the Regional Development of the South Southeast. Published 2021. Available at: https://sursureste.org.mx/en/region/. Accessed April 4, 2023.
10. INEGI, Instituto Nacional de Estadística y Geografía. Información por entidad Yucatán. Available at: https://www.cuentame.inegi.org.mx/monografias/informacion/ yuc/poblacion/diversidad.aspx?tema=me&e=31. Accessed April 4, 2023.
11. Aggarwal A, Unger-Saldaña K, Lewison G, et al. The challenge of cancer in middle-income countries with an ageing population: Mexico as a case study. Ecancermedicalscience 2015;9:536.
12. Flamand L, Moreno C, Arriaga R. Cáncer y desigualdades sociales en México 2020. El El Colegio de México, Red de Estudios Sobre Desigualdades : ITESO, Universidad Jesuita de Guadalajara : Fundación de Alba : Respirando con Valor A.C. : Salvati A.C. de Mexico; 2021:120. Available at: https://desigualdades. colmex.mx/cancer/informe-cancer-desigualdades-2020.pdf. Accessed January 4, 2023.
13. Chávarri-Guerra Y, Villarreal-Garza C, Liedke PE, et al. Breast cancer in Mexico: a growing challenge to health and the health system. Lancet Oncol 2012;13(8): e335–43.
14. Gerson R, Zatarain-Barrón ZL, Blanco C, et al. Access to lung cancer therapy in the Mexican population: opportunities for reducing inequity within the health system. Salud Publica Mex 2019;61(3):352–8. Acceso a la terapia para cáncer de pulmón en la población mexicana: oportunidades para reducir la inequidad en el sistema de salud.

15. Moye-Holz D, Soria Saucedo R, van Dijk JP, et al. Access to innovative cancer medicines in a middle-income country - the case of Mexico. J Pharm Policy Pract 2018;11:25.
16. Maldonado Magos F, Lozano Ruíz FJ, Pérez Álvarez SI, et al. Radiation oncology in Mexico: current status according to Mexico's Radiation Oncology Certification Board. Rep Pract Oncol Radiother 2020;25(5):840–5.
17. Soto-Perez-de-Celis E, Chavarri-Guerra Y. National and regional breast cancer incidence and mortality trends in Mexico 2001-2011: analysis of a population-based database. Cancer Epidemiol 2016;41:24–33.
18. Lopez MS, Baker ES, Maza M, et al. Cervical cancer prevention and treatment in Latin America. J Surg Oncol 2017;115(5):615–8.
19. Armenta-Paulino N, Wehrmeister FC, Arroyave L, et al. Ethnic inequalities in health intervention coverage among Mexican women at the individual and municipality levels. EClinicalMedicine 2022;43:101228.
20. Proyecciones – Instituto Nacional de Estadística. Available at: https://www.ine.gob.gt/proyecciones/. Accessed January 4, 2023.
21. World Bank Country and Lending Groups – World Bank Data Help Desk. https://datahelpdesk.worldbank.org/knowledgebase/articles/906519-world-bank-country-and-lending-groups. Accessed January 4, 2023.
22. World Health Organization. Guatemala: non-communicable diseases data. Geneva: ENT Perfiles de países; 2018. p. 1. Available at: https://cdn.who.int/media/docs/default-source/country-profiles/ncds/gtm-es.pdf?sfvrsn=dd461658_36&download=true. Accessed January 4, 2023.
23. National Program for the Prevention of Non-Communicable Diseases and Cancer (Internet). 2015. p. 1–100. Available at: https://www.iccp-portal.org/system/files/plans/GTM_B3_PLAN%20ESTRAT%C3%89GICO%20NACIONAL%20PARA%20PREVENCI%C3%93N%20Y%20CONTROL%20DE%20ENTs%20170715.pdf. Accessed November 4, 2022.
24. Registro de Cancer del INCAN - GUATEMALA. Available at: https://registrocancerguat.wixsite.com/regcangua. Accessed November 4, 2022.
25. National Plan for the prevention, control and management of cervical cancer 2014-2024. Available at: https://www.paho.org/gut/dmdocuments/PlanCaCU_2014-2024w.pdf. Accessed November 4, 2022.
26. Kihn-Alarcón AJ, Alvarado-Muñoz JF, Orozco-Fuentes LI, et al. Years of potential life lost because of breast and cervical cancers in guatemala. JCO Glob Oncol 2020;6:761–5.
27. Rural population (% of total population) – Guatemala. Available at: https://data.worldbank.org/indicator/SP.RUR.TOTL.ZS?locations=GT. Accessed November 4, 2022.
28. Zubizarreta EH, Poitevin A, Levin CV. Overview of radiotherapy resources in Latin America: a survey by the International Atomic Energy Agency (IAEA). Radiother Oncol 2004;73(1):97–100.
29. Busqueda de Registro de Acreditaciones. Available at: https://formacion.mspas.gob.gt/busqueda. Accessed November 4, 2022.
30. Escuela de Estudios de Postgrado | Facultad de Ciencias Medicas. Available at: https://postgrado.medicina.usac.edu.gt/. Accessed November 4, 2022.
31. INE. Estadisticas. Available at: https://www.ine.gob.hn/V3/. Accessed November 4, 2022.
32. CESPAD, Fiallos S, Mendoza C. Periodismo en Profundidad.Salud en Honduras: sin camas, médicos, enfermeras, equipo, medicinas. Available at: https://

cespad.org.hn/2019/05/24/salud-en-honduras-sin-camas-medicos-enfermeras-equipo-medicinas/. Accessed February 4, 2022.

33. Organización Panamericana de la Salud. Situación de los Programas para la Prevención y el Control del Cáncer Cervicouterino: evaluación rápida mediante encuesta en 12 países de América Latina. Washington, D.C.: OPS; 2010.

34. Pan-American Health Organization. Vacuna contra el Virus del Papiloma Humano (VPH). Available at: https://www.paho.org/es/vacuna-contra-virus-papiloma-humano-vph. Accessed June 5 2023.

35. Fundación Hondureña para el Niño con Cáncer. Campañas educativas. Available at: https://salvamivida.org/la-fundacion/campanas-educativas/. Accessed June 4, 2023.

36. Instituto Nacional de Estadística y Censos y Sistema de Estadística Nacional. Unidad de Estadísticas Demográficas. Panorama demográfico. Available at: https://admin.inec.cr/sites/default/files/2022-12/RePoblacEv-2021a-panorama_demografico_2021.pdf. Accessed June 14, 2023.

37. Underwood E. A world of difference. Science 2014;344(6186):820–1.

38. Sung H, Ferlay J, Siegel RL, et al. Global Cancer Statistics 2020: GLOBOCAN Estimates of Incidence and Mortality Worldwide for 36 Cancers in 185 Countries. CA Cancer J Clin 2021;71(3):209–49.

39. Fantin R, Santamaría-Ulloa C, Barboza-Solís C. Socioeconomic inequalities in cancer mortality: Is Costa Rica an exception to the rule? Int J Cancer 2020; 147(5):1286–93.

40. Arias Ramírez R, Sánchez Hernández L, Rodríguez Morales M. Pobreza y desigualdad en Costa Rica: una mirada más allá de la distribución de los ingresos. Estudios Del Desarrollo Social: Cuba Y América Latina 2023;8(1).

41. Panamerican Health Organization. Cáncer en las Américas: perfiles de país 2013. Washington, DC: OPS; 2014.

42. Contraloría general de la Republica. Impacto fiscal del cambio demográfico: retos para una Costa Rica que envejece. 2019. Available at: https://proyectos.conare.ac.cr/asamblea/Contraloria%20cambio%20demografico%202019.pdf. Accessed June 14, 2023.

43. Costa Rica. Ministerio de Salud. Plan Nacional para la Prevención y Control del Cáncer 2011-2017.-1a. ed. –San José, Costa Rica. El Ministerio, ISBN 978-9977-62-115-9; 2012.

44. Caja Costarricense de Seguridad Social. Fortalecimiento de la atención integral del cáncer en la red oncologica nacional de la CCSS. 2009. Available at: https://platform.who.int/docs/default-source/mca-documents/policy-documents/plan-strategy/CRI-RH-47-01-PLAN-STRATEGY-2009-esp-Fortalecimiento-atencion-Cancer-en-red-Oncologica-CCSS.pdf. Accessed August 8, 2023.

45. Ministerio de Salud Desarrollo Científico y Tecnológico en Salud. Estado actual y perspectivas de la gestión de las tecnologías en Salud. 2007. Available at: https://docs.bvsalud.org/biblioref/2017/06/834153/ddcts_estado_actual_y_perspectivas_de_la_gestion_de_las_tecnolo_BLLqKrK.pdf. Accessed August 8, 2023.

46. Costa Rica. Ministerio de Salud y Ministerio de Deporte y Recreación. Plan nacional de actividad física y salud 2011-2021. Available at: https://www.ministeriodesalud.go.cr/index.php/biblioteca-de-archivos-left/documentos-ministerio-de-salud/ministerio-de-salud/planes-y-politicas-institucionales/planes-institucionales/planes-planes-institucionales/720-plan-nacional-de-actividad-fisica-y-salud-2011-2021/file. Accessed August 8, 2023.

47. Caja Costarricense de Seguro Social. Plan institucional para la atención del cáncer 2015-2018. 2015. Available at: www.ministeriodesalud.go.cr. Accessed June 13, 2023.
48. Bray F, Colombet M, Mery L, et al, editors. Cancer incidence in five continents, vol. XI. IARC Scientific Publication No. 166. . Lyon (France): International Agency for Research on Cancer; 2021. Licence: CC BY-NC-ND 3.0 IGO. Available at: https://publications.iarc.fr/597.
49. Razzaghi H, Quesnel-Crooks S, Sherman R, et al. Leading causes of cancer mortality - caribbean region, 2003-2013. MMWR Morb Mortal Wkly Rep 2016;65(49): 1395–400.
50. Spence D, Argentieri MA, Andall-Brereton G, et al. Advancing cancer care and prevention in the Caribbean: a survey of strategies for the region. Lancet Oncol 2019;20(9):e522–34.
51. Coalition. HC. 2017 Port of Spain NCD summit grid. 2017. Available at: https://www.healthycaribbean.org/pos-ncd-summit-progress-grids/. Accessed online June 1, 2023.
52. Spence D, Dyer R, Andall-Brereton G, et al. Cancer control in the Caribbean island countries and territories: some progress but the journey continues. Lancet Oncol 2019;20(9):e503–21.
53. Current health expenditure (% of GDP). The World Bank. Available at: https://data.worldbank.org/indicator/SH.XPD.CHEX.GD.ZS. Accessed February 20,2023.
54. Sonia Bess Constantén IAA, Elvira Sánchez Sordo. Anuario estadístico de salud. Ministerio de salud pública; 2021. Available at: https://temas.sld.cu/estadisticassalud/2022/10/18/anuario-estadistico-de-salud-2021/. Accessed on March 20, 2023.
55. Goss PE, Lee BL, Badovinac-Crnjevic T, et al. Planning cancer control in Latin America and the Caribbean. Lancet Oncol 2013;14(5):391–436.
56. PHCPI. Cuba Health Workforce Profile. Available at: https://www.improvingphc.org/cuba-health-workforce. Accessed June 4, 2023.
57. Guerrero Cancio MC, Romero Pérez T de la C. Diagnóstico y el tratamiento del cáncer en Cuba. Nucleus (Internet). 1 de julio de 2019 (citado 18 de junio de 2023);0(66):27-1. Disponible en: Available at: http://nucleus.cubaenergia.cu/index.php/nucleus/article/view/687.
58. Ruiz-González LA, Piñera-Castro HJ, Smith-Groba J. Impact of the US blockade on the Cuban health system in the last decade. Rev Cubana Med Mil 2023;52:1.
59. Romero Pérez TAR G, Bermejo Bencomo W. Programa integral para el control del cáncer. Guía de prácticas esenciales; 2017. Available at: http://www.ecimed.sld.cu/2019/06/07/3038/. Accessed June 2, 2023.
60. United Nations Population Division . World Population Prospects 2022. United Nations, Geneva. Available at: https://population.un.org/wpp/. Accessed August 8, 2023.
61. Arps S, Peralta KJ. Living conditions and health care usage of Haitian families in the dominican republic: a comparison of urban and rural/peri-urban households. Global Publ Health 2021;16(1):103–19.
62. Keys HM, Noland GS, De Rochars MB, et al. Perceived discrimination in bateyes of the Dominican Republic: results from the Everyday Discrimination Scale and implications for public health programs. BMC Public Health 2019;19(1):1513.
63. Pan American Health Organization. Plan subregional para la prevención y control del cáncer en centroamérica y República Dominicana. 2008. Available at: https://www.paho.org/es/documentos/resscad-plan-subregional-para-prevencion-control-cancer-centroamerica-republica. Accessed August 8, 2023.

64. Tomiris Estepan SS, Virgilio Rodríguez C. Plan nacional de prevención y control de las enfermedades no transmisibles 2019-2024. Santo Domingo: Ministerio de Salud pública de República Dominicana; 2019.
65. El Nuevo Diario. Gobierno reestructura y aumenta financiamiento a Medicamentos de Alto Costo. Available at: https://elnuevodiario.com.do/gobierno-reestructura-y-aumenta-financiamiento-a-medicamentos-de-alto-costo/. Accessed June 14, 2023.
66. Norwood DA, Montalvan-Sanchez EE, Corral JE, et al. Western Honduras Copán Population-Based Cancer Registry: Initial Estimates and a Model for Rural Central America. JCO Glob Oncol 2021;7:1694–702.
67. United Nations, Department of Economic and Social Affairs, Population Division (2020). World Population Ageing 2019 (ST/ESA/SER.A/444). Available at: https://www.un.org/en/development/desa/population/publications/pdf/ageing/WorldPopulationAgeing2019-Report.pdf. Accessed August 8, 2023.
68. WHO Cancer Country Profiles 2020. Available at: https://www.who.int/teams/noncommunicable-diseases/surveillance/data/cancer-profiles. Accessed June 1, 2023.
69. Strasser-Weippl K, Chavarri-Guerra Y, Villarreal-Garza C, et al. Progress and remaining challenges for cancer control in Latin America and the Caribbean. Lancet Oncol 2015;16(14):1405–38.
70. Soto-Perez-de-Celis E, Chavarri-Guerra Y, Pastrana T, et al. End-of-life care in Latin America. Journal of Global Oncology 2017;3(3):261–70.

State of Cancer Control in South America
Challenges and Advancement Strategies

Ivy Riano, MD[a],*, Ana I. Velazquez, MD, MSc[b,c,1], Lucia Viola, MD[d],
Inas Abuali, MD[e], Kathya Jimenez, MD[f,2], Oyepeju Abioye, MD[g,3],
Narjust Florez, MD[h]

KEYWORDS

- Latin America • South America • Cancer control • Cancer prevention
- Cancer strategies • Cancer screening programs • Primary prevention

KEY POINTS

- Cancer is now the leading cause of death in South American countries, replacing infectious diseases as the main threat to health care.
- Given the increased incidence of cancer in South America, the region faces several challenges in cancer control, largely neglecting the poorest people and widening health inequities.
- Certain cancers in South America are attributable to infections including hepatitis B, human papilloma virus, human immunodeficiency virus, and *Helicobacter pylori*. Since the introduction of some vaccines, certain cancers have decreased in incidence. However, widespread vaccination is limited due to costs, logistics, and misconceptions.

Continued

[a] Division of Hematology and Oncology, Dartmouth Cancer Center, Geisel School of Medicine Dartmouth, One Medical Drive, Lebanon, NH 03766, USA; [b] Division of Hematology/Oncology, Department of Medicine, University of California, San Francisco, San Francisco, CA, USA; [c] Helen Diller Family Comprehensive Cancer Center, University of California, San Francisco, San Francisco, CA, USA; [d] Fundación Neumológica Colombiana, Centro de Tratamiento e Investigación Sobre Cáncer Luis Carlos Sarmiento Angulo (CTIC), Cra. 13b #161 - 85, Bogotá, Colombia; [e] Division of Hematology and Oncology, Massachusetts General Hospital, Harvard Medical School, 55 Fruit Street, Boston, MA 02114, USA; [f] Universidad Evangelica de El Salvador, El Salvador; [g] University of the Witwatersrand, School of Public Health, Johannesburg, South Africa; [h] Dana Farber Cancer Institute, Harvard School of Medicine, 450 Brookline Avenue - DA1230, Boston, MA 02215, USA
[1] Present address: 995 Potrero Avenue, Building 80, San Francisco, CA 94110.
[2] Present address: 48 Zeliff Avenue, Little Falls, NJ 07424.
[3] Present address: 258 Wildwood Street, Apartment 2D, Morgantown, WV 26505.
* Corresponding author.
E-mail address: Ivy.riano@dartmouth.edu
Twitter: @IvyLorena_Md (I.R.); @AnaVManana (A.I.V.); @LuciaViola9 (L.V.); @Inas_md (I.A.); @KathyaJimenezMD (K.J.); @AbioyeOyepeju (O.A.); @NarjustFlorezMD (N.F.)

Hematol Oncol Clin N Am 38 (2024) 55–76
https://doi.org/10.1016/j.hoc.2023.05.013
0889-8588/24/© 2023 Elsevier Inc. All rights reserved.

hemonc.theclinics.com

Continued

- Crucial actions to improve cancer control in South America include the expansion of financial resources for screening programs in rural areas, promotion of financial support for the uninsured, enhancement of pathology and molecular laboratory diagnostics in a timely fashion, and strengthening of national cancer registries.
- There is an urgent need to increase cancer registries in Latin America to improve cancer epidemiology in the region. Thus, obtaining precise demographic data will help establish efficient national cancer control plans to improve the prevention of cancer.

INTRODUCTION

Cancer is a leading cause of disease and death in South American nations.[1] Cancer incidence and mortality rates in South America are disproportionately high compared with the rest of the world, indicating that the region is not well equipped to grapple with these alarming trends.[2,3] By 2030, more than 1 million cancer cases will be diagnosed in Latin America and the Caribbean, and more than 1 million cancer deaths will occur.[4] As cancer is already the leading cause of premature death in the region, and the burden of cancer is predicted to increase in the coming decades, cancer control faces major challenges.[1] Furthermore, each South American country has its own health-care system, access infrastructure, socioeconomic status, geography, environment, cultural, and racial makeup, increasing the difficulty of unifying cancer control measures. Thus, the health-care systems of many countries struggle to provide optimal specialized cancer care for their populations.[5] Recently, the International Agency for Research on Cancer has recommended focusing on relatively inexpensive prevention strategies because policies that tackle tobacco use, obesity, and human papilloma virus (HPV) vaccination could prevent millions of cancer diagnoses in the future.[6] Although the region has made significant strides in tobacco control,[7] preventive measures, such as those targeting diet and physical activity, are slower to advance due to the immense challenges associated with motivating populations to exercise more and consume healthier foods that are often more expensive in urban areas.[1] Moreover, economic and cultural barriers persist in the region with a clear need to plan for the provision of oncological care services and the human health workforce.[6] For these reasons, countries in South America should institute national cancer control programs aimed at preventing cancer, with some urgency. Efforts to improve population-based cancer registries are needed to provide reliable incidence and survival data as a basis for policy-making and resource allocations within cancer care.[8] Several major challenges and strategies for advancing cancer control in South America are discussed in this article.

An Overview of the Epidemiology of Cancer in South America

Cancer is one of the leading causes of death worldwide.[9] The rapid economic growth of South American countries noted during the last decades are accompanied by an increase of unhealthy dietary habits, sedentary lifestyles, smoking and alcohol consumption, environmental carcinogenic pollutants, and population aging, contributing to a disease burden of noncommunicable disorders including cancer.[2] Among noncommunicable diseases, cardiovascular disease and cancer account for more than 75% of the 20.4 million deaths of individuals aged 30 to 70 years worldwide.[10] According to the World Health Organization's (WHO) mortality estimates from 2019, cancer is the first or second leading cause of death before the age of 70 years in 61% of countries (112 of 183 countries).[11] In South America, cancer is the first or second leading cause of death before age 70 in most countries, being the number one cause of death in countries such as Colombia, Peru, and Argentina, and the second leading cause of death in Brazil, Mexico, Venezuela, and Bolivia.[10,12]

According to GLOBOCAN statistics, in 2020 there were 1,095,348 new cancer diagnoses and 521,389 cancer-related deaths in South America.[12–14] By 2040, the number of people diagnosed with a new cancer is expected to increase to 1.81 million per year, a 65.4% increase in new cancer cases in South America, which is a much higher rate than expected in North America (37.9%).[15] Similarly, the number of cancer-related deaths in South America is expected to increase by 77.4% by 2040 (925,000 cancer deaths per year), compared with an expected 49.3% in North America.[15] With the expected increase in cancer cases in the region and its significant burden in mortality before the age of 70 years, cancer represents a significant barrier to increasing life expectancy in South America.

Breast cancer, prostate cancer, colorectal cancer, lung cancer, and stomach cancer are the top 5 most frequent new cancer diagnoses in South America, accounting for almost 50% of new nonmelanoma cancer diagnoses for both women and men (**Fig. 1**).[13] Breast cancer is the most diagnosed cancer type (14.29% of total cases) across both sexes, closely followed by prostate cancer, which represents 14.28% of new cancer cases in the region. However, lung cancer is the leading cause of cancer death (12.91% of total cancer deaths), followed by colorectal cancer (9.98%) and breast cancer (7.99%) (**Fig. 2**).[12–14] As seen in worldwide trends, the top 5 most common new cancer diagnoses and causes of cancer death vary by sex (**Fig. 3**).

During 2020, new cancer cases in South America accounted for 5.7% of all new cancer cases worldwide.[13,14] The overall age-standardized incidence and mortality rates (ASR per 100,000) for South America were 201.4 and 91.5, respectively.[12,13] Compared with other American subregions, South America had higher incidence

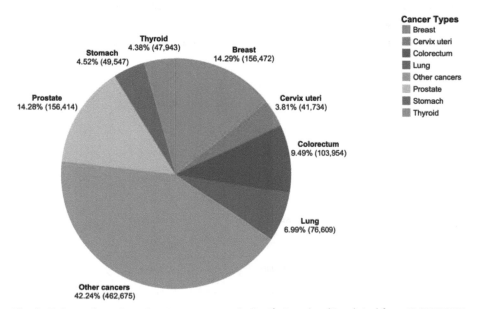

Fig. 1. Estimated number of new cancer cases in South America. (*Reprinted from* GLOBOCAN. Global Cancer Observatory: Cancer Today. Accessed April 1, 2023, http://gco.iarc.fr/today/home. Copyright 2023.)

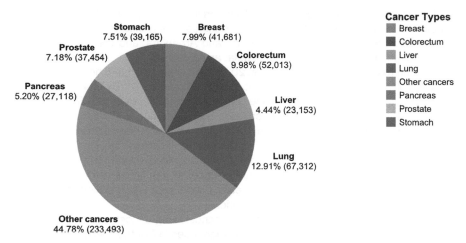

Fig. 2. Estimated number of deaths by type of cancer in South America. (*Reprinted from* GLOBOCAN. Global Cancer Observatory: Cancer Today. Accessed April 1, 2023, http://gco.iarc.fr/today/home. Copyright 2023.)

and mortality rates (ASR per 100,000) for all cancers and both sexes combined than North America and Central America. Overall, the highest country-specific incidence and mortality rates (ASR per 100,000) were seen in Uruguay, at 269.3 and 127.5, respectively. There is also significant variability in country-specific incidence and mortality rates (ASR per 100,000), with Bolivia having the lowest incidence rate (137.5 ASR per 100,000) and Guyana the lowest mortality rate (67.7 ASR per 100,000), nearly half that of Uruguay's.[12,13] In general, countries in Central America had lower specific incidence and mortality (ASR per 100,000) rates than countries in South America; for example, Belize had a 120.9 incidence rate (ASR per 100,000) and Mexico a mortality

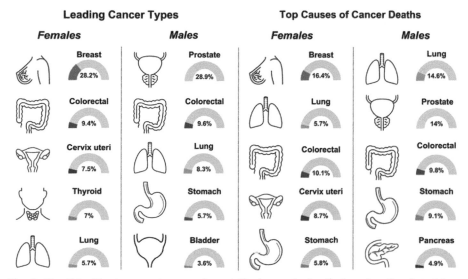

Fig. 3. Top 5 incident cancer types and mortality by sex in South America. *Reprinted from* GLOBOCAN. Global Cancer Observatory: Cancer Today. Accessed April 1, 2023, http://gco.iarc.fr/today/home. Copyright 2023.

rate (ASR per 100,000) of 63.2. Overall, men had higher incidence and mortality rates (ASR per 100,000) than women, except in countries such as Bolivia, Guyana, Ecuador, and Peru, which had greater incidence rates (ASR per 100,000) among women. Peru, Bolivia, and Guyana had higher mortality rates (ASR per 100,000) in women compared with men in the South America regions.[12–14]

By cancer type, prostate cancer and breast cancer in 2020 had the highest incidence and mortality rates (ASR per 100,000) across South America (**Table 1**),[13,14] although geographic variation was seen in such rates. Overall, prostate cancer was the most frequently diagnosed cancer in 25 of 32 countries (78.1%) comprising South and Central America, and breast cancer being the most frequent diagnosed cancer in another 6 countries (18.8%). However, there was more variability in the top cancer type associated with highest mortality rates per country. Indeed, prostate cancer was the leading form of cancer mortality in 17 countries (53%) comprising South America and America, followed by breast cancer in 8 countries (25%), and cervical cancer in 3 countries (9.4%).[12–14] Among men, prostate cancer was the top newly diagnosed cancer in all 32 countries and the leading type of cancer mortality in 17 countries (53.1%), followed by lung cancer (7 countries) and stomach cancer (6 countries). Breast cancer was the most frequent incident cancer in women in all South and Central American countries except Bolivia, where cervical cancer had the highest incidence. Similarly, breast cancer was the leading type of cancer mortality among women (23 of 32 countries; 71.8%), followed by cervical cancer, which was the top cause of death in 7 countries (21.9%).[12–14]

Main Challenges of Cancer Control in South American Countries

In general, South American nations lack resources to respond to the dramatic increase in cancer incidence and disproportionately high mortality rates, highlighting the urgent need to improve cancer control.[2] South America is composed of 12 sovereign countries with diverse health-care systems, socioeconomic, geographic, environmental, and cultural factors, which ultimately affect the access to care. Moreover, the majority of health systems in Latin America is underfunded by government spending and requires high out-of-pocket expenditures.[2] Despite the development of new initiatives to control cancer in South America during the recent decades, several significant challenges persist:

Table 1
Age-standardized incidence and mortality rates (ASR per 100,000) of top 10 cancers in South America.[13]

Type of Cancer	Incidence Rate (ASR per 100,000)	Mortality Rate (ASR per 100,000)
Prostate	59.20	14.20
Breast	51.90	13.50
Colorectum	16.60	8.20
Cervix uteri	14.90	7.60
Lung	12.00	10.50
Thyroid	8.60	0.53
Stomach	8.30	6.40
Corpus uteri	8.20	2.00
Ovary	5.80	3.60
Leukemia	5.40	3.70

Reprinted from GLOBOCAN. Global Cancer Observatory: Cancer Today. Accessed April 1, 2023, http://gco.iarc.fr/today/home. Copyright 2023.

- Fragmented health-care systems: As a result, there is a delay in timely diagnosis and treatment, contributing to advanced-stage disease and high rates of mortality. For instance, low screening rates, late referrals, and not seeking medical attention when symptoms develop contribute to advanced disease at presentation for breast, cervical, and gastric cancer in Latin America. Inequity in health care is typically aggravated by fragmented health-care systems that are inefficient in financing and providing care. When people do present for medical care, families are exposed to impoverishing health payments, resulting in high rates of care abandonment, resulting in poor health outcomes disproportionately affecting the poorest families in the region.[2,16] For instance, in 2008, around a third of Latin Americans were considered at high risk of such impoverishment and catastrophic health expenditures.[2]
- Rural and remote populations: Adverse cancer outcomes are more likely to occur in these populations. Oncologists and cancer experts are often unavailable in these areas and local health centers cannot offer specialized cancer care, including survivorship care. Moreover, a lack of access to medication and affordable transportation can limit access to health care for the poorest populations in rural settings, even when health care is free.[2,17]
- Indigenous populations: The cancer presentation and outcomes of indigenous people in Latin America are more adverse, including more advanced diseases at diagnosis and higher death rates.[18] The way indigenous people interact with modern cancer and health services is influenced by cultural differences. Often, indigenous people need detailed explanations about why they got sick, how their drugs worked, and why they should follow treatment plans; those needs are often overlooked by health providers, or they are too busy to attend to them.[2,19]
- Insufficient cancer screening and early detection programs: According to the International Agency for Research on Cancer, there are around 415 known carcinogens. In South America, the main modifiable risk factors for cancer are alcohol use,[20] tobacco use,[21] obesity,[20] and those related to infectious agents including hepatitis B, human immunodeficiency virus (HIV), *Helicobacter pylori*, and HPV.[22] By reducing these risk factors and protecting the population's health, primary prevention is the most cost-effective way to reduce cancer rates. Main challenges of primary prevention are not only high cost but financial and cultural barriers specific to each patient, inadequate health-care infrastructure, poor laboratory quality, and delays in detecting and treating cancer once the diagnosis is issued.[2,23]
- Deficient population-based cancer registries: Less than 10% of the populations of South America are covered by high-quality cancer registries. Thus, there is a lack of epidemiological data tracking cancer, limiting the ability to create effective cancer prevention plans. Although many countries support cancer registration politically, its sustainability remains questionable.[8]
- Limited molecular testing and diagnostic delays: Studies assessing the quality of cancer diagnosis in South America have demonstrated low concordance rates in cancer diagnostic testing, including cervical cytology, gastric, and prostate biopsy assessments, and immunohistochemistry evaluation for breast cancer.[24] For instance, human epidermal growth factor receptor 2 (HER2) testing has been technically challenging[25] and the drugs are disproportionately expensive despite trastuzumab being on the WHO Essential Medicine list (see later discussion). Such inaccurate testing can lead to misdiagnoses or inappropriate cancer-related treatment, ultimately affecting survival rates. Further, it is difficult to initiate treatment in a timely manner due to pathology result delays.[24]

- Lack of access to high-cost cancer medications: There is a lack of access to expensive medications and technologies within Latin American public health systems, whereas patients with private insurance (or private funds) have access to many costly treatments.[2]
- Shortage of oncology services and specialized training personnel: Patients struggle to find enough medical oncologists, surgical oncologists, and clinical oncology nurses to meet their cancer care needs. Moreover, the majority of oncologists tend to work in their respective capital cities, resulting in significant shortages in smaller towns and rural areas.[26] Additionally, the training of clinical oncologists in Latin America lacks a unified curriculum and each country sets its own requirements. Therefore, educational strategies are needed to train general practice physicians to participate in cancer screening, diagnostics, treatment, and survivorship.[2]
- Insufficient radiotherapy services: Although the process of improving the modernization of radiotherapy equipment varies throughout the region, it is slow and inaccessible to a considerable amount of patients with cancer. There is a current lack of validated clinical protocols and procedural manuals as well as insufficient infrastructure.[27]
- Scarce palliative care services: In the majority of South American countries, funds are directed to primary prevention and curative treatments, rather than palliative therapies. There are several barriers surrounding the adoption of such therapies, including limited available potent analgesics, fear of diversion of opioids to illegal markets, inadequate policies and legislation regarding end-of-life care, and beliefs that palliative care destroys hope, among others.[2,28] Thus, managing cancer pain in Latin America remains challenging.

Hurdles Associated with Available Therapeutic Options

Cancer-directed systemic therapies

The WHO defines essential medicines as those that "satisfy the priority health care needs of a population. They are intended to be available in functioning health systems at all times, in appropriate dosage forms, of assured quality and at prices individuals and health systems can afford."[29] Multiple antineoplastic therapies fall under this list, including cytotoxic drugs, immunomodulators, targeted therapies, and supportive medications utilized in cancer care.

However, due to numerous economic, political, and geographical barriers, equitable access to high-cost cancer therapeutics across all of South America is lacking and fraught with numerous challenges.[30] One report by the Pan American Health Organization (PAHO) estimated that approximately 50% of the Latin American population does not have access to high-cost drugs.[31] With the advent of newer, more expensive targeted and immune therapies, the global oncology gap continues to widen because many of those drugs are not available in the region. Furthermore, when those drugs do become available, they are usually accessible only to the wealthy minority through private insurance programs or on an out-of-pocket basis. One report noted that 32% and 57.7% of cancer medications on the essential medicine list were available in low and middle-income countries (LMIC) and low-income countries (LIC), respectively, only if patients were willing to pay the full costs out of pocket.[32] One such example is trastuzumab, which is not covered by the public health system in Brazil, Chile, or Peru.[33]

Additionally, there is high pricing of cancer drugs in many LMICs as compared with high-income countries (HICs), with wide variability in drug prices across South America and less affordability by patients with low-income levels.[34] A year's worth of adjuvant trastuzumab, for example, can cost US$25,636 in Uruguay, compared with US$61,302 in Brazil.[35]

Surgical oncology and radiotherapy

Multidisciplinary care between medical oncology, radiation oncology, and surgical oncology is required to improve the quality of care and outcomes in a variety of malignancies but is often lacking in many countries in South America.[36] Many patients present with advanced malignancies due to the limited national implementation of screening initiatives, long wait times to access specialties, and significant geographical disparities. In underserved regions of Latin America, for example, there is a shortage of providers able to perform screening tests, colposcopies, cervical biopsies, and loop electrosurgical excision procedures, leading to vastly high rates of cervical cancer.[37] In Peru and Mexico also approximately 50% of patients with breast cancer present with advanced disease.[38] Opportunities to undergo surgical specialty training are limited in many LMICs without formal surgical oncology fellowships, and quality control protocols and surgical data, required to improve surgical techniques, are often lacking.[39] This results in mastectomy being the only surgical option for breast cancer regardless of size of the tumor, which additionally creates a disincentive to earlier detection due to fear of mastectomy.

Similarly, there is a paucity of trained radiation oncologists across the region, and lack of adherence to formalized quality standards.[27] It has been proposed that LMICs could have a greater need for radiotherapy due to their epidemiologic features and advanced disease burden.[40] However, the availability and accessibility of radiotherapy is quite limited in many countries across South America; at one point, there were an estimated 620 radiotherapy centers serving 600 million inhabitants.[41] Although the number of radiation therapy centers are increasing, many lack adequate infrastructure and equipment, with the majority (81%) lacking a simulation system and more than half (55%) lacking a treatment planning system. Many centers also have old machines (>20 years old) with questionable reliability and functionality. In addition, most centers tend to be centralized in urban areas, inaccessible to large segments of the population, and are clustered in few countries, namely Brazil, Mexico, Colombia, and Argentina, whereas other countries such as Haiti have none.[41]

Precision oncology

Decades ago, the mainstay of cancer-directed therapies relied on cytotoxic drugs that inhibit rapidly dividing cancer cells. Those treatments often carried a lower efficacy and broad side effects due to their lack of specific targeting of tumor cells. During the past decade, we have increasingly identified tumor-specific biomarkers along the cancer-care continuum: preventive, diagnostic, predictive, and prognostic. This allowed for the development of targeted therapeutics that has transformed the cancer treatment paradigm by ushering in a new era of personalized precision oncology, from screening, to treatment, to surveillance strategies.

In South America, multiple barriers persist that hinder the successful implementation of personalized medicine and are predominantly related to the region's significant inequities and shortage of cancer-care resources and funding.[42] There is variability among populations in the region who carry different mutations and polymorphisms, and further research is required to formulate appropriate guidelines.[43] Insufficient investment in research and development, in addition to the fragmented infrastructure of health-care facilities and significant delays in obtaining regulatory approvals, are all major obstacles.[44] A small percentage of the gross national income per capita in South America, about 0.12%, is devoted toward cancer care, compared with 0.51% and 1.02% in the United Kingdom and the United State, respectively.[31] Many areas lack specialized oncologists with few educational opportunities and training in conducting clinical research.

Access to Cancer Care and Treatments

Cancer care in South America is riddled with inequities that predominantly affect people of lower socioeconomic status, rural dwellers, and indigenous populations. Affordability is a critical determinant of access to cancer care and subsequent cancer control in this region. Although a few South American countries (eg, Brazil, Costa Rica) are close to achieving universal health care, many other countries are far behind in their quest to bridge the gap between the insured and uninsured. This has resulted in significant disparities in access to care.[45]

Because cancer care is typically highly specialized, this often means that resources (manpower, equipment) are concentrated in urban areas, putting rural dwellers at a significant location disadvantage.[7] This is of particular importance in South America, as a Chilean study reported different cancer types linked to varying environmental influences in rural compared with urban areas.[46] Ripple effects include nonpresentation, late presentation, and poor follow-up, thereby negatively impacting survival.

Fragmentation is a well-known barrier to accessing adequate health care, consequently leading to subpar cancer care in South America. In this region, the problem is 2-pronged: first, an institutional fragmentation of health-care policies ultimately results in delayed implementation of national cancer plans,[45] and second, such fragmentation often results in widely differentiated quality of health-care coverage, for example, comprehensive private insurance coverage/social security systems, inclusive of appropriate cancer care for individuals in formal employment versus public insurance that covers only basic care.[47] This often results in large out-of-pocket payments for patients on public insurance,[33] resulting in vast disparities in outcomes among patients, depending on their socioeconomic and employment status.

As insurmountable as the challenge seems, notable strides regarding the provision of Universal Healthcare Coverage have been made in the region, with countries such as Costa Rica offering almost complete universal health care via its Social Security Administration,[48] the Colombian Ministry of Health collapsing all private insurance schemes into a unified, extended health-care package that covers all cancers, whereas others such as Argentina and Peru continue to make outstanding progress.[33] In addition, Uruguay currently provides radiotherapy and chemotherapy for free, and Chile has developed a national program that standardizes treatment of health conditions including all cancers in children aged younger than 15 years, and 11 cancers in adults.[33] Cross-sectoral collaboration is proposed to reduce segregation between the private and public health-care sector and close critical fragmentation gaps in the region, aimed to reduce inequalities in access to cancer care in the region (**Table 2**).

Importance of Cancer Registers and National Cancer Plans

Some countries in South America have population-based cancer registries, such as Argentina, Brazil, Chile, Colombia, Uruguay, Costa Rica, Puerto Rico, Cuba, Ecuador, Peru, Panama, and Mexico.[49] Peru, in particular, has 2 population-based cancer registries, both of which are members of the International Association of Cancer Registries and collate information from about 33% of the Peruvian populace.[49] Paraguay and Bolivia are also putting new population-based cancer registries in place.[46] In addition, Argentina, Bolivia, Chile, Brazil, Colombia, Costa Rica, Panama, Peru, Uruguay, and Ecuador have established legislative frameworks for the detection, diagnosis, and treatment of breast cancer.[50] For policy-making and resource allocations within cancer care, only population-based cancer registries can provide reliable incidence and survival data. Given the lack of high-quality cancer registries, the Global Initiative for

Table 2 Health-care systems in some countries of South America		
Country	**Type of Insurance**	**National Cancer Care Plan**
Argentina	Public, social security and private *Plan Médico Obligatorio*	Yes, only for specific malignancies such as breast cancer
Brazil	Public ~75% *Sistema Único de Saúde* Private ~25%	Yes, at state level
Bolivia	Universal health coverage model through 3 programs: *Sistema Unico de Salud de Bolivia* *Seguro Universal Materno Infantil* *Seguro Especial para Adultos*	Yes, only for specific malignancies such as breast cancer
Chile	A specific portfolio of diseases (selected by government) is covered to all citizens	Yes *Plan Nacional de Cancer 2018–2028*
Colombia	Social security system with 2 schemes: 1. Contributive scheme, which covers a wide diagnostic test 2. Subsidized scheme, which mainly provides coverage for poor habitants Plan Obligatorio de Salud	Yes *Plan Decenal para el Control del Cáncer*
Paraguay	Paraguay Health National System, which establishes that the system will provide services through the public, private or public–private subsectors, from health insurances and universities *Sistema Nacional de Salud de Paraguay*	Yes *Programa Nacional de Control del Cancer—PRONAC*
Peru	Public health insurance through 2 systems: *Segura Integral de Salud (SIS)* *EsSalud* SIS is regulated by the Peruvian Ministry of Health and is largely aimed at those who are poverty-stricken and have no health coverage	Yes *Plan Esperanza*
Uruguay	Nationally Integrated Health System 1. National health-insurance body (*Fondo Nacional de Salud; FONASA*) 2. National board of health (*Junta Nacional de Salud; JUNASA*) *Plan Integral de Atención a la Salud*	Yes
Venezuela	Contributive government programs 1. Solidario health system with compulsory affiliation 2. Complementary system with voluntary affiliation	In preparation

Cancer Registry Development provides support to improve this situation via the International Agency for Research on Cancer Regional Hub for Latin America. Thus, it is imperative to improve data quality in Latin America, ensuring that the data collected are made available, widely disseminated, and used effectively in cancer control.[8]

According to WHO, many South American nations have programs or standards in place to improve the early detection of symptoms in primary care. High-quality epidemiological data and comprehensive cancer registries are crucial to the success of national cancer care plans' implementation. Currently, Chile and Cuba have successful national plans to follow-up with patients with positive cytology-based cervical cancer screening, reporting up to a 90% rate for high-grade squamous intraepithelial lesions, whereas countries such as Colombia, Peru, and Bolivia have follow-up rates of approximately 60%, with subsequent biopsy and treatment.[51] For HPV vaccination, a 2013 survey by the PAHO showed a 67% national coverage by the governments of Panama and Mexico.[52] National cancer plans for prostate cancer have been prioritized in several South American countries due to the region's increased prostate cancer burden, with resultant development of effective guidelines from the point of detection up until follow-up.[53] Specific programs and directives include Argentina's "Programa Nacional de Consensos Inter-Sociedades, Programa Argentino de Consensos de Enfermedades Oncológicas,"[53] Chile's labor code amendment that allows men aged older than 50 years to take off half of a working day for prostate exams,[54] Peru's Strategic Program for Cancer Prevention and Control, and Uruguay's prostate specific antigen (PSA) and digital rectal examination (DRE) availability in health centers for men aged 40 years and older.[53] For colorectal cancer screening and early detection using immunochemical FOBT and follow-up colonoscopy, national policies have been rolled out in Argentina and Uruguay,[53] Chile,[55] and Cuba.[56] In addition, general bowel cancer screening is made available at the primary health-care level in Brazil, Costa Rica, Ecuador, Cuba, and Argentina.[57] **Table 3** shows an example of a Colombian National Cancer Control Program.

Primary Prevention Initiatives in South America

The most cost-effective strategy for cancer control is the implementation of primary prevention initiatives focused on reducing the main risk factor associated with the disease. Thus, public health priorities are concentrated in establishing screening programs to reduce the cancer burden and respond to the increased morbidity and mortality from advanced disease observed during recent decades.[2] Some of most important detection strategies implemented in South America are briefly described below.

Lung cancer: tobacco control measures

Prevention and control strategies for lung cancer in Central and South America is chiefly focused on the reduction of tobacco smoking, the predominant risk factor for the development of lung cancer worldwide[21]; this risk factor is reported in 75% to 90% of patients with lung cancer.[58]

In line with the above, by 2014, smoke-free policies were implemented in about 13 countries in the region (Argentina, Brazil, Chile, Colombia, Costa Rica, Ecuador, Guatemala, Honduras, Panama, Peru, Suriname, Uruguay, and Venezuela).[59] These policies were enacted to ensure that public spaces are at least 90% smoke-free but because the implemented policies are not fully in concordance with other standards, such as those regarding taxation, few other countries complied with the recommendation.[60]

Some other control strategies used to promote smoking cessation in this region include offering nicotine replacement therapy and the availability of national quit lines, with countries such as Argentina, Mexico, Panama, and Brazil covering the cost of these services.[61] In other countries, although, smoking cessation programs are not covered by insurance or the availability of them is not guaranteed. There is also growing concern about novel forms of tobacco consumption with devices such as electronic nicotine delivery systems. In Colombia, the National Study of Consumption of Psychoactive Substances[62] that included almost 50,000 individuals

Table 3
National program for the control of cancer in Colombia

No.	Strategy	Description
1	Primary prevention: Risk control	• Control of the risk of consumption of alcohol and tobacco products • Promotion of healthy diet • Risk control against occupational carcinogens including ultraviolet radiation • Specific protection to cancer-related viruses
2	Early detection of disease	• Cervical cancer – Breast cancer – Prostate cancer – Colorectal cancer – Childhood Cancer (pediatric acute leukemias)
3	Care and recovery of the damage caused by cancer	• Rehabilitation of patients with cancer • Organization of the supply and demand for cancer services • Quality control in the provision of oncological services
4	Improving the quality of life of patients with cancer and survivors	• Expand types of interventions of palliative care for patients with cancer and cancer survivors
5	Knowledge management and technology for cancer control	• National Cancer Information System and Cancer Observatory
6	Training and development of human talent	• Continuous training and well-being of human talent in oncology

Addressing the rising burden of cancer in Colombia: Challenges & opportunities. An Analysis of Colombia's Health System and Cancer Control Policies. UICC-ICCILA, June 2021. Retrieved from: https://www.uicc.org/sites/main/files/atoms/files/UICC-ICCILA-Colombia-Report-English-June-2021-FA.pdf.

showed that at least 5% of the surveyed population reported having used this type of device at least once in their life. Most Latin American countries do not include these kinds of devices as cigarettes, prohibiting the law to regulate or control access to them.[63]

Screening for lung cancer with low-dose computed tomography saves lives, as demonstrated by the reduction of mortality in high-risk populations with history of smoking exposure in the National Lung Screening Trial and Nelson trial.[64,65] In Latin America, access to lung cancer screening remains low; in a recent anonymous survey, only 32.2% of physicians had access to a lung cancer screening program, which were mainly concentrated in large cities.[66] There is a lack of lung cancer screening policies in the region, related to the availability of clinical trials including Hispanic populations or initiatives developed in individuals located in Latin America, where unique risk factors may be important.

Cervical cancer: human papilloma virus vaccination

HPV vaccination has been identified as a crucial prevention strategy for cervical cancer in South America. In 2020, the WHO launched a global strategy plan that called for all nations to implement primary prevention strategies for cervical cancer, including vaccine delivery platforms (eg, school immunization programs), advocacy and social mobilization efforts to combat vaccine hesitancy, and age-appropriate information regarding safe sexual behaviors to eliminate cervical cancer as a public health concern.[67] Currently, a bivalent vaccine containing HPV types 16 and 18 and a quadrivalent vaccine containing HPV types 6, 11, 16, and 18 antigens are in use in vaccination programs around the world. Between 2011 and 2015, 14 countries in Latin America introduced HPV vaccines into their national immunization programs, and since 2016, the other remaining 27 HPV vaccine introductions have occurred in the region.[68] Currently, 42 countries use the quadrivalent HPV vaccine,[69] and it is estimated that 89% of PAHO Member States will offer HPV vaccination to teenage girls by the end of 2021.[70]

Children aged 9 to 13 years are the target cohort for vaccination, although Colombia and Mexico define it by school grade rather than by age. In general, the vaccination schedule corresponds to that indicated by the vaccine manufacturer, although Colombia and Brazil use an extended schedule with 3 doses at 0, 6, and 60 months; Mexico, Chile, and other countries use 2 doses (0–6 months).[71] The delivery strategy in Uruguay is focused on health centers, whereas the remaining countries use a school-based strategy (Peru, Paraguay, and Colombia) or a combination of schools and health-care centers (Argentina, Brazil, Mexico, and Panama).[72] The HPV vaccine is in addition to cytology-based screening via pap smear and/or HPV testing in almost all South American countries.[72] After the COVID-19 pandemic, a redoubled effort should be made to ensure that HPV vaccine implementation remains a priority within national immunization programs.[68]

Breast cancer: mammography screening
Breast cancer prevention strategies in South America include clinical breast examination (CBE), an economical method that has been noted to facilitate breast cancer detection at earlier stages,[73] and mammography screening, an effective method of lowering breast cancer mortality by up to 25% in women aged 50 to 69 years.[74] Country-specific mammography screening rates vary widely, at 2.3% in Cuba, 22% in Mexico, 25% to 32% in Brazil, 30% in Peru, 32% in Chile, 34% in Costa Rica, 46% in Argentina, and 54% in Colombia,[56,75–77] which is highly correlated with level of education, which tends to be higher in urban areas.[78]

Community-based programs to facilitate early breast cancer detection have been effective in some countries in the region. In the Brazilian municipalities of São Paulo, Barretos, and 19 other adjacent municipalities, for instance, a mammography screening program was able to screen close to 18,000 women with a notable breast cancer detection rate of 4.2 per 1000 and 43% of cases detected at early stages.[79] A mammography screening program in Mexico examined about 97,000 women aged older than 40 years with a detection rate of 2.1 per 1000,[80] whereas Peru's breast cancer awareness program involved a media campaign (television advertisements), where health professionals and community health workers performed CBEs and biopsies as appropriate.[81]

Nonetheless, a Colombian survey of more than 1000 women with breast cancer revealed that breast cancer screening, diagnosis, and treatment was more attainable for women with higher socioeconomic status and robust health insurance compared with lower-income women who have either poor or no health insurance.[81] Moreover, conclusions from the 2008 study on breast cancer in Latin America also demonstrated that hormone receptor and molecular markers were not available for all patients, there was high percentage of mastectomy, surgery is performed by gynecologists or general surgeon in an important number of cases, and clinical epidemiologic and basic research were insufficient. In addition, access to targeted therapies such as trastuzumab, bevacizumab, or lapatinib, important treatment options for patients with advanced breast cancer, were restricted, which leaves patients with few therapeutic alternatives, uncontrolled disease progression, and consequently, poor outcomes.[82]

Most countries in this region follow national recommendations for breast cancer screening, comprising mammography, CBE, and in some countries, breast self-examination. However, variations exist in age at recommended baseline mammography screening, with some starting at 35 years (Panama), 40 years (Uruguay, Colombia, Peru and Costa Rica), whereas most perform annual screening for women aged between 50 and 70 years. Regardless of country specification/parameters, when a woman is considered to be high-risk (eg, with a family history of breast cancer), mammography is recommended from the age of 35 or 40 years.[83]

Prostate cancer: prostate specific antigen screening and digital rectal examination
Prostate cancer detection and prevention strategies in South America is centered around the measurement of PSA and DRE,[84] with confirmation of diagnosis using transrectal ultrasound (TRUS) and TRUS-guided needle biopsy. A couple of studies have been conducted on prostate cancer detection in the region, revealing findings of 6.4% of cases from 2197 men screened in Chile[85] and 12.8% of cases from 973 men screened in Mexico. In the Mexican study, only 44% of the men with abnormal screening test had a prostate biopsy, of which 27% were diagnosed with prostate cancer.[86]

Palliative Care in South America: Barriers for the Appropriate Cancer Pain Management

People living in LMICs have minimal or no palliative care or cancer pain treatment when compared with high-income countries.[87,88] Cancer pain is a symptom that notoriously affects a person's life, generating a gradual deterioration of the quality of life in the physical, mental, spiritual, and economic aspects in most developing countries.[89-91]

Barriers such as economic, ethic, and cultural diversity, poor education, lack of diagnostic and prognostic information provided to patients and families, shortages of strong pain relievers, fear of opioid use, poor regulation of the local health system, and concerns from oncologists of palliative care being used to treat cancer, continue to impede progress in Latin American countries.[2] Thus, the optimal pain treatment is impeded by several barriers that affect both patients and health-care providers, as well as the health-care system.

Inadequate knowledge of pain management
The acceptance of palliative care is severely hampered by the inadequate training of health professionals in LMICs, both during and after they finish their careers.[92] Regular medication for chronic cancer pain, the pathophysiology of cancer pain, the dose, adjuvant medications, addiction, and tolerance have all been identified as areas of knowledge deficiency among physicians.[28]

In a study carried out in Colombia, it was determined that basic and advanced knowledge of the management of the course of treatment was a barrier that greatly influenced the management of cancer pain. They discovered a lack of training in palliative care as well as the common misconception among patients that palliative care is only for those nearing death, and not during their illness.[93] In reality, although, palliative care can be provided in addition to the specific treatments of the disease to improve quality of life.[94]

Nevertheless, not all Latin American countries have palliative education as a specialty or subspecialty. In fact, a recent study revealed that only 6 countries from South America have palliative care training[95] (**Table 4**).

Several references cite Argentina as one of the leaders in palliative care in Latin America, but even so, there are some barriers to its formal development of palliative care, such as the distance of health professionals from the main cities, those resulting

Table 4
Palliative care training in South America

Country	Year of Started Palliative Care Training
Argentina	2006
Brazil	2011
Colombia	1998
Ecuador	2018
Paraguay	2016
Venezuela	2009

from the modalities of education in palliative care currently available, and those related to the delivery of palliative care education in the main health institutions.[96]

Availability and access to pain management
Many factors can influence availability and access, including medical equipment and supply distribution challenges, complex reimbursement systems and legal paperwork, and a lengthy and intricate procedure that all patients must go through.[97]

Opioids formulations cost and availability can vary in every South American country. A study dividing the cost depending on opioid formulation by the International Association for Hospice and Palliative Care in Latin American and Caribbean countries showed that Codeine, immediate release oral morphine (MoIR), controlled release oral morphine, injectable morphine, oral immediate release oxycodone, transdermal fentanyl, and oral methadone were mainly at full cost to patients in Bolivia, Brazil, Ecuador, and Peru, which is truly concerning. The availability was divided as always, usually, half of time, occasionally, and never, and were usually available in South America; only Chile had occasionally availability of MoIR while Colombia and Bolivia had half of time availability for MoIR.[97]

The availability of distributed opioid morphine equivalent (DOME) (Morphine, codeine, fentanyl, hydromorphone, pethidine, and oxycodone) during the years has remained low in Latin American countries, with a growing gap between countries such as the United States and Canada. In a study conducted in Colombia, it was found that DOME availability was insufficient to cover the needs of the population, with some rural areas lacking or having very limited access to these drugs.[98]

Inadequate pain assessment
Even though the literature expresses that there are several pain assessments, a proper method of evaluation is still missing.[99] Pain is a symptom of many different disorders, whether acute or chronic; it is a universal symptom and is the primary symptom in cancer associated with the treatment or progress of a disease, making it critical to examine it and establish a prompt treatment approach.[100] A Brazilian investigation highlighted the importance of pain assessment in palliative care, emphasizing pain severity, clinical characteristics, daily activities, sleep pattern disturbance, triggering events, and relieving factors.[101]

From the patient perspective, fear of opioid drugs is a significant reason why they do not communicate their true suffering to medical professionals, specifically either due to opioid side effects or the possibility of developing an addiction to them.[102] This concept of fear is called "opiophobia." Up to 50% of hospice patients taking strong opioid medications seem to have opiophobia; it is an important barrier that prevents successful communication between patients and health-care workers, prompting inadequate pain management.[103]

Administrative and judicial barriers of prescribing opioids

Institutional barriers such as the absence of contracts or agreements between insurers and providers also results in missed opportunities for care.[93] The health system of South America has a deficit in the epidemiological plan, resulting in failures of rapid prescriptions that thereby delay access to opioid drugs and increases the hospital stay with the deterioration of the patient.[101] Only few countries have developed a palliative care policy and national plan for palliative care management, such as Argentina, Chile, Ecuador, Uruguay, and Venezuela.[104] Such a lack of policy support leaves palliative care without a solid implementation foundation and does not meet the needs of the large number of people who require palliative care services.[105] Overly strict regulation on available forms of drugs, lack of supply and delivery distribution, limitations for the health-care provider in prescribing, and fear of law enforcement intervention in the use of opioids are some of the barriers that continue to prevent quality cancer pain management.[105]

CLINICS CARE POINTS

- In South America, the top 5 most frequent new cancer diagnoses include breast, prostate, colorectal, lung, and stomach cancers, which account for almost 50% of new nonmelanoma cancer diagnoses.

- Breast cancer is the most common cancer diagnosed in women and prostate cancer is in men. Lung cancer is the leading cause of cancer death, followed by colorectal and breast cancer.

- Tobacco use is the most important cancer risk factor in Latin America; it accounts for about one-quarter of all cancer deaths and is associated with several other solid tumor malignancies.

- The main challenges of cancer control in South America include fragmented health-care systems; unavailable oncology services for rural and Indigenous populations; insufficient cancer screening and tailored detection programs; limited molecular testing and diagnostic delays; deficient population-based cancer registries; inaccessibility to high-cost cancer medications; shortage of oncology services; limited trained personnel including medical oncologists, surgical oncologists, and clinical oncology nurses; restricted palliative care services and inadequate cancer pain control; and insufficient investment in research to implement personalized cancer care, among others.

DISCLOSURE

I. Riano, I. Abuali, O. Abioye, and K. Jimenez have nothing to declare. A.I. Velazquez: Advisory: AstraZeneca. Stock Ownership: Corbus Pharmaceuticals. Honoraria: OptumHealth Education, MDOutlook, Curio Science, ObR Oncology, MJH Life Sciences, CMEOutfitters. Travel: DAVA Oncology, Bio Ascend. Research Funding: National Institute on Aging (under award P30AG015272), and National Cancer Institute (under award U54 CA242646-04S2). L. Viola: Advisory board MSD - BMS. Speaker: AZ - BMS - MSD. Travel grants: BMS - Bayer. N. Florez: Consulting/Advisory to Merck, Astrazeneca, Pfizer, DSI, BMS, Novartis, Neogenomics and Janssen.

REFERENCES

1. Piñeros M, Laversanne M, Barrios E, et al. An updated profile of the cancer burden, patterns and trends in Latin America and the Caribbean. The Lancet Regional Health – Americas 2022;13. https://doi.org/10.1016/j.lana.2022.100294.

2. Goss PE, Lee BL, Badovinac-Crnjevic T, et al. Planning cancer control in Latin America and the Caribbean. Lancet Oncol 2013;14(5):391–436.

3. Bray F, Piñeros M. Cancer patterns, trends and projections in Latin America and the Caribbean: a global context. Salud Publica Mex 2016;58(2):104–17.

4. Ferlay J, Shin HR, Bray F, et al. Estimates of worldwide burden of cancer in 2008: GLOBOCAN 2008. Int J Cancer 2010;127(12):2893–917.

5. Spence D, Argentieri MA, Andall-Brereton G, et al. Advancing cancer care and prevention in the Caribbean: a survey of strategies for the region. Lancet Oncol 2019;20(9):e522–34.

6. Soerjomataram I, Bray F. Planning for tomorrow: global cancer incidence and the role of prevention 2020-2070. Nat Rev Clin Oncol 2021;18(10):663–72.

7. Barrios CH, Werutsky G, Mohar A, et al. Cancer control in Latin America and the Caribbean: recent advances and opportunities to move forward. Lancet Oncol 2021;22(11):e474–87.

8. Piñeros M, Abriata MG, de Vries E, et al. Progress, challenges and ways forward supporting cancer surveillance in Latin America. Int J Cancer 2021;149(1): 12–20.

9. WHO. The top 10 causes of death, Available at: https://www.who.int/news-room/fact-sheets/detail/the-top-10-causes-of-death. Accessed April 1, 2023.

10. Bray F, Laversanne M, Weiderpass E, et al. The ever-increasing importance of cancer as a leading cause of premature death worldwide. Cancer 2021; 127(16):3029–30.

11. WHO. Global Health Estimates 2020: Deaths by Cause, Age, Sex, by Country and by Region, 2000-2019, Available at: who.int/data/gho/data/themes/mortality-and-global-health-estimates/ghe-leading-causes-of-death. Accessed April 1, 2023.

12. Sung H, Ferlay J, Siegel RL, et al. Global Cancer Statistics 2020: GLOBOCAN Estimates of Incidence and Mortality Worldwide for 36 Cancers in 185 Countries. CA Cancer J Clin 2021;71(3):209–49.

13. GLOBOCAN. Global Cancer Observatory: Cancer Today, Available at: http://gco.iarc.fr/today/home. Accessed April 1, 2023.

14. Ferlay J, Colombet M, Soerjomataram I, et al. Cancer statistics for the year 2020: An overview. Int J Cancer 2021. https://doi.org/10.1002/ijc.33588.

15. GLOBOCAN. Global Cancer Observatory: Cancer Tomorrow, Available at: http://gco.iarc.fr/today/home. Accessed April 1, 2023.

16. Knaul FM, Wong R, Arreola-Ornelas H, et al. Household catastrophic health expenditures: a comparative analysis of twelve Latin American and Caribbean Countries. Salud Publica Mex 2011;53(Suppl 2):s85–95.

17. World Health Organization. (↱2010)↱. Why urban health matters. World Health Organization. Available at: https://apps.who.int/iris/handle/10665/70230.

18. Pereira L, Zamudio R, Soares-Souza G, et al. Socioeconomic and nutritional factors account for the association of gastric cancer with Amerindian ancestry in a Latin American admixed population. PLoS One 2012;7(8):e41200.

19. Gracey M, King M. Indigenous health part 1: determinants and disease patterns. Lancet 2009;374(9683):65–75.

20. AICR. Food, nutrition, physical activity and the prevention of cancer: a global perspective, Available at: https://www.paho.org/hq/dmdocuments/2011/nutrition-AICR-WCR-food-physical-activ.pdf. Accessed April 2, 2023.

21. World Health Organization. (↱2008)↱. WHO Report on the Global Tobacco Epidemic, 2008: the MPOWER package. World Health Organization. Available at: https://apps.who.int/iris/handle/10665/43818.

22. de Martel C, Ferlay J, Franceschi S, et al. Global burden of cancers attributable to infections in 2008: a review and synthetic analysis. Lancet Oncol 2012;13(6): 607–15.
23. Espinosa de Los Monteros K, Gallo LC. The relevance of fatalism in the study of Latinas' cancer screening behavior: a systematic review of the literature. Int J Behav Med 2011;18(4):310–8.
24. Cendales R, Wiesner C, Murillo RH, et al. [Quality of vaginal smear for cervical cancer screening: a concordance study]. Biomedica 2010;30(1):107–15. La calidad de las citologías para tamización de cáncer de cuello uterino en cuatro departamentos de Colombia: un estudio de concordancia.
25. Perez EA, Suman VJ, Davidson NE, et al. HER2 testing by local, central, and reference laboratories in specimens from the North Central Cancer Treatment Group N9831 intergroup adjuvant trial. J Clin Oncol 2006;24(19):3032–8.
26. Anampa-Guzmán A, Brito-Hijar AD, Gutierrez-Narvaez CA, et al. American Society of Clinical Oncology–Sponsored Oncology Student Interest Groups in Latin America. JCO Global Oncology 2020;(6):1439–45.
27. Grover S, Xu MJ, Yeager A, et al. A systematic review of radiotherapy capacity in low- and middle-income countries. Front Oncol 2014;4:380.
28. Kwon JH. Overcoming barriers in cancer pain management. J Clin Oncol 2014; 32(16):1727–33.
29. Organization WH. WHO model list of essential medicines–22nd list, 2021. Geneva: WHO; 2021.
30. Ruiz R, Strasser-Weippl K, Touya D, et al. Improving access to high-cost cancer drugs in Latin America: Much to be done. Cancer 2017;123(8):1313–23.
31. Pan American Health Organization. Area of Medicines and Health Technologies. Project of Essential Medicines and Biologicals. Access to High-Cost Medicines in the Americas: Situation, Challenges and Perspectives. Washington, DC: PAHO; 2010. Technical Series No. 1 Essential Medicines, Access, and Innovation. Available at: https://www3.paho.org/hq/index.php?option=com_content&view=article&id=2149:2008-el-acceso-medicamentos-alto-costo-americas&Itemid=0&lang=en#gsc.tab=0.
32. World Health Organization. (↱2018)↱. Technical report: pricing of cancer medicines and its impacts: a comprehensive technical report for the World Health Assembly Resolution 70.12: operative paragraph 2.9 on pricing approaches and their impacts on availability and affordability of medicines for the prevention and treatment of cancer. World Health Organization. Available at: https://apps.who.int/iris/handle/10665/277190. License: CC BY-NC-SA 3.0 IGO.
33. Strasser-Weippl K, Chavarri-Guerra Y, Villarreal-Garza C, et al. Progress and remaining challenges for cancer control in Latin America and the Caribbean. Lancet Oncol 2015;16(14):1405–38.
34. Ocran Mattila P, Ahmad R, Hasan SS, et al. Availability, Affordability, Access, and Pricing of Anti-cancer Medicines in Low- and Middle-Income Countries: A Systematic Review of Literature. Front Public Health 2021;9:628744.
35. Pichon-Riviere A, Silva Elias FT, Rivero VG, et al. Early awareness and alert activities in Latin America: current situation in four countries. Int J Technol Assess Health Care 2012;28(3):315–20.
36. Barrios C, Sánchez-Vanegas G, Villarreal-Garza C, et al. Barriers and facilitators to provide multidisciplinary care for breast cancer patients in five Latin American countries: A descriptive-interpretative qualitative study. The Lancet Regional Health-Americas 2022;11:100254.

37. Lopez MS, Baker ES, Maza M, et al. Cervical cancer prevention and treatment in Latin America. J Surg Oncol 2017;115(5):615–8.
38. Justo N, Wilking N, Jönsson B, et al. A review of breast cancer care and outcomes in Latin America. Oncol 2013;18(3):248–56.
39. El Saghir NS, Adebamowo CA, Anderson BO, et al. Breast cancer management in low resource countries (LRCs): consensus statement from the Breast Health Global Initiative. Breast 2011;20(Suppl 2):S3–11.
40. Barton MB, Frommer M, Shafiq J. Role of radiotherapy in cancer control in low-income and middle-income countries. Lancet Oncol 2006;7(7):584–95.
41. Zubizarreta E, Van Dyk J, Lievens Y. Analysis of Global Radiotherapy Needs and Costs by Geographic Region and Income Level. Clin Oncol 2017;29(2):84–92.
42. Calderón-Aparicio A, Orue A. Precision oncology in Latin America: current situation, challenges and perspectives. Ecancermedicalscience 2019;13:920.
43. López-Cortés A, Guerrero S, Redal MA, et al. State of Art of Cancer Pharmacogenomics in Latin American Populations. Int J Mol Sci 2017;18(6). https://doi.org/10.3390/ijms18060639.
44. Rolfo C, Caglevic C, Bretel D, et al. Cancer clinical research in Latin America: current situation and opportunities. Expert opinion from the first ESMO workshop on clinical trials, Lima, 2015. ESMO Open 2016;1(4):e000055.
45. World Cancer Initiative. Cancer preparedness around the world: National readiness for a global epidemic. June 9, 2023. Available at: chrome-extension://efaidnbmnnnibpcajpcglclefindmkaj/https://www.iccp-portal.org/system/files/resources/Cancer_preparedness_around_the_world.pdf.
46. Kielstra P. Cancer control, access and inequality in Latin America: A tale of light and Shadow. Econ Intell Unit 2017;22:e488–500.
47. Atun R, de Andrade LO, Almeida G, et al. Health-system reform and universal health coverage in Latin America. Lancet 2015;385(9974):1230–47.
48. del Rocio Sáenz M., Bermúdez J.L., Acosta M. (2010). Universal coverage in a middle income country: Costa Rica. Geneva (Switzerland): World Health Organization (World Health Report [2010] background paper, No. 11). chrome-extension://efaidnbmnnnibpcajpcglclefindmkaj/https://mronline.org/wp-content/uploads/2021/02/CostaRicaNo11.pdf.
49. Piñeros M, Abriata MG, Mery L, et al. Cancer registration for cancer control in Latin America: a status and progress report. Rev Panam Salud Publica 2017; 41:e2.
50. Lee BL, Liedke PE, Barrios CH, et al. Breast cancer in Brazil: present status and future goals. Lancet Oncol 2012;13(3):e95–102.
51. Murillo R, Wiesner C, Cendales R, et al. Comprehensive evaluation of cervical cancer screening programs: the case of Colombia. Salud Publica Mex 2011; 53(6):469–77.
52. Nogueira-Rodrigues A. HPV Vaccination in Latin America: Global Challenges and Feasible Solutions. American Society of Clinical Oncology Educational Book 2019;39:e45–52.
53. Sierra MS, Soerjomataram I, Antoni S, et al. Cancer patterns and trends in Central and South America. Cancer Epidemiol 2016;44(Suppl 1):S23–42.
54. Jimenez de la Jara J, Bastias G, Ferreccio C, et al. A snapshot of cancer in Chile: analytical frameworks for developing a cancer policy. Biol Res 2015; 48(1):10.
55. Okada T, Tanaka K, Kawachi H, et al. International collaboration between Japan and Chile to improve detection rates in colorectal cancer screening. Cancer 2016;122(1):71–7.

56. González RS. Cancer screening: global debates and Cuban experience. MED-ICC Rev 2014;16(3–4):73–7.
57. Schreuders EH, Ruco A, Rabeneck L, et al. Colorectal cancer screening: a global overview of existing programmes. Gut 2015;64(10):1637–49.
58. Walser T, Cui X, Yanagawa J, et al. Smoking and lung cancer: the role of inflammation. Proc Am Thorac Soc 2008;5(8):811–5.
59. World Health Organization. (ᴦ2015)ᴦ. WHO report on the global tobacco epidemic, 2015: raising taxes on tobacco. World Health Organization. Available at: https://apps.who.int/iris/handle/10665/178574.
60. WHO. WHO report on the global tobacco epidemic 2021: addressing new and emerging products, Available at: https://www.who.int/publications/i/item/9789240032095. Accessed April 1, 2023.
61. WHO. WHO report on the global tobacco epidemic, 2013: enforcing bans on tobacco advertising, promotion and sponsorship, Available at: https://www.who.int/publications/i/item/9789241505871. Accessed April 1, 2023.
62. Ministerio de Justicia y del Derecho C. Estudio nacional de sustancias psicoactivas Colombia 2019, Available at: https://www.unodc.org/documents/colombia/2013/septiembre/Estudio_Nacional_Consumo_1996.pdf. Accessed April 1, 2023.
63. Sóñora G, Reynales-Shigematsu LM, Barnoya J, et al. Achievements, challenges, priorities and needs to address the current tobacco epidemic in Latin America. Tob Control 2022;31(2):138–41.
64. Aberle DR, Adams AM, Berg CD, et al. Reduced lung-cancer mortality with low-dose computed tomographic screening. N Engl J Med 2011;365(5):395–409.
65. de Koning HJ, van der Aalst CM, de Jong PA, et al. Reduced Lung-Cancer Mortality with Volume CT Screening in a Randomized Trial. N Engl J Med 2020;382(6):503–13.
66. Lamot S, Viola L, Benitez S, et al. PP.52 Current status of Lung Cancer Screening in Latin America. J Thorac Oncol 2023;18(3):S29.
67. WHO. Cervical Cancer Elimination Initiative, Available at: https://www.who.int/initiatives/cervical-cancer-elimination-initiative. Accessed March 20, 2023.
68. De Oliveira LH, Janusz CB, Da Costa MT, et al. HPV vaccine introduction in the Americas: a decade of progress and lessons learned. Expert Rev Vaccines 2022;21(11):1569–80.
69. PAHO. 2021 : DTP3 District Coverage - Region of the Americas, Available at: https://ais.paho.org/imm/IM_ADM2_COVERAGE-MAPS-Americas.asp. Accessed March 20, 2023.
70. PAHO. PAHO. Cancer in the Americas. Basic Indicators, 2013, Available at: https://www.paho.org/en/documents/paho-cancer-americas-basic-indicators-2013. Accessed March 20, 2023.
71. Herrero R, González P, Markowitz LE. Present status of human papillomavirus vaccine development and implementation. Lancet Oncol 2015;16(5):e206–16.
72. Murillo R, Herrero R, Sierra MS, et al. Cervical cancer in Central and South America: Burden of disease and status of disease control. Cancer Epidemiol 2016;44(Suppl 1):S121–30.
73. Lauby-Secretan B, Loomis D, Straif K. Breast-Cancer Screening–Viewpoint of the IARC Working Group. N Engl J Med 2015;373(15):1479.
74. Soliman A., Schottenfeld D., Boffetta P, editors. Cancer Epidemiology: Low- and Middle-Income Countries and Special Populations (2013; online edn, Oxford Academic, 1 Feb. 2014), Available at: https://doi.org/10.1093/med/9780199733507.001.0001. Accessed June 9, 2023.

75. Knaul FM, Nigenda G, Lozano R, et al. Breast cancer in Mexico: a pressing priority. Reprod Health Matters 2008;16(32):113–23.
76. Azevedo ESG, Bustamante-Teixeira MT, Aquino EM, et al. [Access to early breast cancer diagnosis in the Brazilian Unified National Health System: an analysis of data from the Health Information System]. Cad Saúde Pública 2014; 30(7):1537–50. Acesso à detecção precoce do câncer de mama no Sistema Único de Saúde: uma análise a partir dos dados do Sistema de Informações em Saúde.
77. Agudelo-Botero M. Niveles, tendencias e impacto de la mortalidad por cáncer de mama en Costa Rica según provincias, 2000-2009. Población y Salud en Mesoamérica 2011;9(1):1–14.
78. de Oliveira EX, Pinheiro RS, Melo EC, et al. [Socioeconomic and geographic constraints to access mammography in Brasil, 2003-2008]. Cien Saude Colet 2011;16(9):3649–64. Condicionantes socioeconômicos e geográficos do acesso à mamografia no Brasil, 2003-2008.
79. Haikel RL Jr, Mauad EC, Silva TB, et al. Mammography-based screening program: preliminary results from a first 2-year round in a Brazilian region using mobile and fixed units. BMC Wom Health 2012;12:32.
80. Rodríguez-Cuevas S, Guisa-Hohenstein F, Labastida-Almendaro S. First breast cancer mammography screening program in Mexico: initial results 2005-2006. Breast J 2009;15(6):623–31.
81. Di Sibio A, Abriata G, Forman D, et al. Female breast cancer in Central and South America. Cancer Epidemiol 2016;44(Suppl 1):S110–20.
82. Cazap E. Breast cancer in Latin America: a map of the disease in the region, 38. American Society of Clinical Oncology Educational Book; 2018. p. 451–6.
83. PAHO. Breast cancer: Country Profiles, Available at: https://www.paho.org/en/topics/breast-cancer. Accessed April 1, 2023.
84. Ilic D, Djulbegovic M, Jung JH, et al. Prostate cancer screening with prostate-specific antigen (PSA) test: a systematic review and meta-analysis. Bmj 2018; 362:k3519.
85. Pow-Sang M, Destefano V, Astigueta JC, et al. Prostate cancer in Latin America. Actas Urol Esp 2009;33(10):1057–61.
86. Gomez-Guerra LS, Martinez-Fierro ML, Alcantara-Aragon V, et al. Population based prostate cancer screening in north Mexico reveals a high prevalence of aggressive tumors in detected cases. BMC Cancer 2009;9:91.
87. Knaul FM, Farmer PE, Krakauer EL, et al. Alleviating the access abyss in palliative care and pain relief-an imperative of universal health coverage: the Lancet Commission report. Lancet 2018;391(10128):1391–454.
88. United Nations Office on Drugs and Crime. World Drug Report 2022, 2022. Available at: https://www.unodc.org/unodc/en/data-and-analysis/world-drug-report-2022.html. Accessed December 14, 2022.
89. Assis MR, Marx AG, Magna LA, et al. Late morbidity in upper limb function and quality of life in women after breast cancer surgery. Braz J Phys Ther 2013; 17(3):236–43.
90. Franceschini J, Jardim JR, Fernandes AL, et al. Relationship between the magnitude of symptoms and the quality of life: a cluster analysis of lung cancer patients in Brazil. J Bras Pneumol 2013;39(1):23–31.
91. Pracucho EM, Lopes LR, Zanatto RM, et al. Profile of patients with gastrointestinal stromal tumors (GIST). Arq Bras Cir Dig 2015;28(2):124–7.

92. Hannon B, Zimmermann C, Knaul FM, et al. Provision of Palliative Care in Low-and Middle-Income Countries: Overcoming Obstacles for Effective Treatment Delivery. J Clin Oncol 2016;34(1):62–8.
93. Uribe C, Amado A, Rueda AM, et al. Barriers to access to palliative care services perceived by gastric cancer patients, their caregivers and physicians in Santander, Colombia. Cien Saude Colet 2019;24(5):1597–607.
94. Hawley P. Barriers to Access to Palliative Care. Palliat Care 2017;10. 1178224216688887.
95. Pastrana T, De Lima L, Stoltenberg M, et al. Palliative Medicine Specialization in Latin America: A Comparative Analysis. J Pain Symptom Manage 2021;62(5): 960–7.
96. Paz Silvia. Palliative Care in Argentina: Barriers, Opportunities and Recommendations for Future Developments. Prog Palliat Care 2004;12(6). https://doi.org/10.1179/096992604225007018.
97. Cleary J, De Lima L, Eisenchlas J, et al. Formulary availability and regulatory barriers to accessibility of opioids for cancer pain in Latin America and the Caribbean: a report from the Global Opioid Policy Initiative (GOPI). Ann Oncol 2013;24(Suppl 11):xi41–50.
98. Pastrana T, De Lima L, Knaul F, et al. How Universal Is Palliative Care in Colombia? A Health Policy and Systems Analysis. J Pain Symptom Manage 2022;63(1):e124–33.
99. Anderson KO. Assessment tools for the evaluation of pain in the oncology patient. Curr Pain Headache Rep 2007;11(4):259–64.
100. Cluxton C. The Challenge of Cancer Pain Assessment. Ulster Med J 2019; 88(1):43–6.
101. Santos LCS MA, Neto João Paulo R, Stefani Stephen D. Access to pain management for cancer patients treated under the Brazilian private healthcare system. J Bras Econ Saúde 2019;11(3). https://doi.org/10.21115/JBES.v11.n3.p255-62.
102. Lara-Solares A, Ahumada Olea M, Basantes Pinos ALA, et al. Latin-American guidelines for cancer pain management. Pain Manag 2017;7(4):287–98.
103. Graczyk M, Borkowska A, Krajnik M. Why patients are afraid of opioid analgesics: a study on opioid perception in patients with chronic pain. Pol Arch Intern Med 2018;128(2):89–97.
104. Clelland D, van Steijn D, Whitelaw S, et al. Palliative Care in Public Policy: Results from a Global Survey. Palliat Med Rep 2020;1(1):183–90.
105. Worldwide Hospice Palliative Care Alliance. Global Atlas of Palliative Care, 2022. Available at: http://www.thewhpca.org/resources/global-atlas-on-end-of-life-care. Accessed December 14, 2022.

Fighting Cancer in Ukraine at Times of War

Erza Selmani, MSc[a,b], Ilir Hoxha, MD, PhD[a,b,c,*], Orest Tril, MD[d,1],
Olga Khan, MD[e], Andriy Hrynkiv, MD[f], Leticia Nogueira, PhD, MPH[g],
Doug Pyle, MBA[h], Mary Chamberlin, MD[c]

KEYWORDS

- Cancer • Treatment • Ukraine • War • Support

KEY POINTS

- Cancer management in low- and middle-income countries is challenging at baseline due to unreliable resources and inequitable access.
- Conflict from military aggressions makes this even more difficult and critical for international humanitarian interventions.
- The after war can potentially have an impact on tobacco consumption increase and unhealthy lifestyles further increasing the risk of disease and malignancy in a vulnerable population.

INTRODUCTION

This article discusses the ongoing war situation in Ukraine and its impact in the health care system highlighting the view from the ground, from the providers remaining in Ukraine. Since February 2022, the war has been damaging and disrupting lives without resolution in sight. Previously known as one of the highest functioning health care systems in the region, the war now has led the Ukrainian health care system to a scarcity of staff and medication, disrupting medical supply chains and health services. The current conditions have not only put a massive strain on the health care system but also have increased the risk of spreading infectious disease and caused major

[a] Evidence Synthesis Group, Ali Vitia Street PN, Prishtina 10000, Kosovo; [b] Heimerer College, Veternik, Prishtina 10000, Kosovo; [c] Geisel School of Medicine at Dartmouth, Dartmouth Hitchcock Medical Center, 1 Medical Center Drive, Lebanon, NH 03756, USA; [d] Regional Oncology Center for Treatment and Diagnostic, St. Haseka, 2a, Lviv 79058, Ukraine; [e] World Bank Ukraine, 1Dniprovskiy Uzviz, Kyiv 01010, Ukraine; [f] Chemotherapy Department, Lviv Regional Cancer Center of Ukraine, Hasheka 2a Street, Lviv 79058, Ukraine; [g] American Cancer Society, 3380 Chastain Meadows Parkway Northwest Suite 200, Kennesaw, GA 30144, USA; [h] American Society of Clinical Oncology (ASCO), 318 Mill Road #800, Alexandria, VA 22314, USA
[1] Present address: St. Haseka, 2a, 79058.
* Corresponding author. Rruga e Shkupit Veternik PN, Prishtina 10000, Kosovo.
E-mail address: ilir@evidencesynthesisgroup.com

Hematol Oncol Clin N Am 38 (2024) 77–85
https://doi.org/10.1016/j.hoc.2023.06.001
0889-8588/24/© 2023 Elsevier Inc. All rights reserved.

excesses of morbidity and mortality related toNCDs such as cancer, diabetes, and cardiovascular disease. The war aftermath can lead to trauma, increase in tobacco consumption, and poor lifestyle choices.

In response to this crisis, several international organizations have provided humanitarian aid and medical supplies to Ukraine, and the Ukrainian government has attempted to import essential medical supplies to ease the situation. Despite the challenges, the country's specialized oncological institutions have shown resilience, and efforts have been made to involve internally displaced persons in cancer screening.

The War in Ukraine

The tension between Russia and Ukraine dates from the early 1990s when Ukraine proclaimed independence from Russia after the fallout of the Soviet Union. Despite corruption scandals, economic mismanagement, and intensifying Russian interference, Ukraine achieved the second-largest economy and population of the 15 Soviet Republics. Conflict began in 2014 with the Russian annexation of Crimea and by the spring of 2021 Russia began locating building up armed troops near Ukraine's borders in Belarus as a training exercise, only to attack Ukraine in late February 2022.[1] This war situation has been damaging and disrupting lives for over a year without resolution in sight.

Prior to the escalation of the conflict into war, Ukraine possessed one of the most robust health care systems in the region, characterized by a relatively high incidence and moderate mortality rates of cancer, along with comparatively higher health expenditures. Based on data provided by the World Health Organization (WHO), Ukraine recorded 169,817 cancer cases and 98,226 deaths in 2018. In contrast, Spain, with a similar population size, reported a considerably higher number of cancer cases (270,363) and deaths (113,584) in the same year.[2,3]

It was predicted at the outset that this conflict will likely result in 9-11 million refugees in the first 6 months [4] creating the first cancer and non-communicable disease humanitarian crisis ever in Ukraine and Europe.

The primary contributing factor behind this stems from the inherent vulnerability of displaced people to non-communicable disease due to limited access to health care, a range of psycho-social and environmental factors affecting their lifestyle behaviors and unhealthy diets.[4]

While others have reported on baseline strategy analysis focusing on the primary receiving countries and their capacity for cancer care,[5] we will be focusing on the view from the ground, from the cancer care providers remaining in Ukraine.

A scarcity of staff and medication typically characterize health and care services in war times, for example the ongoing wars in Afghanistan and Yemen has resulted in a shortage of health services and health care professionals.[6,7] During the Covid-19 pandemic this situation has been further exacerbated leaving Yemen with only 10 doctors per 10,000 patients.[8] Eventually, this causes a complete breakdown with severe consequences for the state of health of the overall population. The lack of access to health care and infrastructure damage to the water and sanitation systems increases the risk of spreading infectious diseases. In South Sudan, the underfunding of the health care system due to the civil war has caused a shortage of basic health services and high burden of infectious diseases such as malaria, pneumonia, and diarrhea.[7,9] On the other hand, the disruption of medical supply chains and health care services can increase mortality and excess illness related to non-communicable diseases such as cancer, diabetes, and cardiovascular disease.

If pre-conflict Ukraine was already managing 13,105 patients with cancer per month,[10] management of delayed presentations, disruption of care as refugees and destroyed infrastructure will inevitably cause major excesses of morbidity and mortality. In 2022, WHO marked COVID-19, measles, infectious diseases, cardiovascular diseases, COPDs, diabetes, and mental health as the key health risks that could result in excess mortality and morbidity in the first three months of the crisis escalation.[11] Being in a war tremendously impacts the general unaffected population's mental status and the aftermath trauma that follows. Kosovo, a nation recovering from the aftermath of armed conflict, exhibits a prevalence of depression ranging from 30% to 60%, surpassing the global range. This is accompanied by a relatively low life expectancy and a heightened incidence of non-communicable diseases (NCDs).[12]

Cancer Situation Pre-war

Ukrainian citizens at baseline have had a government -sponsored universal health care system since 2017, entitling all Ukranians to health care with the option of buying private health insurance. Expensive cancer drugs such as immune-oncology are paid out-of-pocket, and the private sector of health care is quite small compared to other Eastern European countries. In terms of health system capacity, in 2019 and 2020, Ukraine had around 5.4 external beam radiography 24.7 mammographs, 22.3 CT-scanners, 8.9 MRI scanners, and 0.2 PET scanners, PET/CT in every 10,000 patients. At the same time, Ukraine marked 5.8 medical physicists and 396.4 radiologists, while there is no data available regarding the number of radiation oncologists, surgeons, nuclear medicine physicists, and medical and pathology lab scientists.[2]

In Ukraine, there are close to 170,000 new patients with cancer each year. One of the most common cancers in women is breast cancer with 11.2% and a death rate of 8.4%.[2] Even though there was no war in 2016, Ukraine marked around 170,000 premature deaths from NCDs.[2] In 2020, around 84,000 patients with cancer died.[13] Ninety percent of the Ukrainian refugees are women due to the mandate of requiring men aged 18-60 to stay in the country, so the burden of breast and cervical cancers, leading cause of death among women between the age of 18 – 29, falls disproportionately on the refugee health care systems. The absence of the National Screening Program in Ukraine already puts women at risk of late presentations of cervical cancer and high mortality. The highest rate of cancer-related infant deaths is also reported to occur in Ukraine.[13] Brain tumors and leukemia are the most often occurring of oncological diseases with a fatal outcome among children under the age of 17.[a]

Given this circumstance, it is clear that there is a sizable need for cancer care and treatment among Ukrainians, which is an essential consideration for developments in cancer care during wartime.

The Impact of War on Patients with Cancer and the Challenges

Armed conflicts and war attacks have severely affected cancer treatment in the country. More than 5 million people fled the country because of security reasons.[b] Delays in treatment, a shortage of medical supplies, improper therapy administration, and postponed surgeries have all been brought on by infrastructure damage, power outages, and disrupted supply chains across the whole country. As a result, many patients with cancer have started leaving the country in search of safety and the ability to continue receiving treatment [13] in Poland, Italy, Romania,[14] and other neighboring countries. Of course, their challenges did not end once they left the country. The capacity of the

---

[a] Bulletin of the National Cancer Registry of Ukraine, Vol. 23 http://www.ncru.inf.ua/publications/BULL_23/PDF_E/07-stru_sm.pdf.

[b] https://data.unhcr.org/en/dataviz/107.

refugee health care systems to cope with the influx of patients with breast cancer and their knowledge about it presents a significant challenge due to several factors which are also very similar to displaced people from other countries facing conflicts.[15] For instance, those who flew to Italy[13] could not receive any cancer treatment without being vaccinated for COVID-19 first because only one-third of the total Ukrainian population was already vaccinated.[14] Second, there were language barriers in communication and medical records i.e., their medical histories were fragmented and written in the Cyrillic alphabet. Needless to say, their psychological state and cultural and language challenges also impeded their access to health care.[13] The challenges were more pronounced for patients with more advanced cancers due to their need to have access to cross-cutting technology and highly advanced health care services. However, it was not any easier for patients with limited financial resources, patients without a support system (family and friends), and for patients with limited knowledge of health care systems.

This situation has not only impacted the health care system in Ukraine, but it has extended beyond its borders, putting a strain on the health care systems of the countries Ukrainians flew to, considering the medical costs and medical staff misbalance.[14]

The ability to receive chemotherapy drugs, which are purchased on a centralized basis from the state budget, is severely limited by the war. Many warehouses with pharmaceutical products in the center of the country were under threat of destruction. The challenges faced by state-funded chemotherapy programs pre-war such as limited funding, lack of medications, outdated infrastructure, and lack of skilled health care workers were exacerbated once the war started, when access to targeted drugs and immunotherapy decreased, and massive migration within the country further complicated receipt of timely cancer diagnosis and treatment. In the face of competing priorities, internally displaced individuals understandably prioritized safety and shelter while cancer screening or full diagnostics of early forms of cancer was not a priority at that stage.

Looking at previous countries facing ongoing conflict, it can be predicted that after more than a year of conflict in Ukraine, individuals are now being diagnosed with cancer at later stages, which require more complex and more expensive types of antitumor treatment in conditions of limited resources.[16–18]

However, we have to admit the resilience of the system in most specialized oncological institutions in Ukraine, the level of provision of high-quality special care quickly recovered in the center and in areas close to a war zone. According to WHO, there are significant improvements in the overall accessibility to medicines, while at the same time barriers such as the access to health services are decreased. Nevertheless, for patients with chronic diseases there are still challenges with the cost of medicines, cost of treatment, transport, and services unavailable. Notably, the price of some medicines increased but patients could not afford even the original prices. This report from WHO also states that a high percentage of respondents from their study, seek self-treatment instead of going to the GP either because they had knowledge about the condition or due to high costs. The latter is particularly pertinent to the displaced individuals.[19]

There is the capacity for treatment because in pre-war times Ukraine built 8 screening centers in the Lviv region with the support of the World Bank in 2017-2019, purchased modern mammography and radiological equipment for screening and treatment of breast cancer and cervical cancer. There is difficulty in involving internally displaced persons in screening mainly because of the inconsistency of their places of stay, change of care providers, lack of information and patient road maps, and low awareness regarding screening.

There are several other effects that follow the war aftermath. For instance, the war experience significantly impacts soldiers' lifestyles after the war as they tend to develop coping mechanisms associated with detrimental health consequences which can also add to the increase in the prevalence of cancer in the following years. The mental trauma burden experienced during times of conflict disproportionately affects women across multiple domains, encompassing financial implications, caregiving responsibilities, gender-based violence, stigma surrounding mental health help-seeking behaviors, and implications for reproductive health.

This situation has undoubtedly impacted global cancer research, as Ukraine is an important site for many cancer trials.[20]

Country and International Response to New Circumstances for Patients with Cancer

In a limited state capacity, several humanitarian organizations provide essential services such as water and sanitation, and their focus is on transmissible rather than non-communicable disease care, i.e., cancer care. However, several important efforts have been made to address current developments and repercussions in patients with cancer. The rapid mobilization of the UN, WHO, professional societies and the ECO/ASCO Special Network: Impact of the War in Ukraine on Cancer has meant that many patients with cancer, especially children are actively being moved into host cancer centers. For those that stay, Ukrainian oncologists are working beyond capacity to aid their patients and their country during this extraordinary crisis due to the Russian invasion.[21] The National Health Service of Ukraine and the Ministry of Health of Ukraine's websites frequently update information on cancer centers.[20] Certain medical centers in western Ukraine are working at their maximum capacity to provide services to all Ukrainians.

The overload of chemotherapy and radiology departments in western Ukraine was 200%, a significant part of services was provided outpatient, since stay in the hospital was dangerous during air strikes. As of November 2022, around 188 facilities were damaged, among this number cancer centers which have been devastated by air attacks. [c] During the first months of war anticipating the possibility of civilian and military casualties, most hospitals limited the implementation of planned surgical interventions, including oncology surgical procedures, which worsened patients with cancer ' access to timely care. However, cardio-oncological services are primarily available through online consultations.[21] Although there has been a disruption in the logistics of the supply of pharmaceuticals and medical items, the Ukrainian government has attempted to make it easier to import essential medical supplies.[22] As a result of Russia's attacks on energy infrastructure, added difficulties in providing care in oncological institutions, due to the lack of electricity supply, which was critically reflected in complex types of examinations such as (X-ray, CT, MRI) and radiological treatment.

Regarding international efforts, humanitarian action has been taken by several organizations, including WHO,[23] UNICEF,[24] World Bank[d], UNFPA[25] and Red Cross.[26] The World Health Organization (WHO) has delivered tons of emergency and medical supplies as well as equipment to Ukraine including medicines that treat NCDs.[27] The International Medical Corps has developed a program to provide services and medical

---

[c] https://uhc.org.ua/.

[d] https://moz.gov.ua/article/news/ponad-6-tisjach-odinic-suchasnogo-obladnannja-zakupleno-moz-ta-sv itovim-bankom-dlja-medzakladiv-ukraini?fbclid=IwAR0mIAB12CYqMlLxOvcEO_nZJcbLe05iQ2s9 nVf99_JGczyo59qml6e2W9I.

supplies of various types for Ukrainian people in Poland, Moldova and Romania.[28] Poland has created a so-called "green corridor" to provide services for women with gynecologic cancer.[22] Other international cancer organizations have formed collaborations to respond to the crisis. The American Cancer Society (ACS) created with the help of the American Society of Clinical Oncology (ASCO) an international call center to connect medical professionals in Ukraine and the neighboring countries to volunteer oncologists and translators, along with providing translated materials for Ukrainian patients with cancer. ASCO also joined with the European Cancer Organization, which represents European professional and patient organizations, to form a "Special Network" of over a hundred cancer organizations from multiple countries and disciplines to coordinate the cancer community's response to the war in Ukraine. The Network has been linking efforts by patient advocate organizations and NGOs with broader efforts by the World Health Organization and the European Commission, tracking data on care access and resources for Ukrainian patients, and has hosted webinars to share information about the state of cancer care delivery in Ukraine and the border countries. Most recently, the ECO-ASCO Network is working to address the ongoing cancer medicine shortages in Ukraine and considering a network of regional cancer centers to better coordinate information gathering and provision of assistance (Personal communication with Doug Pyle and Julie Gralow, MD of ASCO International, 2023).

What Are the Needs and Recommendations for the Future?

The health care system in Ukraine requires long-term dedication to ongoing support. Including cancer prevention and treatment education in the humanitarian response could be done immediately. Wide support by the state and international organizations of educational programs and the adoption of an operational screening program for the duration of hostilities could facilitate earlier detection of cancer among target populations, which would reduce the cost of early cancer treatment.

Telemedicine should be utilized to its full potential to help patients with cancer manage their treatments and provide health education across the broad population.

Addressing the social determinants of mental health is imperative to treat post-war trauma. This includes addressing housing, unemployment, poverty, and education. Focusing on community-based interventions, psychosocial support, trauma-informed care, and therapy is recommended.

A needs-based priority assessment and policies should be put into place first, according to the literature,[29] albeit this calls on data to be available to make data-driven decisions and policy decisions.[30] According to some authors, effective communication between local stakeholders and foreign organizations is crucial to the success of any activity. Other authors suggest that effective communication between local stakeholders and international organizations is essential so that the initiatives taken are fully efficient. Networking between local institutions in Ukraine with medical centers out of Ukraine to treat sensitive and complex patients is advised. It is recommended for some societies, such as the society of breast surgeons, to collaborate and seize every available opportunity. It would also foster a culture of cooperation that might make the post-war health care system stronger.[31,32]

CLINICS CARE POINTS

- Armed conflicts and war attacks have severely affected cancer treatment in Ukraine and surrounding countries.

- The overload of chemotherapy and radiology departments in western Ukraine was 200%.

About 188 facilities were damaged, among this number are cancer centers which have been devastated by air attacks.

- Wide support by the state and international organizations of educational programs and the adoption of an operational screening program for the duration of hostilities could facilitate.

earlier detection of cancer among target populations, which would reduce the cost of early cancer treatment.

DISCLOSURE

All authors have no financial interests to disclose.

REFERENCES

1. War in Ukraine -Global Conflict Tracker. Council on Foreign Relations, 2022. Available at: https://www.cfr.org/global-conflict-tracker/conflict/conflict-ukraine. Accessed July 1, 2023.
2. Cancer Country Profile Ukraine 2020, World Health Organization, 2020. Available at: https://www.who.int/publications/m/item/cancer-ukr-2020. Accessed July 1, 2023.
3. Cancer Country Profile 2020, Spain. World Health Organization, 2020. Available at: https://www.who.int/publications/m/item/cancer-esp-2020. Accessed July 1, 2023.
4. Hidden in plain sight: The increasing burden of noncommunicable diseases among refugees and migrants, World Health Organization, 2023. Available at: https://www.who.int/news-room/events/detail/2023/03/08/default-calendar/hidden-in-plain-sight--the-increasing-burden-of-noncommunicable-diseases-among-refugees-and-migrants#:~:text=The%20increasing%20prevalence%20of%20NCDs,levels%20of%20health%20literacy%20and. Accessed July 1, 2023.
5. Kizub D, Melnitchouk N, Beznosenko A, et al. Resilience and perseverance under siege: providing cancer care during the invasion of Ukraine. Lancet Oncol 2022; 23(5):1474–5488.
6. Van Hemelrijck M, Fox L, Beyer K, et al. Cancer care for ukrainian refugees: strategic impact assessments in the early days of the conflict. Journal of Cancer Policy 2022;34:100370.
7. Narain K, Rackimuthu S, Essar MY, et al. Call for solidarity: the war may be over in Afghanistan but the health crises continue. J Glob Health 2022;12:03002.
8. Alsabri M, Alsakkaf L, Alhadheri A, et al. Chronic health crises and emergency medicine in war-torn yemen, exacerbated by the COVID-19 Pandemic. WestJEM 2022;23(2):276–84.
9. Wakabi W. South Sudan faces grim health and humanitarian situation. Lancet 2011;377(9784):2167–8.
10. WHO. Public health risk assessment and interventions: conflict and humanitarian crisis in South Sudan, 2013. Available at: https://www.humanitarianresponse.info/sites/www.humanitarianresponse.info/files/documents/files/south_sudan_public_health_risk_assessment_10january2014%20%28F%29.pdf. Accessed July 1, 2023
11. Bytyci-Katanolli A, Merten S, Kwiatkowski M, et al. Non-communicable disease prevention in Kosovo: quantitative and qualitative assessment of uptake and

barriers of an intervention for healthier lifestyles in primary healthcare. BMC Health Serv Res 2022;22(1):647.

12. Ratnayake R, Wittcoff A, Majaribu J, et al. Early experiences in the integration of noncommunicable diseases into emergency primary health care, beni region, democratic republic of the congo. Annals of Global Health 2021;87(1):27.

13. Cavallo Jo., *The Impact of War on Patients with Cancer. The ASCO Post*, 2022. Available at: https://ascopost.com/issues/may-25-2022/the-impact-of-war-on-patients-with-cancer/. Accessed July 1, 2023.

14. Tolia M, Kamposioras K, Symvoulakis EK, et al. Cancer patient care during different war times; is the response too slow? ESMO Open 2022;7(4):100–557.

15. Suphanchaimat R, Kantamaturapoj K, Putthasri W, et al. Challenges in the provision of healthcare services for migrants: a systematic review through providers' lens. BMC Health Serv Res 2015;15(1):390.

16. Massimino M, Casiraghi G, Armiraglio M, et al. Caring for children with cancer evacuated from Ukraine. The Lancet Child& Adolescent Health 2022;6(6):365–6.

17. El Saghir NS, Soto Pérez De Celis E, Fares JE, et al. Cancer care for refugees and displaced populations: middle east conflicts and global natural disasters. American Society of Clinical Oncology Educational Book 2018;(38):433–40.

18. Ongoing humanitarian crisis in Ukraine. Lancet Haematol 2022;9(5). https://doi.org/10.1016/S2352-3026(22)00109-0.

19. World report on the health of refugees and migrants, World Health Organization, 2022. Available at: https://www.who.int/publications/i/item/9789240054462www.who.int. Accessed July 1, 2023.

20. Health needs assessment of the adult population in Ukraine, World Health Organziation, 2022. Available at: https://www.who.int/europe/publications/i/item/WHO-EURO-2023-6904-46670-67870www.who.int. Accessed July 1, 2023.

21. American Assocation for Cancer Research, War in Ukraine Disrupts Trials, Cancer Care. Cancer Discovery 2022;12(5):1178–1178. https://doi.org/10.1158/2159-8290.cd-nd2022-0004.

22. Kovalchuk N, Beznosenko A, Kowalchuk R, et al. While Ukrainian soldiers are fearlessly defending their country, ukrainian oncologists are bravely battling cancer. Advances Rad Onc 2022;7(6):100–965.

23. Shushkevich A. Inside the war: life in Ukraine. Int J Gynecol Cancer 2022;32(5):686–7.

24. After Six Months of War, Ukraine's Life-Saving Health System Prepares for a Challenging Winter Ahead, *World Health Organization*, 2022. Available at: https://www.who.int/europe/news/item/24-08-2022-after-six-months-of-war–ukraine-s-life-saving-health-system-prepares-for-a-challenging-winter-ahead.   Accessed July 1, 2023.

25. Unicef, Stop attacks on health care in Ukraine,2022. Available at: https://www.unicef.org/press-releases/stop-attacks-health-care-ukraine. Accessed July 1, 2023.

26. Zubchenko A., Denmark contributes $3.6 million to protect women and girls' health and rights in Ukraine and Moldova, *Ukraineunorg*, 2022. Available at: https://ukraine.un.org/en/198966-denmark-contributes-36-million-protect-women-and-girls-health-and-rights-ukraine-and-moldova.   Accessed July 1, 2023.

27. IFRC. Preventing a second crisis: health needs extend beyond Ukraine's borders warns IFRC 2022. https://www.ifrc.org/press-release/preventing-second-crisis-health-needs-extend-beyond-ukraine%E2%80%99s-borders-warns-ifrc.   Accessed July 1,2023.

28. Walker L., WHO: Ukraine has received 216 tonnes of emergency and medical supplies, *The Brussels Times*, 2022. Available at: https://www.brusselstimes.com/216541/who-ukraine-has-received-216-tonnes-of-emergency-and-medical-supplies. Accessed July 1, 2023.
29. "War in Ukraine." International Medical Corps, 2023. Available at: https://internationalmedicalcorps.org/emergency-response/war-in-ukraine/. Accessed July 1, 2023.
30. Saab R, Slama S, Mansour A, et al. Cancer care in humanitarian crises n.d. CANCER CONTROL EASTERN MEDITERRANEAN REGION. SPECIAL REPORT 2022;68–71.
31. Sayed RE, Abdul-Sater Z, Mukherji D. Cancer care during war and conflict. Cancer in the Arab World 2022;461–76.
32. Unukovych D. Surgical services during the war in Ukraine: challenges and call for help. Br J Surg 2022;109(9):785–6.

Impact of Prostate Cancer in Eastern Europe and Approaches to Treatment and Policy

Riaz Agahi, PhD[a,b], Fahredin Veselaj, MD, PhD[c,*],
Dafina Ademi Islami, MD[d], Erza Selmani, MSc[b,e], Olga Khan, MS[f],
Ilir Hoxha, MD, PhD[b,g]

KEYWORDS

- Prostate cancer • Eastern Europe

KEY POINTS

- Incidence and mortality rates for prostate cancer are higher in Eastern Europe compared with Western Europe and in some countries, are increasing.
- Screening programs have given mixed results but have been applied in some countries with success.
- Treatment of cancer is hampered by a lack of funds and consequently resources, such as medicines, specialists, and diagnostic or therapeutic equipment.
- Implementation of cancer control plans is in process, and some key areas are health promotion, mitigation of risk factors, and improvement of radiotherapy resources.

INTRODUCTION

The prevalence of cancer continues to rise, with a reported 23.6 million new cases worldwide in 2019 alone.[1] In Central and Eastern Europe, prostate cancer composed 8.5% of total new cases in 2020.[2] Incidence rates are not, however, uniform, and there is variation between countries within the region.[3] Mortality rates for prostate cancer have generally decreased globally,[4] but Eastern European mortality rates remain

[a] Department of Diagnostic Health Sciences, Heimerer College, Prishtina 10000, Kosovo; [b] Evidence Synthesis Group, Ali Vitia Street PN, Prishtina 10000, Kosovo; [c] Faculty of Medicine, Department of Surgery, University of Prishtina, Prishtina 10000, Kosovo; [d] Oncology Clinic, University Clinical Center of Kosovo, Prishtina 10000, Kosovo; [e] Research Unit, Heimerer College, Prishtina, Kosovo; [f] World Bank Ukraine, Kyiv 01010, Ukraine; [g] The Dartmouth Institute for Health Policy and Clinical Practice, Geisel School of Medicine at Dartmouth, Lebanon, NH 03766, USA
* Corresponding author.
E-mail address: fahredin.veselaj@uni-pr.edu

Hematol Oncol Clin N Am 38 (2024) 87–103
https://doi.org/10.1016/j.hoc.2023.06.007
0889-8588/24/© 2023 Elsevier Inc. All rights reserved.

high and are in some countries, increasing.[5,6] Elsewhere, 5-year survival rates as high as 97% have been reported for localized prostate cancer,[7] suggesting that tackling underlying health determinants and augmenting funding and resources for treatment can dramatically reduce mortality in Eastern Europe.

Screening with prostate-specific antigen (PSA) testing has led to a higher observed incidence of prostate cancer as a result of the detection of early or asymptomatic cases. It is worth noting, however, that even in countries without systematic screening programs, such as Estonia or Slovenia, the incidence has increased, and there are still countries where both incidence and mortality have increased. A global study of prostate cancer incidence and mortality data between 2000 and 2019 found an increased incidence in all Eastern European countries included and increased mortality in 14 out of 17 included countries.[4]

Differences in incidence and mortality have been observed between Eastern and Western Europe. Santucci and coworkers identified a steady decline in mortality in Western Europe since 1990, and prostate cancer incidences have increased to 12.7/100,000 (2016) in Eastern Europe.[8] In North Macedonia, for example, life expectancy has increased, but mortality from some conditions, including prostate cancer, has increased.[2] Interregional variation in lifestyle factors may contribute to the mortality gap, but accessibility and quality of care may also be influential.[9]

This review examines prostate cancer in Eastern Europe and includes epidemiology, health system context, diagnosis, and management. Attention will also be given to approaches to improving outcomes in the future. Eastern Europe is considered here to include the following countries: Albania, Belarus, Bosnia and Herzegovina, Bulgaria, Croatia, Czechia, Estonia, Hungary, Kosovo, Latvia, Lithuania, Moldova, Montenegro, North Macedonia, Poland, Romania, Russia, Serbia, Slovakia, Slovenia, and Ukraine.

EPIDEMIOLOGY

Studies and health data published in different sources clearly establish a higher incidence and mortality for prostate cancer in Eastern Europe compared with Western Europe and variability within the region. It consistently ranks as one of the most prevalent forms of cancer across the whole population. Globally, it is the second most common cancer, and it is the most common in Eastern European Baltic states.[10] In Bosnia, to give another example, prostate cancer accounts for 6.1% of new cases (2020) and 4.7% of deaths across both genders.[2] In comparison with the average value for Europe from GLOBOCON 2020 data, most countries in the region have a higher incidence rate (**Fig. 1A**). Albania, Moldova, Romania, and Ukraine all have an incidence below 63.4 per 100,000 population, which is the overall incidence in Europe. Most of the countries have higher mortality than the European total (11.1 deaths per 100,000 population, **Fig. 1B**). Of the countries included, only Albania, Czechia, and Romania have lower prostate cancer mortality than the European total. Between 2000 and 2019, mortality only decreased in Czechia, Poland, and Romania. All Eastern European countries examined showed increasing incidence rates.[4] This may partially reflect increased early diagnosis and partially result from other factors such as variation in patient risk factors and differences in the availability of resources for treatment.[11]

HEALTH SYSTEMS

Prostate cancer prevention and improved treatment can be primarily addressed through health system-related measures, including access to better treatment, reduction in waiting times, standardized guidelines, and adoption of new therapies. All of these measures, while they may improve efficiency in the long term, require short

A

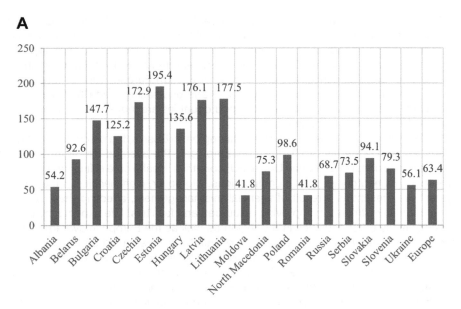

B

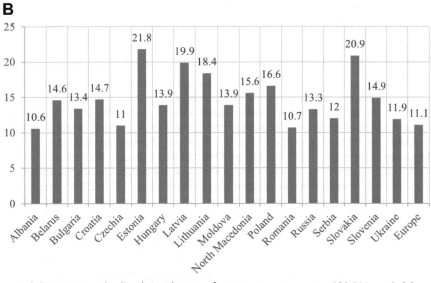

Fig. 1. (*A*) Aage-standardized incidence of prostate cancer per 100,000 and (*B*) age-standardized mortality of prostate cancer per 100,000.

term and sustained financial input. A comparison of health expenditures per capita shows that Eastern European countries generally have lower amounts per person compared with Western Europe while also having increased cancer mortality-to-incidence ratios.[12] For example, Western European gross domestic product (GDP) per capita invested in health has been reported to vary between 7.9% in Luxembourg and 12.0% in the Netherlands; whereas in Eastern Europe lower values have been reported, between 5.6% in Slovenia and 9.3% in Bulgaria.[13]

An inverse correlation between the human development index score for a country and prostate cancer mortality has been observed, as well as the opposite effect for incidence.[4] Economic factors show a considerable association with health outcomes in this case. A study by Zhang, using the Global Burden of Disease data, examined factors at the country level which seem to be influential in incidence, mortality, and disability-adjusted life years (DALYs). The study reported a global decrease in these variables for prostate cancer but an increase in Eastern Europe. Furthermore, there was a correlation between the country's GDP and decreasing mortality.[14] These results imply that more economically developed countries are more able to mobilize resources for screening and treatment.

Health system structures vary widely in the region. In Bosnia, the percentage of GDP spent on health care (as of 2019) exceeds not only the average for South-Eastern Europe but also that of European Union (EU) countries. Health care is financed primarily through mandatory insurance contributions. Moreover, inefficiencies in the health system are present as a result of financial mismanagement, affecting the provision of care and investments in improving resources and facilities. Life expectancy (76.3) is below many other countries in the region as well as the European average (78.3), and cancer is reportedly the main cause of death for those aged 30 to 64 years.[15] Some countries are covered by a National Health Insurance fund, such as Latvia,[16] Bulgaria,[17] or Lithuania, whereas others have compulsory social insurance schemes. In Lithuania, for example, the share of GDP used for public health financing is 7.0%, which is below the EU average (9.9%), although higher than other countries in the region, such as Bulgaria, Poland, and Hungary. Public spending in Lithuania is also supplemented by 32% of out-of-pocket payments, double the EU average.[18]

PATIENT-LEVEL DETERMINANTS

Health system factors are not the only pertinent issue. A study by Thøgersen compared survival rates between indigenous and migrant populations in Norway.[19] Even when accounting for confounders such as socioeconomic factors, comorbidities, and stage at diagnosis, increased mortality was found for Eastern European and Balkan migrants with prostate cancer. A study by the same authors did not report differences in treatment, such as waiting time between groups in prostate cancer.[20]

As the strongest risk factors for prostate cancer are genetic, understanding family history can help in diagnosis, in addition to genetic testing.[21,22] BRCA2 genetic mutations have been identified as risk factors for prostate cancer development, progression, and mortality. For example, carriers of BRCA2 had a strong association with Gleason scores ≥ 7.[23] Germline BRCA2 genetic mutations have a prevalence of approximately 5% to 6% in the patients with prostate cancer.[23–25] Genetic testing and genetic counseling could provide an avenue to improving personalized care and allowing awareness of increased risks for carriers of the relevant mutations, but there is not yet a consistent framework for their utilization in the region. For example, in Poland, although much progress has been made, the legal framework behind genetic testing is still scattered and the quality of genetic testing is yet to be improved.[26] In Bosnia, genetic testing and counseling services are available; however, they lack accessibility and the quality is concerning.[27] Despite its limitations, the health care system in Macedonia demonstrates a commitment to keeping up with advancements in genetic diagnostics and updating legislation pertaining to genetic examinations and research.[28] In Romania, genetic counseling services are still developing, and genetic counseling has not yet gained recognition as a distinct health care profession.[29]

Pollution is also a significant risk factor for a plethora of diseases, including prostate cancer. Levels of pollution are high throughout Eastern Europe.[30] For example, nitrogen oxides (NO_x) and particulate matter (PM) 2.5 pollution are associated with an increased prostate cancer risk.[31] Some of the highest levels of air pollution are in European cities,[32] driven by coal and wood-based power.[33] Policies that aim for cleaner air, water, and soil can help alleviate the burden of prostate cancer.[34]

Although the average age at diagnosis may decline as a result of efforts for early detection, prostate cancer still primarily affects older men.[7] The age profile in several Eastern European countries[35-37] underlines the future potential for increased incidence as the population starts to age. Although this cannot be modified, effort should be made to allocate resources accordingly to ensure a good infrastructure for managing cancer. However, it is worth noting that there is an increasing and worrying trend of prostate cancer diagnoses in younger age groups.[34]

Similar to other cancers, various lifestyle and underlying health effects are associated with the risk of developing prostate cancer, severity, and mortality. Some factors include body mass index (BMI) over 33 kg/m^2, lack of physical activity, diets rich in dairy, calcium, fat or red meat, and smoking. Conversely, diets that were rich in antioxidants had positive effects, both in terms of the risk of developing prostate cancer and in disease progression.[38,39] In the case of smoking,[40] in recent years, there has been a sharp decrease in smoking prevalence in Western or Northern European countries, but only minor decreases in Eastern European countries.[41]

SCREENING AND DIAGNOSIS

The most common method used for screening, or secondary prevention, is PSA testing, often in conjunction with digital rectal examination and confirmed with a biopsy.[42] Systematic screening programs for prostate cancer have been widely implemented, and this is generally associated with an increase in incidence and a decrease in mortality.[4] Screening programs can be considered a double-edged sword. The benefits of early diagnosis are limited by overdiagnosis and overtreatment.[43] It has also been reported that survival times can be artificially inflated by high levels of PSA testing, and thus mortality benefits should be viewed with caution.[44] It has been reported that such screening programs were not associated with any benefit in terms of mortality rate,[45] however, a 16-year follow-up study in Europe found a rate ratio of 0.80 (95%CI 0.72–0.89) for mortality for those who participated in screening.[46]

The implementation of PSA screening varies between countries. In the Baltic states, there has been a difference in approaches and implementation. In Estonia, for example, a government policy has not been adopted, but levels of testing have nevertheless increased. In 2000, 90% of men aged 16 to 64 reported never having been tested, whereas in 2016, this figure was just 50%. In Estonia, testing is determined clinically based on risk factors such as age and in cases of patient request.[47] In Russia, testing has been included in the national health check-up program since 2013.[48] Lithuania introduced systematic screening by PSA testing in 2006. The efficacy of this approach was questionable. For example, survival times may have been artificially inflated by earlier diagnosis rather than increased by improved treatment outcomes.[49] A study of screening data reported that less than 30% of those tested had sufficient life expectancy to benefit from the diagnosis and suggested prescreening by life expectancy to reduce unnecessary treatment and related harms to patients.[50]

A study of Lithuania's PSA screening program showed, as may be expected, an increase in incidence, followed by a decrease, and progressive rises in the incidence of localized cancer, followed by metastasized and distant cancers. In all cases, these incidence increases were followed by decreases. This seems to signal an effective screening program.[51] A study of men tested for prostate cancer by PSA in Kosice, Slovakia, highlights the benefits of PSA testing for early diagnosis but also underlines the possibility of novel biomarkers with higher sensitivity. Screening of 3943 male patients identified 109 low-risk patients, 57 medium-risk patients, and 24 high-risk patients.[52]

Screening programs should avoid opportunistic screening,[44] that is, non-systematic or population-based screening which is offered as a supplementary measure in medical examinations. Although this may seem to be of potential benefit in avoiding overdiagnosis, the opposite has been observed.[53] Indiscriminate testing of asymptomatic men should also be avoided. A rationally developed, well-implemented, and rigorously monitored approach is needed.[52,54] The implementation of systematic screening programs is patchy and controversial and is hampered by a lack of definitive consensus over the benefits of screening. For example, in Croatia's plan for 2020 to 2030, screening for prostate cancer was not considered a priority program to implement, but the possibility was explored within a framework of cost-effectiveness, where a value of €19,000 per quality-adjusted life-year (QALY) was cited.[55]

Most promising seems to be a risk-adapted approach which is focused on screening in higher risk men. Guidelines prepared by the European Association of Urology (EAU) in collaboration with the European Association of Nuclear Medicine (EANM), the European Society for Radiotherapy and Oncology (ESTRO), the European Society of Urogenital Radiology (ESUR), and the International Society of Geriatric Oncology (SIOG) recommend screening in men above 50 years old and younger men with BRCA genetic mutations. It was also recommended that men with less than 15 years of life expectancy not be screened due to minimal potential benefits to diagnosis.[43] Such measures should be taken in consultation between the clinician and patient regarding the potential risks and benefits of such a procedure. The use of biopsy for the stratification of patients into high-, intermediate-, or low-risk cases is needed to identify the correct course of treatment.[11] Less invasive liquid biopsies can also be used for this purpose.[34,56]

In addition to screening using PSA or a combination of PSA and digital rectal examinations, novel biomarkers can also be used.[57,58] Techniques such as The Decipher Prostate Genomic Classifier can provide information that determines the course of treatment, potentially using genetic information to decide between surveillance and intervention.[59] It has been suggested that a more personalized approach may be beneficial, building individualized patient profiles, which can include risk factors, comorbidities, phenotypic data, and other clinical factors.[34]

MANAGEMENT AND TREATMENT

Screening must account for some portion of declining mortality by virtue of earlier diagnosis, but nevertheless, some effect from treatment approaches is likely.[60] Variation in mortality may be explained by differences in management, including the availability of treatment.[61,62] Moreover, there is limited information regarding which management approaches are most preferred in Eastern Europe.

Approaches to treatment should be harmonized with the specific needs of the patient, including the the level of risk. Traditionally, early prostate cancer treatment can be seen as involving three main approaches: watchful waiting/active surveillance, radiotherapy, and radical prostatectomy, including variations within these approaches.[63] These can also be supplemented with pharmacologic reagents. A full examination of treatment options and indications for treatments is beyond the scope of this review. One example of clinical guidelines is those of the Croatian Urology Society.[64] In general, clinical guidelines are needed to provide a standard of care when physician preferences can vary widely.[65]

Watchful waiting or active surveillance can be considered an alternative to surgical procedures or radiotherapy, which can be applied in low-risk cases. This has the obvious benefit of avoiding surgical procedures or radiotherapy. However, Tomašković and coworkers reported that according to the relevant criteria, 38.1% of patients who may qualify for active surveillance displayed negative histopathological markers.[66] This underlines the need for attention from clinicians and policymakers as to the appropriate indications for an approach to prostate cancer management. A study from Serbian researchers compared radical prostatectomy patients with a similarly sized and staged group of patients whose symptoms were monitored. There was improved urinary and sexual function, and no significant improvement observed in quality of life demonstrating the importance of careful shared decision-making discussions between patients and providers, as the data can be confusing and depend on the primary endpoints.[67] For example, a study of health insurance claims in Hungary reported that radical prostatectomy is a beneficial procedure compared with other approaches, both in terms of health system cost and survival after 12 year follow-up.[68]

It is clear that resources are needed for effective treatment. Radiotherapy is widely indicated for prostate cancer and can be especially useful for early prostate cancer in conjunction with hormone therapy.[6] However, the use of radiotherapy is often curtailed by the lack of availability. A study examining the use of radiotherapy throughout the whole of Europe for all cancers showed that less than 1.3 radiotherapy machines per million population in Albania and low availability of machines elsewhere. In Eastern European countries assessed therein, there was a range of quality, with 80% to 90% of resources meeting optimal utilization in Czechia but below 60% in Albania and Estonia.[69] In Serbia, for example, significant delays in the initiation of radiotherapy have been reported, and only 39.3% of patients with prostate cancer were able to initiate therapy within a month of being diagnosed. The Ministry of Health, therefore, acquired new linear accelerators for treatment with the aim of reducing delays by 2022.[70]

Data from the International Cancer Control Partnership, published in 2020,[71] include equipment for external beam radiotherapy, MRI and PET scanners, radiologists and surgeons, and public cancer centers (**Table 1**). There is considerable variability in the density of each resource per 10,000 patients with cancer. For example, six countries have less than one PET scanner for 10,000 patients, meaning that these patients are treated with less accurate information. One example of such issues is in Slovenia. Although not poorly equipped in comparison to other countries in the region (Slovenia has the most MRI scanners per patient of all countries included), this lack of diagnostic equipment was identified as a weakness in health care settings as it falls below the European average.[44] A paucity of equipment can also lead to long waiting times and thus inferior outcomes and quality of life. In comparison with the mortality ratio cited above, it does not seem that any specific resource is necessarily directly related to mortality. As such, although resources and equipment are essential to combating prostate cancer, the provision of extra equipment, staff, or facilities does not, in and of itself, inherently lead to improved outcomes.

Access to drugs is also a potential issue.[63] When there are newly available drugs, a mechanism is needed to ensure they can be available to patients promptly. For examples, a study of newly approved oncological medications throughout Europe found the slowest implementation in Serbia, Slovakia, Poland, Romania, Hungary and Croatia.[72] Even for established, approved medications, there are limitations in access in some countries. One study carried out in Bosnia reported delays in treatment caused by a lack of availability of cancer drugs. Of the six drugs studied, only docetaxel was freely

Table 1
Cancer treatment resources in Eastern Europe

	Amount of Resources per 10,000 Patients with Cancer					
Country	External Beam Radiotherapy	MRI Scanners	PET or PET/CT Scanners	Radiologists	Surgeons	Public Cancer Centers
Albania	6.0	14.5	1.2	36.2	n/a	1.2
Belarus	7.6	10.6	0.7	161.3	1520.1	2.6
Bosnia and Herzegovina	7.0	20.2	1.4	131.4	191.2	16.0
Bulgaria	9.0	15.8	1.7	141.3	1656.1	9.9
Croatia	7.1	18.2	2.0	312.8	828.7	2.0
Czechia	9.3	17.0	2.4	229.2	1289.6	9.3
Estonia	7.8	23.5	3.9	200.9	246.6	2.6
Hungary	5.5	7.9	0.9	n/a	452.6	3.7
Latvia	7.4	11.1	0.0	246.5	866.8	4.1
Lithuania	7.3	21.4	1.2	218.9	1485.5	3.7
Moldova	2.0	7.2	2.0	196.3	368.4	0.7
Montenegro	8.5	21.1	0.0	211.3	n/a	4.2
North Macedonia	5.1	12.8	3.8	294.6	977.3	6.4
Poland	8.0	24.8	1.4	136.1	320.7	2.2
Romania	6.4	21.7	1.4	206.3	1097.2	0.4
Serbia	6.5	12.3	0.4	n/a	n/a	0.8
Slovakia	6.8	17.4	2.7	n/a	342.3	4.1
Slovenia	7.4	25.2	2.2	199.0	631.7	1.5
Ukraine	5.4	8.9	0.2	396.4	n/a	1.6

available, whereas cabazitaxel, abiraterone, and enzalutamide could be obtained if the cost was covered by patient out-of-pocket payments. Ketoconazole and radium-223 were not available at all.[73] Therefore, improvements in the accessibility of medications and insurance coverage are needed to optimize treatment plans. A study comparing the availability of the same medications in multiple countries showed that almost all medications are freely available in almost all Western European countries, whereas availability was lower in Eastern European countries. For example, only one of the six medications was available in Kosovo and Albania, while in some cases, access to medication was only possible by paying the full cost out of pocket.[74] Of these medications, docetaxel and abiraterone and enzalutamide were all included in WHOs list of essential medicines.[75] However, this does not seem to be a guarantee that will safeguard their availability.

To circumvent the challenges associated with newly approved medications, the Health Insurance Institute in Slovenia now includes a board to help introduce medicines newly approved by the European Medicines Agency. Slovenia also aims to offset the costs of medication by the use of generics. A patient who has been prescribed a medication other than the generic version can either use the generic drug or pay the difference out of pocket.[76]

One example of pharmaceutical treatment for prostate cancer is androgen deprivation therapy with gonadotropin-releasing hormone agonists or antagonists. Although associated with significant side effects,[77] studies of physicians in various countries have identified a higher preference for androgen deprivation therapy (ADT) prescription in doctors in Eastern Europe (Czechia, Poland, and Hungary).[78] Although there is a lack of evidence of its benefit,[79] many clinicians prefer continuous ADT in cases where clinical tests such as Gleason score or PSA testing return high values, whereas intermittent ADT seems to be favored as a method to improve patient quality of life.[78] However, funding deficiencies can often impede the use of medications.

THE WAY FORWARD

The question remains of how to improve cancer care in Eastern Europe. The effort is needed not only to reduce inequality in outcomes relative to the standards of Western Europe but to increase the rate of development in an absolute sense. Assuming parity with Western Europe, an estimated 55,000 cancer deaths could have been avoided in Eastern Europe.[8]

Eastern Europeean countries need to adopt a systematic approach to the problem. An illustrative example is the EUs Beating Cancer Plan.[80] A related strategy was recently approved by Romania for implementation between 2023 and 2026.[81] Some of the main areas addressed therein are prevention, early detection, quality of care, and improving quality of life for patients. There is the potential for adapting elements of the "Choosing Wisely" campaign developed in the United States,[82] perhaps in harmony with using the European Society for Medical Oncology (ESMO) guidelines which are applied by many countries in the region, and these guidelines could be considered as a standard of care where national regulations are lacking.[74]

In total, €4 billion has been earmarked for the EU plan. Countries outside of the EU must therefore secure or allocate funding to adopt a systematic approach to reducing the impact of prostate cancer. Allocating funding requires a structured, value-driven approach, envisaging the system as a whole rather than just one aspect, such as drug availability. In some countries, reliance on out-of-pocket payments needs to be reduced by increasing public funding where necessary. Funding can also be given to developing more cost-effective health systems. One example of this is reducing reliance on hospital stays by improving outpatient services.[12]

Tailored approaches are needed to implement a rational and efficient screening process, monitor population prevalence, and allocate the necessary resources for treatment. In setting priorities, evidence-based approaches are needed, and the efficacy of these approaches must be continuously monitored.[83,84]

Reduction of the burden of disease, in the final analysis, does not occur in a vacuum. Instead, the downstream causes need to be addressed. New strategies must be adopted throughout the region. Many countries already have national cancer control programs (NCCPs), and these should be implemented and altered if necessary.[12] It is worth noting that tailored measures to tackle prostate cancer tend to be missing from these programs, which signals a potential shortcoming in such policies in light of the high burden of the disease.[85] Of course, there is a large degree of overlap between cancer risk factors, and for this reason, many cancer prevention programs will affect multiple causes of mortality.

Existing NCCPs aim extensively at health promotion, primary prevention, and improving health literacy.[86] Prevention measures have been identified as one of the highest priorities in reducing cancer inequality.[87] Lifestyle-related determinants were included in planning, such as promoting education on diet and anti-tobacco goals.[88–90] Another example of an approach to tackling underlying determinants of health and risk factors for a variety of NCDs was in Bosnia. A World Health Organization (WHO) project aimed to reduce risk factors in the population, focusing on measures such as steering reform, improving health system functioning, educational initiatives, and tobacco control.[91] In a study of tobacco control measures in 36 European states, 9 of the bottom 14 countries were in Eastern Europe,[92] indicating that countries within the region have considerable work to do in order to promote smoking cessation. Notably, studies have shown that men who had quit smoking over 10 years ago had similar risks to those who had never smoked, suggesting that smoking cessation measures could be effective in lowering the burden of prostate cancer.[39]

Considerable improvements in outcomes are associated with early detection, and treatment where necessary.[93] Additional attention should be given to the implementation of screening programs as a form of secondary prevention.[90] Novel treatment approaches, such as personalized or targeted medicine, should be considered. One example of this is PARP inhibitors in patients with *BRCA1/2*. Such approaches have shown promise in clinical trials, including in patients with castration-resistant prostate cancer.[63]

Attention must also be given to resource allocation. There are frequent new developments in cancer therapy, and it is difficult to plan in advance which therapies will be most effective or recommended for broad usage. There is also a gap between implementation in trials and in clinical settings.[69] In this regard, funding for research is essential. A study by Begum and coworkers mapped research efforts in Central and Eastern Europe and Central Asia.[94] The findings of this study revealed that researchers in Poland were the most prolific of the countries studied. They reported that the most common theme of research was cancer biology discovery and novel therapies, and often research priorities were directed towards EU collaboration rather than national or regional needs. The investigators identified other areas where research was less common, such as screening or radiation oncology. In addition, epidemiologic research, including studies with a socioeconomic focus, could aid in policy and implementation and ensure an affordable and high standard of care. Research that involves patient advocacy groups should be used,[95] and in general, a more patient-centered approach that values quality of life must be adopted.

The importance of regional collaboration cannot be overstated. High-quality registries, including tumor registries and potentially regional or subregional registries, would be invaluable.[94] Regarding the monitoring of prostate cancer within the countries, all countries have a national cancer registry, with the exception of Albania.[96,97] The establishment and consolidation of reliable registries for cancer data is a vital task in observing patterns in morbidity and mortality.[98,99] Thereby, it is also possible to assess the impact of previous interventions and to develop evidence-based approaches and resource allocation. In the process of literature review for this article, there was a lack of consistent information throughout the region on treatment and outcomes.

Another example of the benefits of registry data is in prioritizing patients for new therapies. The establishment of a center for Hadron therapy in South-Eastern Europe is planned for 2029 to 2030, and having accurate data can allow not only the selection of patients for this cutting-edge treatment but sufficient information to develop selection criteria ahead of time.[100]

Cancer care is multidisciplinary and multinational. For this reason, diverse stakeholders should be involved in decision-making and strategy.[95] Furthermore, those working to tackle cancer in Eastern European countries should make the use of existing guidelines regarding case management. Guidelines such as those from EAU-EANM-ESTRO-ESUR-SIOG are helpful resources in this regard, as they are regularly updated and give detailed information on handling-specific indications.[43,101]

SUMMARY

Prostate cancer is among the most prevalent cancers globally and within Eastern Europe, where there are also higher levels of mortality compared with Western Europe. Cancer control plans exist in most countries in the region. Prostate cancer should be identified as a high public health priority for devising and implementing optimal screening initiatives. Our review has identified that a lack of resources and deficiencies in health system function hamper progress in ameliorating the burden of prostate cancer. Regional cooperation is needed as well as drawing on guidelines and findings from elsewhere. Health institutions also need to be aware of the latest developments and set up training for providers and updated health care delivery systems that allow swift adoption.

CLINICS CARE POINTS

- Interregional variation in lifestyle factors as well as accessibility and quality of care may contribute to the mortality gap from prostate cancer in Eastern Europe.
- Prostate cancer prevention and improved treatment can be primarily addressed through health system-related measures, including access to better treatment, reduction in waiting times, standardized guidelines, and adoption of new therapies.
- As the strongest risk factors for prostate cancer are genetic, understanding family history can help in diagnosis, in addition to genetic testing.
- Systematic screening programs for prostate cancer have been widely implemented, and this is generally associated with an increase in incidence and a decrease in mortality. The benefits of early diagnosis are limited by overdiagnosis and overtreatment.
- Clinical guidelines for treatment of prostate cancer are needed to provide a standard of care when physician preferences can vary widely.

DISCLOSURE

No external funding was received for this study. I. Hoxha has stock and other ownership interests at LifestylediagnostiX. No other potential conflicts of interest were reported.

REFERENCES

1. Global Burden of Disease 2019 Cancer Collaboration. Cancer Incidence, Mortality, Years of Life Lost, Years Lived With Disability, and Disability-Adjusted Life Years for 29 Cancer Groups From 2010 to 2019: A Systematic Analysis for the Global Burden of Disease Study 2019. JAMA Oncol 2022;8(3):420–44.
2. Sung H, Ferlay J, Siegel RL, et al. Global Cancer Statistics 2020: GLOBOCAN Estimates of Incidence and Mortality Worldwide for 36 Cancers in 185 Countries. CA Cancer J Clin 2021;71(3):209–49.
3. Vrdoljak E, Wojtukiewicz MZ, Pienkowski T, et al. Cancer epidemiology in Central and South Eastern European countries. Croat Med J 2011;52(4):478–87.
4. Wang L, Lu B, He M, Wang Y, Wang Z, Du L. Prostate Cancer Incidence and Mortality: Global Status and Temporal Trends in 89 Countries From 2000 to 2019. Front Public Health. 2022;10. Available at: https://www.frontiersin.org/articles/10.3389/fpubh.2022.811044. Accessed June 4, 2023.
5. Culp MB, Soerjomataram I, Efstathiou JA, et al. Recent Global Patterns in Prostate Cancer Incidence and Mortality Rates. Eur Urol 2020;77(1):38–52.

6. Trama A, Foschi R, Larrañaga N, et al. Survival of male genital cancers (prostate, testis and penis) in Europe 1999-2007: Results from the EUROCARE-5 study. Eur J Cancer Oxf Engl 1990 2015;51(15):2206–16.

7. Dragomir M, Pizot C, Macacu A, et al. Global burden of prostate cancer: regional disparities in incidence, mortality, and survival. J Health Inequalities 2020;6(1):63–74.

8. Santucci C, Patel L, Malvezzi M, et al. Persisting cancer mortality gap between western and eastern Europe. Eur J Cancer 2022;165:1–12.

9. Jeziorski K. Reducing the cancer mortality gap between Western and Eastern Europe. A long way off. Eur J Cancer 2022;172:96–7.

10. De Silva F, Alcorn J. A Tale of Two Cancers: A Current Concise Overview of Breast and Prostate Cancer. Cancers 2022;14(12):2954.

11. Bray F, Kiemeney LA. Epidemiology of prostate cancer in europe: patterns, trends and determinants. In: Bolla M, van Poppel H, editors. Management of prostate cancer: a multidisciplinary approach. Switzerland: Springer International Publishing; 2017. p. 1–27. https://doi.org/10.1007/978-3-319-42769-0_1.

12. Vrdoljak E, Bodoky G, Jassem J, et al. Cancer Control in Central and Eastern Europe: Current Situation and Recommendations for Improvement. Oncol 2016;21(10):1183–90.

13. Ades F, Senterre C, de Azambuja E, et al. Discrepancies in cancer incidence and mortality and its relationship to health expenditure in the 27 European Union member states. Ann Oncol Off J Eur Soc Med Oncol 2013;24(11):2897–902.

14. Zhang W, Cao G, Wu F, et al. Global Burden of Prostate Cancer and Association with Socioeconomic Status, 1990–2019: A Systematic Analysis from the Global Burden of Disease Study. J Epidemiol Glob Health 2023. https://doi.org/10.1007/s44197-023-00103-6.

15. Health systems in action: Bosnia and Herzegovina | European Observatory on Health Systems and Polices. Available at: https://eurohealthobservatory.who.int/publications/i/health-systems-in-action-bosnia-and-herzegovina-2022. Accessed June 5, 2023.

16. Latvia: health system summary | European Observatory on Health Systems and Policies. Available at: https://eurohealthobservatory.who.int/publications/i/latvia-health-system-summary. Accessed June 5, 2023.

17. Bulgaria: health system summary | European Observatory on Health Systems and Policies. Available at: https://eurohealthobservatory.who.int/publications/i/bulgaria-health-system-summary. Accessed June 5, 2023.

18. Lithuania: Country Health Profile 2021| European Observatory on Health Systems and Policies. Available at: https://eurohealthobservatory.who.int/publications/m/lithuania-country-health-profile-2021. Accessed June 5, 2023.

19. Thøgersen H, Møller B, Robsahm TE, et al. Differences in cancer survival between immigrants in Norway and the host population. Int J Cancer 2018;143(12):3097–105.

20. Thøgersen H, Møller B, Åsli LM, et al. Waiting times and treatment following cancer diagnosis: comparison between immigrants and the Norwegian host population. Acta Oncol Stockh Swed 2020;59(4):376–83.

21. Janavičius R, Rudaitis V, Mickys U, et al. Comprehensive BRCA1 and BRCA2 mutational profile in Lithuania. Cancer Genet 2014;207(5):195–205.

22. Gandaglia G, Leni R, Bray F, et al. Epidemiology and Prevention of Prostate Cancer. Eur Urol Oncol 2021;4(6):877–92.

23. Nyberg T, Frost D, Barrowdale D, et al. Prostate Cancer Risks for Male BRCA1 and BRCA2 Mutation Carriers: A Prospective Cohort Study. Eur Urol 2020;77(1): 24–35.
24. Pritchard CC, Mateo J, Walsh MF, et al. Inherited DNA-Repair Gene Mutations in Men with Metastatic Prostate Cancer. N Engl J Med 2016;375(5):443–53.
25. Oh M, Alkhushaym N, Fallatah S, et al. The association of BRCA1 and BRCA2 mutations with prostate cancer risk, frequency, and mortality: A meta-analysis. Prostate 2019;79(8):880–95.
26. Nguyen-Dumont T, Karpinski P, Sasiadek MM, et al. Genetic testing in Poland and Ukraine: should comprehensive germline testing of BRCA1 and BRCA2 be recommended for women with breast and ovarian cancer? Genet Res 2020;102:e6.
27. AKA Philip C. Genetic counseling and preventive medicine in Bosnia and Herzegovina. Calif West Int Law J 2020;50.
28. Sukarova - Angelovska E, Petlichkovski A. Genetics in Macedonia-Following the international trends. Mol Genet Genomic Med 2018;6(1):9–14.
29. Ciucă A, Moldovan R, Băban A. Developing genetic counselling services in an underdeveloped healthcare setting. J Community Genet 2021;12(4):539–48.
30. Meisner C, Gjorgjev D, Tozija F. Estimating health impacts and economic costs of air pollution in the Republic of Macedonia. South East Eur J Public Health 2023. https://doi.org/10.56801/seejph.vi.63.
31. Youogo LMAK, Parent ME, Hystad P, et al. Ambient air pollution and prostate cancer risk in a population-based Canadian case-control study. Environ Epidemiol 2022;6(4):e219.
32. Europe's air quality status 2023 — European Environment Agency. Available at: https://www.eea.europa.eu/publications/europes-air-quality-status-2023. Accessed June 12, 2023.
33. Jagiełło P, Struzewska J, Jeleniewicz G, et al. Evaluation of the Effectiveness of the National Clean Air Programme in Terms of Health Impacts from Exposure to PM2.5 and NO2 Concentrations in Poland. Int J Environ Res Public Health 2023; 20(1):530.
34. Kucera R, Pecen L, Topolcan O, et al. Prostate cancer management: long-term beliefs, epidemic developments in the early twenty-first century and 3PM dimensional solutions. EPMA J 2020;11(3):399–418.
35. Teoh JYC, Hirai HW, Ho JMW, et al. Global incidence of prostate cancer in developing and developed countries with changing age structures. PLoS One 2019;14(10):e0221775.
36. Ritchie H, Roser M. Age Structure. Our World Data. Published online September 20, 2019. Available at: https://ourworldindata.org/age-structure. Accessed June 4, 2023.
37. Population structure and ageing. Available at: https://ec.europa.eu/eurostat/statistics-explained/index.php?title=Population_structure_and_ageing. Accessed June 4, 2023.
38. Geybels MS, Neuhouser ML, Wright JL, et al. Coffee and tea consumption in relation to prostate cancer prognosis. Cancer Causes Control CCC 2013; 24(11). https://doi.org/10.1007/s10552-013-0270-5.
39. Peisch SF, Van Blarigan EL, Chan JM, et al. Prostate cancer progression and mortality: a review of diet and lifestyle factors. World J Urol 2017;35(6):867–74.
40. Brookman-May SD, Campi R, Henríquez JDS, et al. Latest Evidence on the Impact of Smoking, Sports, and Sexual Activity as Modifiable Lifestyle Risk Factors for Prostate Cancer Incidence, Recurrence, and Progression: A Systematic

Review of the Literature by the European Association of Urology Section of Oncological Urology (ESOU). Eur Urol Focus 2019;5(5):756–87.

41. Islami F, Torre LA, Jemal A. Global trends of lung cancer mortality and smoking prevalence. Transl Lung Cancer Res 2015;4(4):327–38.

42. Naji L, Randhawa H, Sohani Z, et al. Digital Rectal Examination for Prostate Cancer Screening in Primary Care: A Systematic Review and Meta-Analysis. Ann Fam Med 2018;16(2):149–54.

43. Mottet N, van den Bergh RCN, Briers E, et al. EAU-EANM-ESTRO-ESUR-SIOG Guidelines on Prostate Cancer—2020 Update. Part 1: Screening, Diagnosis, and Local Treatment with Curative Intent. Eur Urol 2021;79(2):243–62.

44. Zadnik V, Zagar T, Lokar K, et al. Trends in Population-based Cancer Survival in Slovenia. Radiol Oncol 2021;55(1):42–9.

45. Ilic D, Neuberger MM, Djulbegovic M, et al. Screening for prostate cancer. Cochrane Database Syst Rev 2013;2013(1):CD004720.

46. Hugosson J, Roobol MJ, Månsson M, et al. A 16-yr Follow-up of the European Randomized study of Screening for Prostate Cancer. Eur Urol 2019;76(1):43–51.

47. Innos K, Baburin A, Kotsar A, et al. Prostate cancer incidence, mortality and survival trends in Estonia, 1995–2014. Scand J Urol 2017;51(6):442–9.

48. Patasius A, Innos K, Barchuk A, et al. Prostate cancer incidence and mortality in the Baltic states, Belarus, the Russian Federation and Ukraine. BMJ Open 2019; 9(10):e031856.

49. Krilaviciute A, Smailyte G, Brenner H, et al. Cancer survival in Lithuania after the restoration of independence: Rapid improvements, but persisting major gaps. Acta Oncol 2014;53(9):1238–44.

50. Gondos A, Krilaviciute A, Smailyte G, et al. Cancer surveillance using registry data: Results and recommendations for the Lithuanian national prostate cancer early detection programme. Eur J Cancer 2015;51(12):1630–7.

51. Patasius A, Smailyte G. Changing Incidence and Stage Distribution of Prostate Cancer in a Lithuanian Population—Evidence from National PSA-Based Screening Program. Int J Environ Res Public Health 2019;16(23):4856.

52. Vargovčák M, Dorko E, Rimárová K, et al. Prostate cancer screening - is it time to change approach? Cent Eur J Public Health 2022;30(Supplement):S11–5.

53. Arnsrud Godtman R, Holmberg E, Lilja H, et al. Opportunistic Testing Versus Organized Prostate-specific Antigen Screening: Outcome After 18 Years in the Göteborg Randomized Population-based Prostate Cancer Screening Trial. Eur Urol 2015;68(3):354–60.

54. Cancer screening · Cancon. Available at: https://cancercontrol.eu/archived/guide-landing-page/guide-cancer-screening.html. Accessed June 5, 2023.

55. Croatia National Cancer Control Plan | ICCP Portal. Available at: https://www.iccp-portal.org/news/croatia-national-cancer-control-plan. Accessed June 5, 2023.

56. Crocetto F, Russo G, Di Zazzo E, et al. Liquid Biopsy in Prostate Cancer Management-Current Challenges and Future Perspectives. Cancers 2022; 14(13):3272.

57. Athanasiou A, Tennstedt P, Wittig A, et al. A novel serum biomarker quintet reveals added prognostic value when combined with standard clinical parameters in prostate cancer patients by predicting biochemical recurrence and adverse pathology. PLoS One 2021;16(11):e0259093.

58. Nagy B, Bhattoa Harjit P, Kappelmayer J. [Routine laboratory diagnostics of prostate cancer: Past, present and the future]. Magy Onkol 2019;63(1):16–25.

59. R I A, Shamsudeen S, Leslie SW. Prostate Cancer Tissue-Based Biomarkers. In: StatPearls. StatPearls Publishing; 2023. Available at: http://www.ncbi.nlm.nih.gov/books/NBK587345/. Accessed June 4, 2023.

60. Bray F, Lortet-Tieulent J, Ferlay J, et al. Prostate cancer incidence and mortality trends in 37 European countries: An overview. Eur J Cancer 2010;46(17):3040–52.

61. Neupane S, Bray F, Auvinen A. National economic and development indicators and international variation in prostate cancer incidence and mortality: an ecological analysis. World J Urol 2017;35(6):851–8.

62. Smailyte G, Aleknaviciene B. Incidence of prostate cancer in Lithuania after introduction of the Early Prostate Cancer Detection Programme. Publ Health 2012;126(12):1075–7.

63. The prostate cancer landscape in Europe: Current challenges, future opportunities. Cancer Lett 2022;526:304–10.

64. Solarić M, Grgić M, Omrcen T, et al. [Clinical guidelines for diagnosing, treatment and monitoring patients with prostate cancer–Croatian Oncology Society and Croatian Urology Society, Croatian Medical Association]. Lijec Vjesn 2013;135(11–12):298–305.

65. Surcel CI, Sooriakumaran P, Briganti A, et al. Preferences in the management of high-risk prostate cancer among urologists in Europe: results of a web-based survey. BJU Int 2015;115(4):571–9.

66. Tomašković I, Ulamec M, Tomić M, et al. Validation of Epstein Biopsy Criteria for Insignificant Prostate Cancer in Contemporary Cohort of Croatian Patients. Coll Antropol 2015;39(3):709–11.

67. Dragićević SM, Krejović-Marić SP, Hasani BH. Evaluation of quality of life after radical prostatectomy-experience in Serbia. Med Glas Off Publ Med Assoc Zenica-Doboj Cant Bosnia Herzeg 2012;9(2):388–92.

68. Brodszky V, Varga P, Gimesi-Országh J, et al. Long-term costs and survival of prostate cancer: a population-based study. Int Urol Nephrol 2017;49(10):1707–14.

69. Lievens Y, Borras JM, Grau C. Provision and use of radiotherapy in Europe. Mol Oncol 2020;14(7):1461–9.

70. Oncology Financing: Evidence from Country Experiences to Inform the Global Challenge. ThinkWell. Available at: https://thinkwell.global/projects/oncology-financing/. Accessed June 5, 2023.

71. WHO Cancer Country profiles 2020 | ICCP Portal. Available at: https://www.iccp-portal.org/news/who-cancer-country-profiles-2020. Accessed June 5, 2023.

72. Uyl-de Groot CA, Heine R, Krol M, et al. Unequal Access to Newly Registered Cancer Drugs Leads to Potential Loss of Life-Years in Europe. Cancers 2020;12(8):2313.

73. Kurtovic-Kozaric A, Vranic S, Kurtovic S, et al. Lack of Access to Targeted Cancer Treatment Modalities in the Developing World in the Era of Precision Medicine: Real-Life Lessons From Bosnia. J Glob Oncol 2017;4. https://doi.org/10.1200/JGO.2016.008698. JGO.2016.008698.

74. Cherny N, Sullivan R, Torode J, et al. ESMO European Consortium Study on the availability, out-of-pocket costs and accessibility of antineoplastic medicines in Europe. Ann Oncol Off J Eur Soc Med Oncol 2016;27(8):1423–43.

75. eEML - Electronic Essential Medicines List. Available at: https://list.essentialmeds.org/. Accessed June 12, 2023.

76. EU Country Cancer Profiles 2023 - OECD. Available at: https://www.oecd.org/health/eu-cancer-profiles.htm. Accessed June 4, 2023.

77. Schmitz-Dräger BJ, Bismarck E, Grammenos D, et al. Lifestyle aspects in a contemporary middle-European cohort of patients undergoing androgen deprivation therapy for advanced prostate cancer: data from the non-interventional LEAN study. Br J Nutr 2022;1–8. https://doi.org/10.1017/S0007114522003452.

78. Liede A, Hallett DC, Hope K, et al. International survey of androgen deprivation therapy (ADT) for non-metastatic prostate cancer in 19 countries. ESMO Open 2016;1(2):e000040.

79. Perera M, Roberts MJ, Klotz L, et al. Intermittent versus continuous androgen deprivation therapy for advanced prostate cancer. Nat Rev Urol 2020;17(8): 469–81.

80. A cancer plan for Europe. Available at: https://commission.europa.eu/strategy-and-policy/priorities-2019-2024/promoting-our-european-way-life/european-health-union/cancer-plan-europe_en. Accessed June 5, 2023.

81. Systems I. Legea nr. 293/2022 pentru prevenirea şi combaterea cancerului. Lege5. Available at: https://lege5.ro/Gratuit/gezdsmzzguyte/legea-nr-293-2022-pentru-prevenirea-si-combaterea-cancerului. Accessed June 5, 2023.

82. Leighl NB, Nirmalakumar S, Ezeife DA, et al. An Arm and a Leg: The Rising Cost of Cancer Drugs and Impact on Access. Am Soc Clin Oncol Educ Book Am Soc Clin Oncol Annu Meet 2021;41:1–12.

83. Angelis A, Linch M, Montibeller G, et al. Multiple Criteria Decision Analysis for HTA across four EU Member States: Piloting the Advance Value Framework. Soc Sci Med 1982 2020;246:112595.

84. Rachev B, Wilking N, Kobelt G, et al. Budget projections and clinical impact of an immuno-oncology class of treatments: Experience in four EU markets. J Cancer Policy 2021;28:100279.

85. Albreht T. Quality management in (prostate) cancer care: what do European cancer control plans tell us? World J Urol 2021;39(1):37–9.

86. Crawford-Williams F, March S, Goodwin BC, et al. Interventions for prostate cancer survivorship: A systematic review of reviews. Psycho Oncol 2018;27(10): 2339–48.

87. Dancing to new tunes to reduce inequalities in cancer prevention and care in central and South Eastern Europe. Available at: https://apps.who.int/iris/handle/10665/338918. Accessed June 4, 2023.

88. Albreht T, Martin-Moreno JM, Jelenc M, et al. (Eds.). (2015). European guide for quality national cancer control programmes. Ljubljana: National Institute of Public Health.

89. Jelenc M, Weiderpass E, Fitzpatrick P, et al. Developments in National Cancer Control Programmes in Europe – Results From the Analysis of a Pan-European Survey. Cancer Control 2021;28. 10732748210415.

90. Espina C, Soerjomataram I, Forman D, et al. Cancer prevention policy in the EU: Best practices are now well recognised; no reason for countries to lag behind. J Cancer Policy 2018;18:40–51.

91. Tackling noncommunicable diseases in Bosnia and Herzegovina (2018). Available at: https://www.who.int/europe/publications/m/item/tackling-noncommunicable-diseases-in-bosnia-and-herzegovina-(2018). Accessed June 4, 2023.

92. Willemsen MC, Mons U, Fernández E. Tobacco control in Europe: progress and key challenges. Tob Control 2022;31(2):160–3.

93. Kenessey I, Szőke G, Dobozi M, et al. Comparison of Cancer Survival Trends in Hungary in the Periods 2001-2005 and 2011-2015 According to a Population-Based Cancer Registry. Pathol Oncol Res 2022;28:1610668.

94. Begum M, Lewison G, Jassem J, et al. Mapping cancer research across Central and Eastern Europe, the Russian Federation and Central Asia: Implications for future national cancer control planning. Eur J Cancer Oxf Engl 1990 2018; 104:127–36.

95. Thallinger C, Belina I, Comanescu A, et al. Limitations of cancer care in Central and South-Eastern Europe: results of the international conference organized by the Central European Cooperative Oncology Group (CECOG). J Health Inequalities 2020;6(2):139–52.

96. Existence of population-based cancer registry. Available at: https://www.who. int/data/gho/data/indicators/indicator-details/GHO/existence-of-population-based-cancer-registry. Accessed June 5, 2023.

97. Berisha M, Miftari-Basholli F, Ramadani N, et al. Impact of the National Population Register in Improving the Health Information System of Malignant Diseases in Kosova. Acta Inform Medica 2018;26(1):62–6.

98. Vrdoljak E, Torday L, Sella A, et al. Insights into cancer surveillance in Central and Eastern Europe, Israel and Turkey. Eur J Cancer Care 2013;24. https://doi.org/10.1111/ecc.12149.

99. Znaor A, van den Hurk C, Primic-Zakelj M, et al. Cancer incidence and mortality patterns in South Eastern Europe in the last decade: Gaps persist compared with the rest of Europe. Eur J Cancer 2013;49(7):1683–91.

100. Ristova MM, Gershan V, Schopper H, et al. Patients With Cancer in the Countries of South-East Europe (the Balkans) Region and Prospective of the Particle Therapy Center: South-East European International Institute for Sustainable Technologies (SEEIIST). Adv Radiat Oncol 2021;6(6):100772.

101. Cornford P, van den Bergh RCN, Briers E, et al. EAU-EANM-ESTRO-ESUR-SIOG Guidelines on Prostate Cancer. Part II—2020 Update: Treatment of Relapsing and Metastatic Prostate Cancer. Eur Urol 2021;79(2):263–82.

The Impact of Climate Change on Global Oncology

Leticia Nogueira, PhD, MPH[a],*, Narjust Florez, MD[b]

KEYWORDS

- Climate change • Cancer • Disparities • Disaster • Emergency preparedness
- Environmental justice

KEY POINTS

- Climate-driven disasters can damage medical infrastructure, disrupt supply chains, hamper transportation, and interrupt access to life-saving cancer care (from prevention to survivorship care).
- Due to discriminatory policies and practices built on settler colonialism structures, such as austerity measures imposed on former exploited territories that are already grappling with environmental degradation from historical and current extractive economic practices (agriculture, mining, fossil fuel extractions, and so forth), the same communities already experiencing barriers in access to cancer care are also the most vulnerable to the threats of climate change.
- Our continuous reliance on fossil fuels is a shared cause of climate change and increased exposure to environmental hazards in communities targeted for marginalization.
- Engaging in climate change mitigation and adaptation efforts is a fundamental component of professionals committed to reducing the burden of cancer.

INTRODUCTION

Settler colonialism is defined as a system of oppression that involves the appropriation of indigenous life, land, and culture, with the goal of replacing these with settler life and culture. Settler colonialism created a structure of unbalanced resources and hazard distribution,[1,2] which is reflected in global patterns of health disparities, including premature deaths due to cancer. Health disparities are deleterious health differences affecting those subjected to systemic discriminatory or exclusionary social and/or economic obstacles to health[3,4] and includes global differences in premature cancer deaths.[5]

Cancer is one of the leading causes of death in Latin America and the Caribbean.[6] The most frequently discussed approaches for addressing the cancer burden have

a Surveillance and Health Equity Sciences, American Cancer Society, Palm Harbor, FL, USA;
b Medical Oncology, DFCI, Boston, MA, USA
* Corresponding author. 3380 Chastain Meadows Parkway NW, Suite 200, Kennesaw, GA 30144.
E-mail address: leticia.nogueira@cancer.org

Hematol Oncol Clin N Am 38 (2024) 105–121
https://doi.org/10.1016/j.hoc.2023.07.004   hemonc.theclinics.com

focus on access to screening, availability of diagnostics, delivery of high-quality cancer treatment and supportive care (psychological and survivorship care).[6–8] However, environmental exposures, including air pollution and water and soil contamination, are often overlooked as modifiable factors that worsen cancer risk (through increased exposure to carcinogens) and outcomes (through exposure to other health hazards and disruptions in access to cancer care).[9] For example, air pollution emitted from burning of fossil fuels, a well-established carcinogen,[10,11] is responsible for 1 in 5 deaths worldwide.[12]

Consumption of fossil fuels is also driving climate change, the most pressing environmental hazard of our time,[13,14] with significant implications for cancer control efforts.[9,15] For example, climate change alters the frequency and behavior of extreme weather events,[16] rendering it more difficult for communities to prepare for and respond to increasingly unpredictable circumstances (**Fig. 1**). For instance, warmer atmospheric temperatures increase the water capacity and decrease the speed of hurricanes and tropical storms,[16,17] resulting in unprecedented flooding when these systems stall after making landfall.[18]

Climate-driven extreme weather events can damage medical infrastructure (facilities, electronic medical records, and so forth),[19] break supply chains (such as damage from Hurricane Maria leading to IV bag shortages in the United States),[9] and disrupt transportation of medical staff and patients to health-care facilities,[20] leading to interruptions in access to potentially life-saving cancer care.[21] Patients with lung cancer in the United States whose facility was affected by a hurricane disaster during radiation treatment had worse overall survival than similar patients who completed treatment in the absence of disasters.[22] Cancer prevention and screening are also affected by climate-driven disasters. For example, human papillomavirus (HPV) vaccination

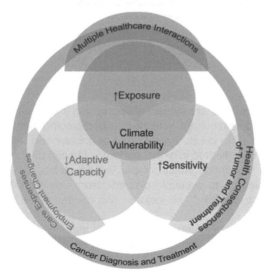

Fig. 1. Climate change and cancer. The physical, psychological, and socioeconomic consequences of cancer diagnosis and treatment exacerbate vulnerability to climate change due to increased risk of *exposure* (time spent outdoors commuting to medical appointments), increased *sensitivity* (cardiorespiratory sensitivities, inhibited thermoregulation as a side effect of some cancer treatment drugs increases sensitivity to extreme temperatures, immunosuppression increases sensitivity to infections common during flooding events, and so forth), and decreased *adaptive capacity* (inability to afford using air conditioner during heat waves, evacuating or stockpiling food, and so forth).

decreased significantly in the months after Hurricane Maria made landfall in Puerto Rico,[23] and Hurricane Harvey flooded several chemical plants, oil refineries, and Superfund sites in the Houston ship channel, releasing large amounts of carcinogens and other environmental toxicants in the community.[24] Cervical cancer screening rates were also affected by climate-driven disasters in Puerto Rico.[25]

In addition to disruptions in access to care, individuals diagnosed with cancer are at an increased risk to the health threats invoked by climate change due to the physical, psychological, and socioeconomic consequences of cancer diagnosis and treatment (see **Fig. 1**).[9] For example, some cancer treatment modalities can result in a weakened immune system, which makes individuals more vulnerable to infections during flooding events.[26,27] Further, the psychological consequences of cancer diagnosis and treatment (stress, anxiety, depression, and so forth)[28,29] are similar to the psychological consequences of exposure to disasters (posttraumatic stress, anxiety, and depression),[30] leading to compounding mental health risks when patients with cancer and survivors are exposed to disasters.[31,32] Cancer diagnosis and treatment can also have socioeconomic consequences resulting from care-related expenses as well as changes in the ability of individuals diagnosed with cancer to maintain employment and income levels during and after cancer treatment.[33,34]

Moreover, our continuous reliance on fossil fuels is a shared cause of climate change and increased exposure to environmental hazards (including carcinogens), which undermine cancer control efforts. For example, individuals residing near natural gas extraction sites are exposed to air contaminated with benzene,[35–38] polycyclic aromatic hydrocarbons (PAHs),[39,40] and fine particulate matter,[41–44] all of which are established human carcinogens.[11,45,46] Crude oil processing, too, includes separation, distillation, and various types of cracking, blending, and extractions,[47] which can release benzene, arsenic, lead, chromium, PAHs, cadmium, and nickel into surrounding communities.[48,49]

In this commentary, we discuss how climate change threatens numerous steps of the cancer care continuum, how the unbalanced distribution of hazards and resources exacerbates cancer disparities and climate vulnerabilities, and how oncology professionals may work to mitigate such inequities, through identifying and implementing solutions with climate mitigation, cancer control, and health equity cobenefits. Throughout the article, we use content and language in line with environmental justice principles. We use terminology (such as "communities targeted for marginalization") that centers the conditions imposed on communities as the root cause of disparities and avoids further oppressing these communities by implying that these are defining characteristics (as terms such as "marginalized communities" would).

CLIMATE CHANGE VULNERABILITY

Vulnerability to climate hazards is determined by differing levels of *exposure, sensitivity*, and *adaptive capacity* in the population.[50] As mentioned above, the physical, psychological, and socioeconomic consequences of cancer diagnosis and treatment can influence vulnerability to climate change. In addition to medical conditions, some sociopolitical structures also influence the determinants of climate vulnerability, placing some groups of people at higher risk for the threats of climate change. For example, a history of settler colonialism resulted in the current sociopolitical and economic structures that perpetuate the colonial reliance on extraction and dispossession for the production of capital and accumulation of wealth among privileged minorities.[2] These neocolonial structures of power and market practices uphold disparities in the distribution of hazards and resources, resulting in increased vulnerability (ie, increased exposure, increased sensitivity, and decreased adaptive capacity)[51] to the threats posed by climate change among individuals from communities targeted for marginalization.[52,53]

The compounding challenges posed by increased exposure, increased sensitivity, and decreased adaptive capacity among individuals diagnosed with cancer who are members of communities targeted for marginalization were exemplified by the impact of Hurricane Maria on cancer care in Puerto Rico,[54] as well as by the global challenges observed throughout the 2017 Hurricane season.[18]

Systemic disinvestment in the Puerto Rican community enabled the complete collapse of the electrical grid, communication infrastructure, and transportation network when Hurricane Maria made landfall.[54] Access to cancer care was disrupted throughout the island,[55] and without access to food, water, and shelter,[20] patients would not have been able to tolerate treatment, even if it was available.[56] Transferring care to other localities was problematic, too, due to geographic restrictions in state-sponsored health insurance coverage and out-of-network costs in private-sponsored insurance.[19] For each component of vulnerability to climate hazards (exposure, sensitivity, and adaptive capacity), we will discuss the compounding challenges posed by cancer and the historical influence of colonialism.

Exposure

Exposure is defined as human contact with environmental hazards.[50] Cancer prevention, screening, diagnosis, treatment, and survivorship care require several interactions with medical facilities, which increase the risk of exposure to climate-driven disasters.[9]

As such, the threats posed by exposure to climate-driven disasters vary by geographic region.[57,58] Disruptions in access to care due to hurricanes, for instance, are a prevalent threat for individuals residing in coastal areas and island territories in the Atlantic and Pacific tropical basins[59,60] because these geographic areas are more likely to be affected by hurricanes,[61] whereas wildfire activity, which is closely tied to temperature and drought (both altered by climate change), is increasing and expanding eastward in the United States,[62] leading to unanticipated circumstances in these affected communities.[63] Similarly, with climate-driven weakening of the temperature differential that stabilizes the polar vortex,[64] severe ice and snow storms are becoming more frequent, intensified, and posing threats (such as power outages) to communities farther south.[65]

However, geographic location is not the only factor contributing to the risk of exposure to environmental hazards.[66] Due to discriminatory policies and practices,[67] hazardous and polluting infrastructure is frequently sited in proximity to communities targeted for marginalization,[52,68] who have been deprived of the resources and political power necessary to oppose these developments.[69–73] For example, in the United States, regulatory governmental agencies are more likely to waive established environmental and public health safety criteria for siting of hazardous waste facilities in predominantly Black and Latinx communities.[74]

When disaster strikes, the hazards posed by extreme weather events are compounded by the hazards posed by environmental contaminants released from such polluting infrastructure.[24,75–78] For example, Hurricane Harvey's record water capacity (which climate change made 3.5 times more likely)[79] flooded chemical plants, oil refineries, and Superfund sites, releasing vast amounts of carcinogens and other contaminants into the surrounding predominantly Black and Latinx communities.[80,81] In the aftermath of Harvey, the Texas General Land Office (the state government entity responsible for distributing the US$9.3 billion in federal aid for communities could rebuild and better prepare for the next storm) implemented discriminatory practices that restricted access to these resources in predominantly Black and Latinx communities,[82] who still continue to be at higher risk of exposure to environmental hazards.[78]

Sensitivity

Sensitivity refers to the degree to which climate hazards affect humans.[50] Chronic diseases, such as cancer, and the side effects of its treatments, can increase sensitivity to the health hazards of climate change.[83] For example, some chemotherapy agents can inhibit thermoregulation, making patients with cancer more vulnerable to heatwaves.[84] Immunosuppression, another common side effect of cancer treatment, also increases the risk of infections, which are common during flooding events.[26,27]

Inequities in the distribution of health hazards and resources leads to disparities in prevalence of chronic health conditions associated with increased sensitivity to the threats of climate change in communities targeted for marginalization.[4,54] For example, colonial violence (including land theft, imposition of the reservation system, and damage of existing food systems) resulted in dramatic shifts in food consumption (including increased consumption of unhealthy food items distributed initially through rations and later through the commodity food program) among native peoples.[85,86] Similarly, systemic disinvestment resulted in limited access to healthy food outlets in predominantly Black neighborhoods.[87] Lack of access to health resources (such as nutritional foods), combined with increased exposure to health hazards (including hazardous infrastructure, as mentioned above, as well as a concentration of tobacco and alcohol outlets),[88–90] resulted in an increased prevalence of chronic health conditions among individuals in communities targeted for marginalization.[91]

Exacerbated sensitivity due to the increased prevalence of chronic health conditions (such as diabetes and chronic kidney disease)[92] among individuals in Puerto Rico,[93] for example, was a main contributor to the significant increase in illness and mortality in these populations in the aftermath of the 2017 Hurricane Maria.[94]

Adaptive Capacity

Adaptive capacity is the ability to cope with climate hazards.[50] Costs associated with cancer treatment and survivorship care, combined with challenges to participate in the workforce, are some of the ways in which a cancer diagnosis is associated with decreased adaptive capacity through increased financial hardship.[34] For example, financial hardship makes it harder for individuals to prepare and respond to disasters, such as securing the resources necessary for evacuating, stockpiling food, or improving housing infrastructure (using air conditioner during heatwaves or installing special air filters during wildfires).[50,95]

Similarly, individuals from communities targeted for marginalization have diminished adaptive capacity due to inequities in distribution of social, cultural, and economic capital and power.[96] For example, the economic and social circumstances imposed by austerity measures in Puerto Rico,[97] such as the Jones Act, which requires all maritime vessels arriving in Puerto Rico to come from US territories, increases prices of goods imported to the island by approximately 25% compared with mainland, one of the main factors contributing to the estimated 43% of individuals in Puerto Rico living under the US federal poverty line.[98] These policies, built on colonial laws,[99] also limit the ability of other nations to provide aid when disaster strikes, restricting the amount of resources that can be mobilized during crises and complicating disaster preparedness and response in the territory.[99]

In the United States, aid provided by the Federal Emergency Management Agency (FEMA), the government agency responsible for responding to and recovering from crises, is especially relevant for individuals diagnosed with cancer.[19] However, discriminatory policies and practices in FEMA's response and resource allocation abound,[54] with privileged communities being more likely to receive federal assistance following a disaster,[100] exacerbating disparities in adaptive capacity in the United States.

Similar inequities in adaptive capacity exist between countries.[68] As explained by Mia Mottley, the Prime Minister of Barbados, at the 26th Conference of Parties on climate (COP26), a history of colonialism created the current structure of economic dependence on tourism and imported goods that hinders the adaptive capacity of island territories in the Atlantic tropical basins (such as Puerto Rico, Barbados, and the Bahamas).[54,59,68] As mentioned previously, these territories are already at increased risk of exposure to climate-driven disasters,[101] and a legacy of settler colonialism structures of power and market forces resulted in former colonies being less likely to have access to the resources required for completing essential climate adaptation projects.[102,103]

Importantly, because communities targeted for marginalization are affected first and most from the threats of climate change, the solutions proposed by individuals in these communities are crucial for global climate mitigation and adaptation strategies.

PROPOSED SOLUTIONS

In November 2022, the United Nation agreed to establish a loss and damage fund in which historically exploitative economies would pay into to help exploited nations cope with the threats of climate change. Although major hurdles remain (eg, there is no guarantee exploitative economies will contribute to the fund, which exploited economies will receive the funds first, how will the money be used), this is an important step toward recognizing how to mitigate ways in which current structures of power perpetuate disparities in climate vulnerability.[2]

Of note, solutions proposed within the settler colonialism framework, such as those relating to carbon credit (through projects that enable land theft and force displacement of native populations)[2] and the new green agricultural revolutions (which enable environmental degradation through deforestation, contamination of soil and water with pesticides and fertilizers, as well as displacement and impoverishment of native communities),[104] will continue to exploit the vulnerabilities of disenfranchised communities,[105] propagate environmental injustice and health disparities,[106] and institutionalize exposure to environmental contaminants.[107] For example, all climate models uphold overconsumption of energy and goods by the privileged.[108] In order to sustain this overconsumption, proposed solutions (such as expanding rare mineral mining,[109] carbon credit, and carbon capture) will continue to amplify cancer disparities through disproportionate exposure to environmental hazards, increased sensitivity, and decreased adaptive capacity of individuals from exploited communities.[2]

Therefore, it is crucial that we center environmental justice and health equity in our climate mitigation and adaptation efforts.[103,110,111] One important component of just environmental and public health efforts (which include global climate treaties and large national policies but also climate-relevant efforts at our own institutions, communities, and personal lives), involves shifting from pathologized narratives of vulnerable populations as powerless (ie, needing solutions prescribed onto them) toward valuing the ingenious strategies and solutions coming from these communities because these solutions present potential benefits for the entire population.[51,53]

THE ROLE OF ONCOLOGISTS IN IDENTIFYING AND IMPLEMENTING SOLUTIONS

Given the significant threats posed by climate change to cancer control efforts, engaging in climate change mitigation and adaptation efforts is a fundamental component of all oncology-related professional activities (**Fig. 2**).

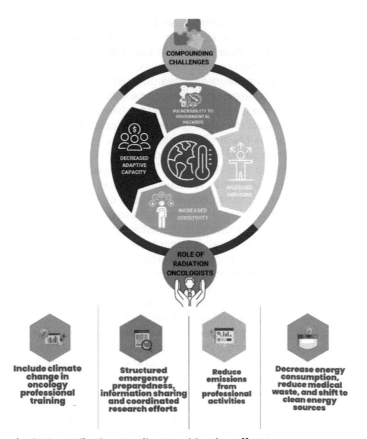

Fig. 2. Oncologists' contributions to climate mitigation efforts.

First, including climate change in all oncology professional training (from basic research to mental health,[31,112] from undergraduate programs to professional conferences)[113] would facilitate recognition of contemporary climate threats and accelerate knowledge advancement at the speed needed to tackle such a rapidly evolving crisis.[114]

Second, information sharing is extremely important. Structured approaches for sharing emergency preparedness and response information, including insights from postdisaster evaluation, are required to build on lessons learned from previous experiences and continuously improve climate adaptation efforts that protect the health and safety of patients, caregivers, and health-care providers.[19,55,115] Here again, lessons learned from communities affected first and most by the threats of climate change are vital. For example, the modifications in radiation oncology regimens that were developed to cope with electricity scarcity in the aftermath of Hurricane Maria in Puerto Rico were later adopted throughout the continental United States when the health-care system was overwhelmed with the demands of the coronavirus disease 2019 pandemic.[32,55]

Third, coordinated interdisciplinary multi-institutional research efforts focused on emergency preparedness for patients with chronic health conditions is urgently needed. For example, patients with cancer in Puerto Rico reported receiving no emergency preparedness plan information before Hurricane Irma or Hurricane Maria made landfall.[20] There is currently no ongoing research or funding opportunities for research focused on cancer-specific emergency preparedness, and less than 25% of National cancer Institute Designated Cancer Centers in the United States provide any emergency preparedness information on their websites.[116]

Importantly, emergency preparedness research must center the patients' needs (ie, patient-centered research questions and outcome measures) instead of centering specific cancer treatment modalities (ie, surgery vs, chemotherapy, vs, radiation therapy). For example, individuals undergoing breast and colorectal cancer treatment in Puerto Rico when Hurricane Maria hit reported that lack of access to basic needs (food, water, and shelter) resulted in patients choosing to delay resuming treatment even as health-care services were reinstated,[117] which was also reported by oncologists, who noted that without access to basic needs and under the severe physical and psychological stressors present in the aftermath of Hurricane Maria,[98] patients would not be able to withstand treatment even if it was available.[56] Further, Hurricane Maria was one of the deadliest disasters in US history due partly to interruptions in access to medical care, such as breathing machines, which failed when power was lost.[118] Since Hurricane Maria struck Puerto Rico and Hurricane Dorian struck the Bahamas (with similar detrimental consequences),[112] both nations have made strides in the construction of storm-resistant solar power installations, which would have allowed residents to maintain food and medicines safely refrigerated and have continuous access to medical devices that require electricity.

Therefore, centering the patients' needs and engaging with communities that have been developing expertise on adaptation to climate hazards for decades (ie, impacted first and most),[83] are both important for advancing knowledge on how to better protect the health and safety of cancer patients during disasters. Such patient-centered and inclusive research initiatives would avoid perpetuating disparities in epistemic power (ie, how ideas developed by a few privileged individuals shape efforts and interventions),[119] promote interdisciplinary collaboration (different oncology specialties working together to improve patient health instead of competing for resources), and expand the pool of knowledge available to identify solutions relevant to the entire population. For example, the strategy championed in Puerto Rico and the Bahamas to developed community-owned cooperatively managed microgrids, informed the recent waiver issued by the Centers for Medicare and Medicaid Services allowing health-care facilities to use microgrids as emergency power sources in the United States. Unlike diesel-power generators, microgrids do not rely on transportation of fuel (improving institutional resilience), have lower emissions, and decrease exposure of nearby communities to air pollution from burning diesel.

Oncology professionals can contribute to these climate mitigation and adaptation efforts, such as enhancing emergency preparedness efforts and reducing emissions from our professional activities.[114] This is especially relevant for oncologists residing in the United States. In fact, the United States remains the largest historical emitter of greenhouse gases,[120] and emissions from the US health-care system alone surpass emissions from the entire United Kingdom.[121] The UK National Health Service has been leading efforts in delivering environmentally responsible health-care services, and more than 50 countries committed to decreasing emissions at the COP26 meeting.[122] It is hopeful that recent legislation advancements in the United States, such as the Inflation Reduction Act, provide incentives and a path for reducing emissions from health care.[123]

Oncologists are well positioned to champion efforts that reduce emissions from health care because climate mitigation strategies have health cobenefits through reduction in exposure to fossil-fuel pollution in the population.[42,124,125] Such efforts include reducing energy consumption in health-care facilities (improving energy efficiency, implementing occupation-based strategies for heating, ventilation, and air conditioning, and so forth); conducting procurement and waste audits (such as those aimed at reducing plastic consumption); seeking environmentally responsible food manufacture, shipment, and waste options, and so forth.[9] Further, engaging and funding research innovation that ameliorates cost, environmental impact, and accessibility of cancer care (such as screening and diagnostic procedures) has tremendous climate and cancer control potential.[119]

Additionally, decreasing energy consumption, reducing medical waste, and other climate mitigation strategies also cut cost and are financially beneficial.[126] Gundersen Health, the first health-care system in the United States to achieve energy independence, also reduced waste management costs 10-fold by implementing sustainable practices.[126] At the University of Minnesota Medical Center, a waste reduction initiative that began by removing unnecessary items from IV port kits for chemotherapy, was later scaled up to the Operating Room, removing unused items from surgery kits with net savings of US$104,000 annually. Albert Einstein Hospital in Brazil significantly reduced institutional emissions and costs by diminishing the use of nitric oxide and fluorinated anesthetic gases that worsen the greenhouse effect more than a 1000-fold compared with carbon dioxide.

Finally, the siting of fossil fuel infrastructure is an environmental justice issue especially relevant to cancer control because it contributes to increased cancer risk (through increased exposure to carcinogens), worse cancer outcomes (through disruptions in access to care and increased exposure to health hazards),[22] and intensifies climate change (through greenhouse gas emissions).[127,128] Therefore, championing efforts to diminish our reliance on fossil fuels within the oncology profession,[129] such as decreasing consumption of petrochemical derivatives,[121] including plastics used in research and clinical care,[130,131] can decrease exposure to hazardous compounds that disproportionately impact communities targeted for marginalization,[52,132,133] and have implications for the entire population.[134] Further, adding a "climate lens" to basic science, epidemiologic, community, or clinical oncology research (eg, biomarkers of exposure, intermediate cancer outcomes, health consequences of exposure to pollution and proximity to fossil fuel infrastructure)[135–138] can expand the evidence base that informs decisions on whether to support local development of fossil fuel infrastructure.[77,139] Finally, supporting environmentally responsible policies, such as the global plastic treaty and the Clean Air Act in the United States,[140,141] is imperative for advancing cancer control and health equity efforts globally.[124]

SUMMARY

Climate change threatens cancer control efforts throughout the globe. Climate-driven extreme weather events lead to disruptions in access to cancer care, and individuals diagnosed with cancer are a vulnerable population to the health hazards of climate change. A legacy of settler colonialism in current power structures perpetuates inequities in the distribution of health hazards and resources through increased exposure, increased sensitivity, and reduced adaptive capacity, compounding the vulnerabilities of patients with cancer in communities targeted for marginalization. Therefore, engaging in climate mitigation and adaptation efforts, including enhancing emergency preparedness efforts and reducing emissions from the health-care system, are fundamental components of oncologists' missions in the era of climate change.

CLINICS CARE POINTS

- Climate-driven disasters can result in disruptions in access to cancer care.
- Individuals diagnosed with cancer are a vulnerable population to the health threats of climate change due to the physical, psychological, and socioeconomic consequences of cancer diagnosis and treatment.
- There are no cancer-specific emergency preparedness resources for patients, caregivers, or providers.

DISCLOSURE

Nothing to disclose.

REFERENCES

1. Wolfe P. Settler colonialism and the elimination of the native. J Genocide Res 2006;8(4):387–409.
2. Sultana F. The unbearable heaviness of climate coloniality. Political Geography; 2022. p. 102638.
3. Alcaraz KI, Wiedt TL, Daniels EC, et al. Understanding and addressing social determinants to advance cancer health equity in the United States: a blueprint for practice, research, and policy. CA Cancer J Clin 2020;70(1):31–46.
4. Nogueira L, White KE, Bell B, et al. The role of behavioral medicine in addressing climate change-related health inequities. Translational Behavioral Medicine 2022;12(4):526–34.
5. Singh D, Vignat J, Lorenzoni V, et al. Global estimates of incidence and mortality of cervical cancer in 2020: a baseline analysis of the WHO Global Cervical Cancer Elimination Initiative. Lancet Glob Health 2023;11(2):e197–206.
6. Piñeros M, Laversanne M, Barrios E, et al. An updated profile of the cancer burden, patterns and trends in Latin America and the Caribbean. Lancet Reg Health Am 2022;13.
7. Bandi P, Minihan AK, Siegel RL, et al. Updated review of major cancer risk factors and screening test use in the United States in 2018 and 2019, with a focus on smoking cessation. Cancer Epidemiol Biomarkers Prev 2021;30(7):1287–99.
8. Miller KD, Nogueira L, Devasia T, et al. Cancer treatment and survivorship statistics, 2022. CA Cancer J Clin 2022.
9. Nogueira LM, Yabroff KR, Bernstein A. Climate change and cancer. CA Cancer J Clin 2020;70(4):239–44.
10. International Agency for Research on Cancer, Air Pollution and Cancer. IARC monographs on the evaluation of carcinogenic risks to humans, 2013. 161.
11. International Agency for Research on Cancer, Outdoor Air Pollution. IARC monographs on the evaluation of carcinogenic risks to humans, 2015. 109.
12. Vohra K, Vodonos A, Schwartz J, et al. Global mortality from outdoor fine particle pollution generated by fossil fuel combustion: results from GEOS-Chem. Environ Res 2021;195:110754.
13. Intergovernmental Panel on Climate Change, I., Pörtner HO, Roberts DC, et al. Climate change 2022: impacts, adaptation and vulnerability. Cambridge University Press; 2022.
14. The Lancet O. Climate crisis and cancer: the need for urgent action. Lancet Oncol 2021;22(10):1341.

15. Hiatt RA, Beyeler N. Cancer and climate change. Lancet Oncol 2020;21(11): e519–27.
16. Kossin JP. A global slowdown of tropical-cyclone translation speed. Nature 2018;558(7708):104–7.
17. Kossin JP, Knapp KR, Olander TL, et al. Global increase in major tropical cyclone exceedance probability over the past four decades. Proc Natl Acad Sci U S A 2020;117(22):11975–80.
18. Shultz JM, Kossin JP, Ettman C, et al. The 2017 perfect storm season, climate change, and environmental injustice. Lancet Planet Health 2018;2(9):e370–1.
19. Ortiz AP, Calo WA, Mendez-Lazaro P, et al. Strengthening resilience and adaptive capacity to disasters in cancer control plans: lessons learned from Puerto Rico. Cancer Epidemiol Biomarkers Prev 2020;29(7):1290–3.
20. Calo WA, Rivera M, Mendez-Lazaro PA, et al. Disruptions in oncology care confronted by patients with gynecologic cancer following Hurricanes Irma and Maria in Puerto Rico. Cancer Control 2022;29. 10732748221114691.
21. Man RX, Lack DA, Wyatt CE, et al. The effect of natural disasters on cancer care: a systematic review. Lancet Oncol 2018;19(9):e482–99.
22. Nogueira LM, Sahar L, Efstathiou JA, et al. Association between declared hurricane disasters and survival of patients with lung cancer undergoing radiation treatment. JAMA 2019;322(3):269–71.
23. Colón-López V, Díaz-Miranda OL, Medina-Laabes DT, et al. Effect of Hurricane Maria on HPV, Tdap, and meningococcal conjugate vaccination rates in Puerto Rico, 2015-2019. Hum Vaccin Immunother 2021;17(12):5623–7.
24. Ratnapradipa D, Cardinal C, Ratnapradipa KL, et al. Implications of Hurricane Harvey on environmental public health in Harris County, Texas. J Environ Health 2018;81(2):24–33.
25. Ortiz AP, Gierbolini-Bermúdez A, Ramos-Cartagena JM, et al. Cervical cancer screening among medicaid patients during natural disasters and the COVID-19 pandemic in Puerto Rico, 2016 to 2020. JAMA Netw Open 2021;4(10): e2128806.
26. Chow NA, Toda M, Pennington AF, et al. Hurricane-associated mold exposures among patients at risk for invasive mold infections after hurricane Harvey - Houston, Texas, 2017. MMWR Morb Mortal Wkly Rep 2019;68(21):469–73.
27. Kontoyiannis DP, Shah EC, Wurster S, et al. Culture-documented invasive mold infections at MD Anderson Cancer Center in Houston, Texas, Pre–and Post–Hurricane Harvey. In: Open forum infectious diseases. Oxford University Press US; 2019.
28. Niedzwiedz CL, Knifton L, Robb KA, et al. Depression and anxiety among people living with and beyond cancer: a growing clinical and research priority. BMC Cancer 2019;19(1):943.
29. Walker ZJ, Xue S, Jones MP, et al. Depression, anxiety, and other mental disorders in patients with cancer in low- and lower-middle-income countries: a systematic review and meta-analysis. JCO Glob Oncol 2021;7:1233–50.
30. Shultz JM, Galea S. Mitigating the mental and physical health consequences of Hurricane Harvey. JAMA 2017;318(15):1437–8.
31. Espinel Z, Galea S, Kossin JP, et al. Climate-driven Atlantic hurricanes pose rising threats for psychopathology. Lancet Psychiatr 2019;6(9):721–3.
32. Espinel Z, Nogueira LM, Gay HA, et al. Climate-driven Atlantic hurricanes create complex challenges for cancer care. Lancet Oncol 2022;23(12):1497–8.
33. Altice CK, Banegas MP, Tucker-Seeley RD, et al. Financial hardships experienced by cancer survivors: a systematic review. J Natl Cancer Inst 2017;109(2).

34. Yabroff KR, Dowling EC, Guy GP Jr, et al. Financial hardship associated with cancer in the United States: findings from a population-based sample of adult cancer survivors. J Clin Oncol 2016;34(3):259–67.

35. Hecobian A, Clements AL, Shonkwiler KB, et al. Air toxics and other volatile organic compound emissions from unconventional oil and gas development. Environ Sci Technol Lett 2019;6(12):720–6.

36. Hildenbrand ZL, Mach PM, McBride EM, et al. Point source attribution of ambient contamination events near unconventional oil and gas development. Sci Total Environ 2016;573:382–8.

37. Khalaj F, Sattler M. Modeling of VOCs and criteria pollutants from multiple natural gas well pads in close proximity, for different terrain conditions: a Barnett Shale case study. Atmos Pollut Res 2019;10(4):1239–49.

38. Marrero JE, Townsend-Small A, Lyon DR, et al. Estimating emissions of toxic hydrocarbons from natural gas production sites in the Barnett Shale Region of Northern Texas. Environ Sci Technol 2016;50(19):10756–64.

39. Paulik LB, Donald CE, Smith BW, et al. Emissions of polycyclic aromatic hydrocarbons from natural gas extraction into air. Environ Sci Technol 2016;50(14): 7921–9.

40. Paulik LB, Hobbie KA, Rohlman D, et al. Environmental and individual PAH exposures near rural natural gas extraction. Environ Pollut 2018;241:397–405.

41. Banan Z, Gernand JM. Evaluation of gas well setback policy in the Marcellus Shale region of Pennsylvania in relation to emissions of fine particulate matter. J Air Waste Manag Assoc 2018;68(9):988–1000.

42. Fann N, Baker KR, Chan EAW, et al. Assessing human health PM(2.5) and ozone impacts from U.S. Oil and Natural Gas Sector Emissions in 2025. Environ Sci Technol 2018;52(15):8095–103.

43. Long CM, Briggs NL, Bamgbose IA. Synthesis and health-based evaluation of ambient air monitoring data for the Marcellus Shale region. J Air Waste Manag Assoc 2019;69(5):527–47.

44. Roohani YH, Roy AA, Heo J, et al. Impact of natural gas development in the Marcellus and Utica shales on regional ozone and fine particulate matter levels. Atmos Environ 2017;155:11–20.

45. International Agency for Research on Cancer. Some non-heterocyclic polycyclic aromatic hydrocarbons and some related exposures. IARC (Int Agency Res Cancer) Monogr Eval Carcinog Risks Hum 2010;92:1–853.

46. International Agency for Research on Cancer, Benzene. IARC Monographs on the Evaluation of Carcinogenic Risks to Humans, 2018. 120.

47. Bozlaker A, Peccia J, Chellam S. Indoor/outdoor relationships and anthropogenic elemental signatures in airborne PM2.5 at a high school: impacts of petroleum refining emissions on Lanthanoid enrichment. Environmental Science & Technology 2017;51(9):4851–9.

48. Brantley HL, Thoma ED, Eisele AP. Assessment of volatile organic compound and hazardous air pollutant emissions from oil and natural gas well pads using mobile remote and on-site direct measurements. J Air Waste Manag Assoc 2015;65(9):1072–82.

49. Schreiber MF, Cozzarelli IM. Arsenic release to the environment from hydrocarbon production, storage, transportation, use and waste management. J Hazard Mater 2021;411:125013.

50. Balbus JM, Malina C. Identifying vulnerable subpopulations for climate change health effects in the United States. J Occup Environ Med 2009;51(1):33–7.

51. Lampis A, Brink E, Carrasco-Torrontegui A, et al. Reparation ecology and climate risk in Latin-America: Experiences from four countries. Frontiers in Climate 2022;4.
52. Bullard RD, Mohai P, Saha R, et al. Toxic wastes and race at twenty 1987–2007: Grassroots struggles to dismantle environmental racism in the United States. 2007.
53. Gilio-Whitaker D. As long as grass grows: the indigenous fight for environmental justice, from colonization to standing rock. Boston (MA): Beacon Press; 2019.
54. Garcia-Lopez GA. The multiple layers of environmental injustice in contexts of (Un)natural Disasters: the case of Puerto Rico Post-Hurricane Maria. Environ Justice 2018;11(3):101–8.
55. Gay HA, Santiago R, Gil B, et al. Lessons learned from Hurricane Maria in Puerto Rico: practical measures to mitigate the impact of a catastrophic natural disaster on radiation oncology patients. Pract Radiat Oncol 2019;9(5):305–21.
56. Lopez-Araujo J, Burnett OL 3rd. Letter from Puerto Rico: the state of radiation oncology after Maria's Landfall. Int J Radiat Oncol Biol Phys 2017;99(5):1071–2.
57. National Oceanic and Atmospheric Administration, N. Billion dollar weather and climate disasters. 2023; Available at: https://www.ncei.noaa.gov/access/billions/. Accessed June 20, 2023.
58. Sharpe JD, Wolkin AF. The epidemiology and geographic patterns of natural disaster and extreme weather mortality by race and ethnicity, United States, 1999-2018. Public Health Rep 2021. 333549211047235.
59. Gould WA, Díaz EL, Álvarez-Berríos NL, et al. US Caribbean: Impacts, Risks, and Adaptation in the United States: Fourth National Climate Assessment, Volume II. 2018 Available at: https://nca2018.globalchange.gov/downloads/NCA4_Ch20_US-Caribbean_Full.pdf.
60. Méndez-Lázaro P, Peña-Orellana M, Padilla-Elías N, et al. The impact of natural hazards on population vulnerability and public health systems in tropical areas. J Geol Geosci 2014;3:114–20.
61. Shultz JM, Kossin JP, Shepherd JM, et al. Risks, health consequences, and response challenges for small-island-based populations: observations from the 2017 Atlantic Hurricane Season. Disaster Med Public Health Prep 2019; 13(1):5–17.
62. Schoennagel T, Balch JK, Brenkert-Smith H, et al. Adapt to more wildfire in western North American forests as climate changes. Proc Natl Acad Sci U S A 2017; 114(18):4582–90.
63. Radeloff VC, Helmers DP, Kramer HA, et al. Rapid growth of the US wildland-urban interface raises wildfire risk. Proc Natl Acad Sci U S A 2018;115(13): 3314–9.
64. Cohen J, Agel L, Barlow M, et al. Linking Arctic variability and change with extreme winter weather in the United States. Science 2021;373(6559):1116–21.
65. Flores NM, McBrien H, Do V, et al. The 2021 Texas Power Crisis: distribution, duration, and disparities. J Expo Sci Environ Epidemiol 2023;33(1):21–31.
66. Environmental Protection Agency, E. Climate Change and Social Vulnerability in the United States: A Focus on Six Impacts. 2021; Available at: https://www.epa.gov/cira/social-vulnerability-report. Accessed June 20, 2023.
67. Gattey E. Global histories of empire and climate in the Anthropocene. Hist Compass 2021;19(8):e12683.
68. Ferdinand M. Decolonial ecology: thinking from the Caribbean World. Paris: John Wiley & Sons; 2021.

69. Auyero J, Hernandez M, Stitt ME. Grassroots activism in the belly of the beast: a relational account of the campaign against urban fracking in Texas. Soc Probl 2017;66(1):28–50.

70. Bergquist P, Mildenberger M, Stokes LC. Combining climate, economic, and social policy builds public support for climate action in the US. Environ Res Lett 2020;15(5):054019.

71. Casey JA, Cushing L, Depsky N, et al. Climate justice and California's methane superemitters: environmental equity assessment of community proximity and exposure intensity. Environ Sci Technol 2021;55(21):14746–57.

72. Krieger N. Climate crisis, health equity, and democratic governance: the need to act together. J Public Health Policy 2020;41(1):4–10.

73. Campbell HE, Peck LR, Tschudi MK. Justice for all? A cross-time analysis of toxics release inventory facility location. Rev Pol Res 2010;27(1):1–25.

74. Taylor DE. Toxic communities: environmental racism, industrial pollution, and residential mobility. New York: NYU Press; 2014.

75. Horney JA, Casillas GA, Baker E, et al. Comparing residential contamination in a Houston environmental justice neighborhood before and after Hurricane Harvey. PLoS One 2018;13(2):e0192660.

76. Kiaghadi A, Rifai HS. Physical, chemical, and microbial quality of floodwaters in Houston following Hurricane Harvey. Environ Sci Technol 2019;53(9):4832–40.

77. Johnston J, Cushing L. Chemical exposures, health, and environmental justice in communities living on the fenceline of industry. Curr Environ Health Rep 2020;7(1):48–57.

78. Anenberg SC, Kalman C. Extreme weather, chemical facilities, and vulnerable communities in the U.S. Gulf Coast: A Disastrous Combination. Geohealth 2019;3(5):122–6.

79. Risser MD, Wehner MF. Attributable human-induced changes in the likelihood and magnitude of the observed extreme precipitation during hurricane Harvey. Geophys Res Lett 2017;44(24):12457–64.

80. Friedrich MJ. Determining health effects of hazardous materials released during Hurricane Harvey. JAMA 2017;318(23):2283–5.

81. Environmental Protection Agency, E. National priorities list (npl) sites-by state. 2020; Available at: https://www.epa.gov/superfund/national-priorities-list-npl-sites-state. Accessed June 20, 2023.

82. U.S. Department of Housing and Urban Development. Letter Finding Noncompliance with Title VI and Section 109. 2021; Available at: https://www.houstontx.gov/mayor/press/2022/hud-glo-discriminates.pdf. Accessed June 20, 2023.

83. Rudolph L, Harrison C, Buckley L, et al. Climate change, health, and equity: a guide for local health departments. Public Health Institute; 2018. Available at: https://www.apha.org/-/media/files/pdf/topics/climate/climate_health_equity.ashx. Accessed June 20, 2023.

84. Hassan AM, Nogueira L, Lin YL, et al. Impact of heatwaves on cancer care delivery: potential mechanisms, health equity concerns, and adaptation strategies. J Clin Oncol 2023;Jco2201951.

85. Warne D, Wescott S. Social determinants of American Indian Nutritional Health. Curr Dev Nutr 2019;3(Suppl 2):12–8.

86. Whyte K. Indigenous food systems, environmental justice, and settler-industrial states. 2016 Available at: https://kylewhyte.marcom.cal.msu.edu/wp-content/uploads/sites/12/2018/07/IP_Food_Systems__EJ_and_Settler_States1-1-16.pdf.

87. Hilmers A, Hilmers DC, Dave J. Neighborhood disparities in access to healthy foods and their effects on environmental justice. Am J Public Health 2012; 102(9):1644–54.
88. García-Pérez J, Fernández de Larrea-Baz N, Lope V, et al. Residential proximity to industrial pollution sources and colorectal cancer risk: a multicase-control study (MCC-Spain). Environ Int 2020;144:106055.
89. Lee JG, Henriksen L, Rose SW, et al. A systematic review of neighborhood disparities in point-of-sale tobacco marketing. Am J Public Health 2015;105(9): e8–18.
90. Trangenstein PJ, Gray C, Rossheim ME, et al. Alcohol outlet clusters and population disparities. J Urban Health 2020;97(1):123–36.
91. Eddie R, Curley C, Yazzie D, et al. Practicing tribal sovereignty through a tribal health policy: implementation of the healthy Diné Nation Act on the Navajo nation. Prev Chronic Dis 2022;19:E78.
92. Vaidyanathan A, Malilay J, Schramm P, et al. Heat-related deaths - United States, 2004-2018. MMWR Morb Mortal Wkly Rep 2020;69(24):729–34.
93. Méndez-Lázaro PA, Pérez-Cardona CM, Rodríguez E, et al. Climate change, heat, and mortality in the tropical urban area of San Juan, Puerto Rico. Int J Biometeorol 2018;62(5):699–707.
94. Santos-Lozada AR, Howard JT. Use of death counts from vital statistics to calculate excess deaths in Puerto Rico following Hurricane Maria. JAMA 2018; 320(14):1491–3.
95. Nogueira LM, Crane TE, Ortiz AP, et al. Climate change and cancer. Cancer Epidemiol Biomarkers Prev 2023;32(7):869–75.
96. Boeckmann M, Zeeb H. Justice and equity implications of climate change adaptation: a theoretical evaluation framework. Healthcare (Basel) 2016;4(3).
97. Joseph SR, Voyles C, Williams KD, et al. Colonial neglect and the right to health in puerto rico after Hurricane Maria. Am J Public Health 2020;110(10):1512–8.
98. Méndez-Lázaro PA, Bernhardt YM, Calo WA, et al. Environmental stressors suffered by women with gynecological cancers in the aftermath of Hurricanes Irma and María in Puerto Rico. Int J Environ Res Public Health 2021;18(21).
99. Rodríguez-Díaz CE. Maria in Puerto Rico: natural disaster in a colonial archipelago. Am J Public Health 2018;108(1):30–2.
100. Domingue SJ, Emrich CT. Social vulnerability and procedural equity: exploring the distribution of disaster aid across counties in the United States. Am Rev Publ Adm 2019;49(8):897–913.
101. Shultz JM, Sands DE, Kossin JP, et al. Double environmental injustice - climate change, Hurricane Dorian, and the Bahamas. N Engl J Med 2020;382(1):1–3.
102. Lustgarten A. Across the Caribbean, soaring national debt is a hidden but decisive aspect of the climate crisis, hobbling countries' ability to protect themselves from disaster. One island's leader is fighting to find a way out. 2022; Available at: https://www.propublica.org/article/mia-mottley-barbados-imf-climate-change. Accessed June 20, 2023.
103. Levy BS, Patz JA. Climate change, human rights, and social justice. Ann Glob Health 2015;81(3):310–22.
104. Carlisle L. Healing grounds: climate, justice, and the deep roots of regenerative farming. Washington, DC: Taylor & Francis; 2022.
105. Bullard RD. Environmental justice in the 21st century: race still matters. Phylon 2001;49(3/4):151–71.
106. Whyte K. Against crisis epistemology. Hokowhitu B, et al, editor. Routledge handbook of critical indigenous studies. 2021. 52–64.

107. McGhee H. The sum of us: what racism costs everyone and how we can prosper together. New York: One World; 2022.

108. Tessum CW, Apte JS, Goodkind AL, et al. Inequity in consumption of goods and services adds to racial-ethnic disparities in air pollution exposure. Proc Natl Acad Sci U S A 2019;116(13):6001–6.

109. Penn I, Lipton E, Angotti-Jones G. The lithium gold rush: inside the race to power electric vehicles. The New York Times 2021. Available at: https://www.nytimes.com/2021/05/06/business/lithium-mining-race.html. Accessed June 20, 2023.

110. Ebi KL, Hess JJ. Health risks due to climate change: inequity in causes and consequences. Health Aff 2020;39(12):2056–62.

111. Climate Justice Alliance. Just Transition Principles. 2020; Available at: https://climatejusticealliance.org/wp-content/uploads/2019/11/CJA_JustTransition_highres.pdf. Accessed June 20, 2023.

112. Shultz JM, Sands DE, Holder-Hamilton N, et al. Scrambling for safety in the eye of Dorian: mental health consequences of exposure to a climate-driven hurricane. Health Aff 2020;39(12):2120–7.

113. Zotova O, Pétrin-Desrosiers C, Gopfert A, et al. Carbon-neutral medical conferences should be the norm. Lancet Planet Health 2020;4(2):e48–50.

114. Sherman JD, MacNeill AJ, Biddinger PD, et al. Sustainable and Resilient Health Care in the Face of a Changing Climate. Annu Rev Public Health 2022.

115. Johnson M, Parada H Jr, Ferran K, et al. Perceptions of preparedness, timing of cancer diagnosis, and objective emergency preparedness among gynecological cancer patients in Puerto Rico before and after Hurricane Maria. J Cancer Policy 2023;36:100415.

116. Espinel Z, Shultz JM, Aubry VP, et al. Protecting vulnerable patient populations from climate hazards: the role of the Nations' Cancer Centers. J Natl Cancer Inst 2023.

117. Colón-López V, Sánchez-Cabrera Y, Soto-Salgado M, et al. 'More stressful than cancer': treatment experiences lived during hurricane maria among breast and colorectal cancer patients in Puerto Rico. Res Sq 2023.

118. Kishore N, Marqués D, Mahmud A, et al. Mortality in Puerto Rico after Hurricane Maria. N Engl J Med 2018;379(2):162–70.

119. Mutebi M, Dehar N, Nogueira LM, et al. Cancer groundshot: building a robust cancer control platform in addition to launching the cancer moonshot. Am Soc Clin Oncol Educ Book 2022;42:1–16.

120. Olhoff A, Christensen JM. Emissions Gap Report 2020. 2020; Available at: https://www.unep.org/emissions-gap-report-2020. Accessed June 20, 2023.

121. Dzau VJ, Levine R, Barrett G, et al. Decarbonizing the U.S. Health sector - A call to action. N Engl J Med 2021;385(23):2117–9.

122. Singh H, Eckelman M, Berwick DM, et al. Mandatory reporting of emissions to achieve net-zero health care. N Engl J Med 2022;387(26):2469–76.

123. Herzog A. The Inflation Reduction Act brings new opportunities for health care's climate action. 2022; Available at: https://noharm.medium.com/the-inflation-reduction-act-brings-new-opportunities-for-health-cares-climate-action-f47a14202c5. Accessed June 20, 2023.

124. Haines A, Ebi K. The imperative for climate action to protect health. N Engl J Med 2019;380(3):263–73.

125. Eckelman MJ, Sherman J. Environmental impacts of the U.S. Health Care System and effects on public health. PLoS One 2016;11(6):e0157014.

126. Gundersen Health. Leading the way toward a sustainable, healthy future. 2023; Accessed; Available at: https://www.gundersenenvision.org/.
127. Adgate JL, Goldstein BD, McKenzie LM. Potential public health hazards, exposures and health effects from unconventional natural gas development. Environ Sci Technol 2014;48(15):8307–20.
128. Emanuel RE, Caretta MA, Rivers L 3rd, et al. Natural gas gathering and transmission pipelines and social vulnerability in the United States. Geohealth 2021;5(6). e2021GH000442.
129. Bouley T, Roschnik S, Karliner J, et al. Climate-smart healthcare: low-carbon and resilience strategies for the health sector. 2017; Available at: http://documents.worldbank.org/curated/en/322251495434571418/pdf/113572-WP-PUBLIC-FINAL-WBG-Climate-smart-Healthcare-002.pdf. Accessed June 20, 2023.
130. Sherman JD, MacNeill A, Thiel C. Reducing pollution from the health care industry. JAMA 2019;322(11):1043–4.
131. Landrigan PJ, Raps H, Cropper M, et al. The Minderoo-Monaco commission on plastics and human health. Ann Glob Health 2023;89(1):23.
132. Banzhaf S, Ma L, Timmins C. Environmental justice: the economics of race, place, and pollution. J Econ Perspect 2019;33(1):185–208.
133. Donaghy TQ, Healy N, Jiang CY, et al. Fossil fuel racism in the United States: how phasing out coal, oil, and gas can protect communities. Energy Res Social Sci 2023;100:103104.
134. Ash M, Boyce JK, Chang G, et al. Is environmental justice good for white folks? Industrial air toxics exposure in Urban America. Soc Sci Q 2013;94(3):616–36.
135. Fowlie M, Walker R, Wooley D. Climate policy, environmental justice, and local air pollution. Berkeley: University of California; 2020.
136. Garcia-Gonzales DA, Shonkoff SBC, Hays J, et al. Hazardous air pollutants associated with upstream oil and natural gas development: a critical synthesis of current peer-reviewed literature. Annu Rev Public Health 2019;40:283–304.
137. Pullen Fedinick K, Yiliqi I, Lam Y, et al. A cumulative framework for identifying overburdened populations under the toxic substances control act: formaldehyde case study. Int J Environ Res Public Health 2021;18(11).
138. Raheja G, Harper L, Hoffman A, et al. Community-based participatory research for low-cost air pollution monitoring in the wake of unconventional oil and gas development in the Ohio River Valley: empowering impacted residents through community science. Environ Res Lett 2022;17(6):065006.
139. Peters E, Salas RN. Communicating statistics on the health effects of climate change. N Engl J Med 2022.
140. Salas RN, Friend TH, Bernstein A, et al. Adding a climate lens to health policy in the United States. Health Aff 2020;39(12):2063–70.
141. Park H, County F, County W. Local Policies for Environmental Justice: A National Scan. 2019; Accessed; Available at: https://www.nrdc.org/sites/default/files/local-policies-environmental-justice-national-scan-tishman-201902.pdf.

Breast Cancer in India
Screening, Detection, and Management

Prarthna V. Bhardwaj, MBBS[a], Renuka Dulala, MD[b],
Senthil Rajappa, MD[c], Chandravathi Loke, MD[a],*

KEYWORDS

• Breast cancer • India • Global oncology • Cancer in India

KEY POINTS

• Breast cancer is the most common cancer in urban Indian women and the second most common cancer in all Indian women, following cervical cancer. It tends to occur in younger women at a more advanced stage and with a more aggressive course compared with Western women.

• The lack of population-based breast cancer screening programs and delay in seeking a medical consult due to financial and social reasons, including lack of awareness and fear related to a cancer diagnosis, results in delayed diagnosis.

• Limited access to high-quality multimodality treatment facilities, few large treatment facilities, and financial constraints result in compromised quality of care to patients with established cancer.

• Care of breast cancer remains heterogeneous across the country.

INTRODUCTION

The epidemiology of breast cancer differs in Indian women compared with those of the Western world. Over 100,000 new patients with breast cancer are estimated to be diagnosed in India annually.[1] With rising awareness and incidence, breast cancer is the most common cancer in urban Indian women and the second most common in rural Indian women, following cervical cancer.[1–3] The projected cancer burden in India for 2021 was 26.7 million Disability-Adjusted Life Years (disability-adjusted life year is a measure of overall disease burden, expressed as the number of years lost due to ill-health, disability, or early death) and is expected to increase to 29.8 million by 2025. Further, in 2016, over 40% of the total cancer burden was contributed by seven leading cancer sites, with breast cancer being the second most common cancer

[a] Division of Hematology-Oncology, University of Massachusetts Chan Medical School - Baystate, 759 Chestnut Street, Springfield, MA 01199, USA; [b] Division of Hematology-Oncology, Holyoke Medical Center, 575 Beech Street, Holyoke, MA 01040, USA; [c] Department of Medical Oncology, Basavatarakam Indo-American Cancer Hospital and Research Institute, Road no. 10, Banjara Hills, Hyderabad, Telangana 500034, India
* Corresponding author. 759 Chestnut Street, Springfield, MA 01199.
E-mail address: Chandravathi.loke@baystatehealth.org

Hematol Oncol Clin N Am 38 (2024) 123–135
https://doi.org/10.1016/j.hoc.2023.05.014
0889-8588/24/© 2023 Elsevier Inc. All rights reserved.

(10.5%).[4] The incidence-to-mortality ratio is high for breast cancer in India attributed to late-stage presentation, inadequate medical facilities, lack of awareness, and lack of routine mammography screening.[5,6]

Generally, breast cancer has been reported to occur a decade earlier in Indian women compared with their Western counterparts, although this is difficult to compare directly due to the lack of screening mammograms in India. More than 80% of diagnosed Indian patients are younger than 60 years, with an average age of 48 to 53 years, and a higher proportion of women diagnosed with breast cancer in India are premenopausal (~40% to 50%) compared with women in the United States.[7–9] In fact, a considerable proportion (11% to 26%) of Indian women with breast cancer are younger than 35 years, and these young patients tend to have higher grade and receptor-negative tumors.[10] Based on the largest data set of early-stage breast cancer from three Indian centers, the median age at the time of diagnosis was 53 years. In this study, 11.8% of patients were diagnosed with stage I breast cancer, 66.8% were diagnosed with stage II cancer, and 21.64% with stage III cancer. Of these patients, 55.2% were hormone receptor-positive, 24.2% triple-negative, and 20.6% human epidermal growth factor receptor 2 (HER-2)-positive.[11]

As a subcontinent with wide ethnic, cultural, religious, economic, and linguistic diversity, health care facility patterns are heterogeneous across the country. Illiteracy, lack of awareness, financial constraints, lack of surgical options other than mastectomy, and social stigma associated with a cancer diagnosis are some reasons why women often do not present for early medical care, resulting in most women being treated at locally advanced and metastatic stages.[9]

Early and multiple childbirths, marriage at an early age, and breastfeeding all children for an extended period (up to 2 years) are common in most Indian households, although the educated urban class is moving away from this practice. In addition, other factors such as a sedentary lifestyle, increased tobacco/alcohol consumption, and increasing incidence of metabolic syndrome and obesity have likely contributed to the rising incidence of breast cancer.[12]

Detection of Breast Cancer in India

Population-based, organized breast cancer screening services are almost nonexistent in low- and middle-income countries (LMICs) like India, making the benefits of screening, early detection, and multidisciplinary programs not available uniformly throughout the country. Indeed, breast cancer awareness programs are concentrated in larger cities, but have not yet reached remote and rural parts of the country.[13] Even among health care professionals, awareness about warning signs, risk factors, and screening practices of breast cancers is less than satisfactory.[14] Screening uptake tends to be higher in older women in urban residences, having higher education, employment, and health insurance, and those using electronic media.[15,16] The lack of governmental support for screening, diagnosis, and treatment costs are other major deterrents to obtaining timely medical care. Resultingly, most patients self-detect their disease at a stage when it presents with a palpable lump or with secondary changes related to chest wall changes or distant metastases.

Various screening modes in India include mammograms, breast self-examination (BSE), and clinical breast examination (CBE).

Mammography screening is a complex undertaking requiring substantial resources and infrastructure in LMICs. Although mammograms have demonstrated breast cancer-specific mortality reduction in women of ages 50 to 69 years in developed countries, it may not be as effective in LMICs with a lower incidence and younger population structure that results in younger age at diagnosis. The per capita spending on health in India is approximately $81.[17] This is less than Medicare reimbursement of a digital mammogram at $135,[18] making mammography screening not a cost-effective solution for most Indian women.[19] The potential for overdiagnosis and overtreatment associated with mammography is likely to overburden the health care system, too, which is already facing a resource crunch.

BSE is a reasonable and feasible approach to early detection and reduction of breast cancer mortality in India and other developing countries.[20–22] Studies have also suggested that BSE can be used to create breast health awareness among women, allowing trained female health workers to play a promising role in disseminating this knowledge among women to carry out BSE.[23] BSE in India is concentrated among wealthier populations defined by place of residence, religion, age, employment, and marital status presently.[24]

CBE is a simple and less expensive screening tool that seems promising. There are two randomized controlled trials on CBE screening versus no screening from the Indian subcontinent.[25,26] Among these, CBE was conducted by trained primary health care workers in Mumbai, India, demonstrating significant downstaging of breast cancers in all age groups and a 30% reduction in mortality among women greater than 50 years of age at the end of 20 years without any concerns for overdiagnosis.[23,27] However, such mortality benefit was not observed in women younger than 50 years, pointing toward less sensitivity of CBE in younger women and other potentially undetermined biological factors. Furthermore, whether incorporating CBE as a sole method of screening at a population level translates into an actual decrement in patient mortality is yet to be established. However, its benefits have been deemed to be similar to mammograms and are less expensive.[28]

A cost-effectiveness analysis was performed for breast cancer in India based on a microsimulation screening analysis model that included an evaluation of CBE and mammography screening among various age groups and at different time intervals based on projected costs, its benefits in terms of mortality reduction, and its effectiveness vis-a-vis cost.[29] Accordingly, in India, 2-yearly CBE screening was projected to be a cost-effective breast cancer screening method, meeting the World Health Organization criterion. If changed to yearly screening, though, its benefit in terms of cost-effectiveness would not be retained but would be as efficacious as biennial mammography screening for reducing breast cancer mortality among ages 40 to 60 years while incurring only half the net costs. The estimated cost-effectiveness of CBE screening for breast cancer in India compares favorably with mammography in developed countries.[19]

Cultural and Socioeconomic Barriers

Screening and management of breast cancer in India are intricately linked to cultural and social factors. Women from low socioeconomic families and those having low income and less education may not seek medical care on discovering a breast lump. This is often due to a lack of awareness regarding what the lump represents, the social stigma of being rejected by the community or partner, the prevailing taboo of not discussing the topic of cancer openly, fear of loss of the breast when surgical options other than mastectomy are not available, and reliance on non-allopathic therapies.[30–32] Studies have found fatalistic attitudes as one of the barriers to the uptake of breast cancer screening, in which Indian women often believe that events are governed by the doctrine of fate.[33] Indeed, studies regarding health-seeking attitudes of women have suggested that Indians mainly reported emotional rather than a logistic or practical barrier to seeking medical help among women across all socioeconomic groups.[21,34] Even among educated women, uptake of breast cancer screening is unsatisfactory despite knowing the risk factors, signs and symptoms, and availability of screening tools.[35,36]

In a populous country with limited health care professionals, Accredited Social Health Activist (ASHA) women, trained nonmedical health personnel from the same or nearby community who can quickly establish rapport with patients, have high acceptance as educators in rural communities.[37,38] The involvement of ASHA in breast cancer screening programs could overcome several obstacles faced by women in remote parts of the country with limited access to health care, including shyness and hesitation during examination by a male physician and the need for a male to escort them to a health care facility.[38]

In urban communities, increased awareness programs can be a feasible and acceptable way of ensuring compliance with screening.[39–41] Numerous other initiatives, including those by nongovernmental organizations including "Helping Hand 4 Cancer Care," Prashanti Cancer Care Mission Pune, The Cancer Patients Aid Association, and "Maina Foundation" are considered to be socially and culturally acceptable and cost-effective solutions for breast cancer detection and management in urban settings.[42,43]

Genetic Testing in India

India harbors a young breast cancer population with a higher prevalence of triple-negative breast cancer,[44] suggesting a high projected burden of hereditary breast cancer; the incidence of pathogenic variants causing breast cancer has ranged from 18% to 36%.[45–47] Potential prevention opportunities remain undefined though due to lack of population and hospital-based studies. The National Comprehensive Cancer Network criteria are universally followed, including in Indian centers, but have not been formally validated in the Indian setting. The effectiveness of pretest and posttest counseling performed by a medical oncologist has shown the feasibility of mainstreaming genetic testing, an urgent need in LMICs due to a shortage of trained cancer genetic counselors and the potential therapeutic implications.[45] In addition to lack of research, cost and scarcity of resources remain barriers to routine implementation of such germline testing.[48]

Treatment Patterns: Surgical and Medical

A critical barrier to optimal breast cancer treatment is a workforce shortage. India seems to have around 8000 oncologists including surgical, radiation, and medical oncologists with the number of oncologists being lower in semi-urban and rural areas.[49–51] Further, although nearly 70% of the Indian population lives in rural areas, about 95% of cancer treatment facilities exist in the country's urban areas, and nearly 60% of specialist facilities are in Southern and Western India, whereas over 50% of the population lives in the Northern, Central, and Eastern regions.[52] Regarding diagnostics, there is an absence of uniform standardization of basic procedures such as fixation and processing and hence non-uniform reporting of receptor subtypes of breast cancer. The results of HER-2 testing across states are also non-uniform as economics drive testing protocols too. No study has accurately determined the economic burden of the disease among Indian patients; however, costs are expected to be high due to high out-of-pocket expenditures in both the public and private sectors. A 2016 study from North India revealed that obtaining treatment from the private sector was more expensive than the public sector, with costs increasing with older age and a higher stage of diagnosis.[53] The typical out-of-pocket expenditure for breast cancer in 2014 was INR 29,066 in the public sector but INR 84,320 in the private sector (USD 1715.82 and USD 4977.56, respectively, at 2014 purchasing power parity).

Nearly half of low-income households in rural settings used borrowings, the sale of assets, and contributions from friends and relatives to pay for treatment expenditures related to breast cancer. Finally, more than 50% of patients from low-income households spent greater than 20% of their annual household expenditure on breast cancer treatment, resulting in catastrophic payments.[54]

Expenditures have increased due to expensive infrastructure, new technology-based research costs, and newer therapies. The cost of targeted therapy on the WHO Essential Medicine List for Stage I HER2 positive breast cancer, for example, is projected to be comparable to approximately 10 years of average yearly income in India.[55,56] Although work remains to be done, national public health insurance schemes such as "Ayushman Bharat" have aligned cancer care and payments with the National Cancer Grid (NCG) guidelines. NCG is a network of major cancer centers, research institutes, patient groups, and charitable institutions across India, mandated to establish uniform standards for prevention, diagnosis, and treatment of cancer. This has resulted in a significant decrease in the cost burden borne by women from lower socioeconomic groups. In addition, there are several drug-patient assistance programs from pharmaceutical companies such as Roche, Novartis, Dr Reddy's, and so forth, which help follow patient-centric care from the start to the end.

Breast surgery

Compared with high-income countries (HICs), patients from India have more advanced tumors with higher likelihood of lymph node involvement.[57] Breast-conserving surgery (BCS) has been demonstrated to be safe and feasible in a limited resource setting, leading surgeons to offer this, albeit mainly to women with smaller tumors.[10] BCS was initially carried out primarily at larger high-volume centers with mammography and radiation facilities, though this was short-lived due to the lack of breast surgeons, specifically.[58,59] Overall, rates of breast conservation surgery seem to be lower than HICs; however, rates remain variable across the country.[57,59,60] Less BCS has largely been due to the need for a preoperative mammography, which is available only in a limited fashion in rural areas. In a study by Nadkarni and colleagues, 38 out of 735 women would have been wrongly planned for BCS based on clinical findings alone without a mammogram. Of the 38 patients, 13 had multicentric disease that was non-palpable and 25 had extensive microcalcifications.[61] Furthermore, quite a few women decline BCS and tend to choose mastectomies due to fear of recurrence, potential need for repeat surgeries, fear of radiation, and a predetermined opinion formed by the patient or her family, irrespective of the pros and cons of various available surgical options.[62] Other factors for low uptake of BCS include limited access to neoadjuvant therapies, late presentations, inappropriate initial surgical management, and poor quality of pathology reporting on biopsy and surgical specimens.[9]

Regarding axillary management, complete axillary dissection remains the standard treatment in cases of node-positive breast cancer per the NCG guidelines.[63] Low axillary sampling (LAS) has been compared with sentinel lymph node biopsy in clinically node-negative breast cancer and has been known to be as accurate in predicting axillary nodal status,[64] but its success depends on the availability of appropriate radiation and other adjuvant therapies.

Radiotherapy

Radiation oncologists previously offered standard dose fractionation of 50 Gy/25 fraction regimens for radiation therapy, but using hypo-fractionated radiotherapy (40 Gy in 15 fractions over 3 weeks) irrespective of BCS or mastectomy showed similar overall survival, disease-free survival, and locoregional recurrence-free survival as standard fractionation.[65,66] For a limited resource country like India with limited access to radiotherapy, the use of this 3-week regimen allows treatment of one extra patient for every two patients treated, compared with the standard 5-week regimen. This is also logistically more advantageous for patients, resulting in improved compliance. Resulting, most centers have now shifted to hypo-fractionated radiation therapy. Postmastectomy radiation is not widely offered, despite the improvement in survival for locally advanced breast cancers.

Systemic therapies
A wide variety of chemotherapy regimens are in use. Most agree that anthracycline-based combination chemotherapy is the appropriate first-line chemotherapy for most patients based on the acknowledgment that anthracycline-based regimens are superior when compared with cyclophosphamide-methotrexate-5FU combination. Anthracycline and taxane-based therapies are widely available, including under the Ayushman Bharat scheme. Neoadjuvant chemotherapy has also been used, although the most common indication remains locally advanced breast cancer, for which anthracycline and taxane-based regimens are commonly used. The reported rates of pathologic complete response in the Indian setting most recently seems to be consistent with that of the western population.[67]

Limited access to anti-HER-2 therapy has been reported by several centers in India,[68,69] though this has improved in recent years with the availability of biosimilars and active philanthropic support.[70,71]

In determining adjuvant chemotherapy for hormone receptor–positive and HER-2-negative early-stage breast cancers, the utility of genomic tests such as Oncotype Dx, MammaPrint, Prosigna, and Endopredict have allowed for de-escalation of therapy with oncotype Dx and MammaPrint being validated in large prospective trials.[72–74] However, few patients in LMICs have access to these genomic assays due to exorbitant costs, putting many women with ER-positive tumors at risk for overtreatment with toxic chemotherapy. None of the widely available genomic assays recommended in international guidelines have been validated for use among Indians, though CanAssist Breast Test (an immunohistochemistry [IHC]-based test that when combined with tumor size, nodal status, and tumor grade generates a score for every patient) has been proposed to optimize treatment decision for chemotherapy use among hormone receptor-positive and HER-2-negative early-stage breast cancer in India based on consensus guidelines.[75,76] This is based on data available from retrospective studies that demonstrate the test being prognostic for distant recurrences.[77–79] Of note, there are several critiques to this method, as an IHC-based assay is seemingly inferior to RNA-based assay in terms of reliability. In addition, Akhade and colleagues question the method used to develop the consensus guidelines and the lack of prospective trials to guide decision-making.[80]

Small single-institution studies have demonstrated that neoadjuvant therapies available for HER-2-positive breast cancers have similar pathologic complete rates compared with the Western world.[81] However, the current cost of dual HER-2-based adjuvant therapy in the Indian market is approximately INR 3,000,000 (USD $38,720), nearly six times the annual per capita income adjusted for purchasing power (USD $6371).[82] The use of biosimilars has decreased the cost of the therapy significantly without compromising on efficacy and is gaining popularity in several institutions.[83]

Endocrine therapy
Adjuvant hormonal therapy protocols in India are similar to those of the West.[63] Increasingly, physicians agree that patients with high-risk cancer should be offered extended endocrine therapy.[84]

Metastatic breast cancer

Although 5% to 10% of patients present with de novo metastatic breast cancer in the West, this number is between 5% and 25% for women in India.[9,57] Hormone receptor-positive status, oligo-metastasis, and good performance status were associated with more favorable outcomes.[7] Discordance in receptor status at the time of metastases is present in 21% of hormone receptor and 15% of HER-2 receptor status with the recommendation to repeat biomarker studies at metastatic recurrence, consistent with international guidelines.[85] Based on an open-label randomized control trial based at the Tata Memorial Center in Mumbai, there is no evidence to suggest locoregional treatment of primary tumor results in a survival benefit among patients with metastatic breast cancer.[86]

The use of comprehensive genomic profiling in India is mainly limited to urban centers, as only 15% of patients with breast cancer in a large multicenter study in India underwent next-generation sequencing.[87] Of such, none with breast cancer received targeted therapy. Despite the promise of precision medicine, the uptake of comprehensive genomic profiling remains limited due to cost of sequencing, lack of access to specific targeted therapies, and the economic burden of using targeted therapy in a country with high out-of-pocket expenditure. The NCG of India guidelines do not presently enlist most targeted therapies as essential.[63]

Breast Cancer Survivorship

There is a paucity of data available related to breast cancer survivorship in India. For follow-up of patients with early-stage breast cancer, surveillance practices vary across different settings. Astoundingly, a survey of 158 medical oncologists in India showed that 90% of them felt a CBE to be an uncomfortable practice for patients and physicians.[88] Nearly 40% of them ordered screening chest x-rays and ultrasounds of the abdomen for routine surveillance of early-stage breast cancer. A bone density scan was recommended by approximately 50% of the physicians for patients on aromatase inhibitors, highlighting the disparity between scientific recommendations and real-world follow-up practices in LMICs.

A study on the physical, social, psychological, and economic concerns of Indian adult cancer survivors revealed that most of the survivors experienced fatigue (52%) and loss of appetite (27%). A high percentage also reported significant financial setbacks, receiving no financial assistance during or after treatments. Social anxiety, post-traumatic stress disorder, and depression were common.[89] Another hospital-based cross-sectional study among North Indian breast cancer survivors demonstrated that the most significant factors negatively impacting quality of life were emotional distress, cancer-related fatigue, and premature menopause resulting in sexual dysfunction.[90] Although various consensus guidelines are now available in India in efforts to improve the consistency of care for breast cancer,[63,91] survivorship care remains poorly studied.

Despite the standard treatment guidelines enacted by the NCG for management of cancers and the free treatment being provided by the government under the Ayushman Bharat Health scheme for low socioeconomic backgrounds, disparities exist in lack of access and uniformity of care due to the limited oncology work force, lack of universal insurance coverage, high cost of care (especially in the private sector), lack of drug access programs for patients without the means to pay for therapy, and low health literacy. There is ample evidence that following standard treatment guidelines results in outcomes similar to Western countries.[11] Although generic and biosimilar drugs have increased availability of cancer drugs, access to newer targeted therapies and monoclonal antibodies remains very limited. Better implementation of the standard cost-effective, value-based management guidelines, price regulation, investing in development of indigenous pharmaceutical research into cancer medicines, and greater budget allocation for health care, may significantly improve treatment outcomes.[92]

SUMMARY

The management of breast cancers continues to evolve in India amid the increasing burden of the disease. Greater emphasis on awareness and early detection is necessary to reduce the burden of mortality. Emphasis should also be placed on standardizing pathologic testing and reporting so that patients may obtain appropriate treatment. Standardization of surgical, radiation, and oncologic care using cost-effective solutions should also be investigated. With standardized management, outcomes like those of developed countries can be expected. Finally, clinical trials geared towards a more diverse population in different LMICs like India should be undertaken.

CLINICS CARE POINTS

- In the jargon of challenges of breast cancer control, prioritizing implementation of a cost-effective, risk-stratified national cancer screening program for early detection of breast cancer is the need of the hour.
- The availability of government provided health care schemes and biosimilars in treatment of breast cancers have decreased the cost burden of breast cancer in India.
- Efforts should be directed toward decreasing stigma, improving awareness and promoting health literacy among patients and their providers.
- The global cancer community at large should strive toward bridging the gap between care delivery in low- and middle-income countries and high-income countries to make cancer care more equitable across the globe.

DISCLOSURE

P.V. Bhardwaj has stock options with Doximity. Other authors have nothing to disclose.

REFERENCES

1. Agarwal G, Pradeep PV, Aggarwal V, et al. Spectrum of breast cancer in Asian women. World J Surg 2007;31(5):1031–40.
2. Mathur P, Sathishkumar K, Chaturvedi M, et al. Cancer Statistics, 2020: Report From National Cancer Registry Programme, India. JCO Glob Oncol 2020;6: 1063–75.
3. Chaturvedi M, Sathishkumar K, Lakshminarayana SK, et al. Women cancers in India: Incidence, trends and their clinical extent from the National Cancer Registry Programme. Cancer Epidemiol 2022;80:102248.
4. Kulothungan V, Sathishkumar K, Leburu S, et al. Burden of cancers in India - estimates of cancer crude incidence, YLLs, YLDs and DALYs for 2021 and 2025 based on National Cancer Registry Program. BMC Cancer 2022;22(1):527.
5. Dikshit R, Gupta PC, Ramasundarahettige C, et al. Cancer mortality in India: a nationally representative survey. Lancet Lond Engl 2012;379(9828):1807–16.

6. The burden of cancers and their variations across the states of India: the Global Burden of Disease Study 1990–2016. Lancet Oncol 2018;19(10):1289–306.

7. Gogia A, Deo SVS, Sharma D, et al. Clinicopathologic Characteristics and Treatment Outcomes of Patients With Up-Front Metastatic Breast Cancer: Single-Center Experience in India. J Glob Oncol 2019;5:1–9.

8. Gogia A, Raina V, Deo SVS, et al. Triple-negative breast cancer: An institutional analysis. Indian J Cancer 2014;51(2):163.

9. Agarwal G, Ramakant P. Breast Cancer Care in India: The Current Scenario and the Challenges for the Future. Breast Care 2008;3(1):21–7.

10. Dinshaw KA, Sarin R, Budrukkar AN, et al. Safety and feasibility of breast conserving therapy in Indian women: two decades of experience at Tata Memorial Hospital. J Surg Oncol 2006;94(2):105–13.

11. Doval DC, Radhakrishna S, Tripathi R, et al. A multi-institutional real world data study from India of 3453 non-metastatic breast cancer patients undergoing up-front surgery. Sci Rep 2020;10:5886.

12. Paymaster JC, Gangadharan P. Some observations on the epidemiology of cancer of the breast in women of Western India. Int J Cancer 1972;10(3):443–50.

13. Chopra R. The Indian scene. J Clin Oncol Off J Am Soc Clin Oncol 2001;19(18 Suppl):106S–11S.

14. Bajaj K, Ravi A, Thakur U, et al. Awareness about breast cancer in first-year junior residents at a tertiary care institute in India: A cross-sectional study. Med J Armed Forces India 2021;77(Suppl 1):S208–14.

15. Changkun Z, Bishwajit G, Ji L, et al. Sociodemographic correlates of cervix, breast and oral cancer screening among Indian women. PLoS One 2022;17(5): e0265881.

16. Pal A, Taneja N, Malhotra N, et al. Knowledge, attitude, and practice towards breast cancer and its screening among women in India: A systematic review. J Cancer Res Ther 2021;17(6):1314–21.

17. World Health Organization. World health statistics 2010. World Health Organization; 2010. Available at: https://apps.who.int/iris/handle/10665/44292. Accessed October 27, 2022.

18. Available at: reimbursement-information-for-mammo-cad-and-digital-breast-tomosynthesis.pdf. https://www.gehealthcare.com/en-my/-/jssmedia/files/reimbursement/reimbursement-information-for-mammo-cad-and-digital-breast-tomosynthesis.pdf?rev=-1&hash=19570FB31A0A23B44FE0869CD9F1592A. Accessed November 10, 2022.

19. Zelle SG, Baltussen RM. Economic analyses of breast cancer control in low- and middle-income countries: a systematic review. Syst Rev 2013;2:20.

20. RamBihariLal Shrivastava S, Saurabh Shrivastava P, Ramasamy J. Self Breast Examination: A Tool for Early Diagnosis of Breast Cancer. Am J Public Health Res 2013;1(6):135–9.

21. Vidyarthi A, Soumya A, Choudhary S, et al. Barriers to Breast Cancer Screening In Young Indian Women: A Tale of Two Cities. Asian J Exp Sci 2013;27:29–35.

22. Somdatta P, Baridalyne N. Awareness of breast cancer in women of an urban re-settlement colony. Indian J Cancer 2008;45(4):149.

23. Mittra I, Mishra GA, Dikshit RP, et al. Effect of screening by clinical breast examination on breast cancer incidence and mortality after 20 years: prospective, cluster randomised controlled trial in Mumbai. BMJ 2021;372:n256.

24. Negi J, Nambiar D. Intersectional social-economic inequalities in breast cancer screening in India: analysis of the National Family Health Survey. BMC Wom Health 2021;21:324.

25. Mittra I, Mishra GA, Singh S, et al. A cluster randomized, controlled trial of breast and cervix cancer screening in Mumbai, India: methodology and interim results after three rounds of screening. Int J Cancer 2010;126(4):976–84.

26. Sankaranarayanan R, Ramadas K, Thara S, et al. Clinical breast examination: preliminary results from a cluster randomized controlled trial in India. J Natl Cancer Inst 2011;103(19):1476–80.

27. Shastri SS, Mittra I, Mishra GA, et al. Effect of VIA screening by primary health workers: randomized controlled study in Mumbai, India. J Natl Cancer Inst 2014;106(3):dju009.

28. Gyawali B, Shimokata T, Honda K, et al. Should low-income countries invest in breast cancer screening? Cancer Causes Control CCC 2016;27(11):1341–5.

29. Okonkwo QL, Dralsma G, der Kinderen A, et al. Breast cancer screening policies in developing countries: a cost-effectiveness analysis for India. J Natl Cancer Inst 2008;100(18):1290–300.

30. Maggi RM, Johnson AR, Agrawal T. Community perceptions and individual experiences of breast cancer in communities in and around Bangalore, India: a qualitative study. J Psychosoc Oncol 2022;40(2):234–46.

31. Rai A, Sharda P, Aggarwal P, et al. Study of Diagnostic Delay among Symptomatic Breast Cancer Patients in Northern India: A Mixed-Methods Analysis from a Dedicated Breast Cancer Centre. Asian Pac J Cancer Prev APJCP 2022; 23(3):893.

32. Daniel S, Venkateswaran C, Singh C, Hutchinson A, Johnson MJ. "So, when a woman becomes ill, the total structure of the family is affected, they can't do anything…" Voices from the community on women with breast cancer in India: a qualitative focus group study. Support Care Cancer 2022;30(1):951–63.

33. Charkazi A, Samimi A, Razzaghi K, et al. Adherence to Recommended Breast Cancer Screening in Iranian Turkmen Women: The Role of Knowledge and Beliefs. ISRN Prev Med 2013;2013:581027.

34. Mahalakshmi S, Suresh S. Barriers to Cancer Screening Uptake in Women: A Qualitative Study from Tamil Nadu, India. Asian Pac J Cancer Prev APJCP 2020;21(4):1081–7.

35. Subba SH, Parida SP, Sahu DP, et al. Knowledge and attitude towards, and the utilisation of cervical and breast cancer screening services by female healthcare professionals at a tertiary care hospital of Eastern India: A cross-sectional study. Niger Postgrad Med J 2022;29(1):63–9.

36. Bodapati SL, Babu GR. Oncologist perspectives on breast cancer screening in India- results from a qualitative study in Andhra Pradesh. Asian Pac J Cancer Prev APJCP 2013;14(10):5817–23.

37. Rao RSP, Nair S, Nair NS, et al. Acceptability and effectiveness of a breast health awareness programme for rural women in India. Indian J Med Sci 2005;59(9): 398–402.

38. Memon F, Saxena D, Puwar T, et al. Can urban Accredited Social Health Activist (ASHA) be change agent for breast cancer awareness in urban area: Experience from Ahmedabad India. J Fam Med Prim Care 2019;8(12):3881–6.

39. Kulkarni SV, Mishra GA, Dusane RR. Determinants of Compliance to Breast Cancer Screening and Referral in Low Socio-Economic Regions of Urban India. Int J Prev Med 2019;10:84.

40. Dahiya N, Basu S, Singh MC, et al. Knowledge and Practices Related to Screening for Breast Cancer among Women in Delhi, India. Asian Pac J Cancer Prev APJCP 2018;19(1):155–9.

41. Gadgil A, Sauvaget C, Roy N, et al. Breast Cancer Awareness among Middle Class Urban Women–a Community-Based Study from Mumbai, India. Asian Pac J Cancer Prev APJCP 2015;16(15):6249–54.
42. Maina Foundation. Available at: https://mainafoundation.org/. Accessed November 10, 2022.
43. D M. Helping Hands For Cancer Care. Dr. Suresh Advani. Available at: https://drsureshadvani.in/helping-hands-for-cancer-care/. Accessed November 10, 2022.
44. Sandhu GS, Erqou S, Patterson H, et al. Prevalence of Triple-Negative Breast Cancer in India: Systematic Review and Meta-Analysis. J Glob Oncol 2016; 2(6):412–21.
45. Mittal A, Deo SVS, Gogia A, et al. Profile of Pathogenic Mutations and Evaluation of Germline Genetic Testing Criteria in Consecutive Breast Cancer Patients Treated at a North Indian Tertiary Care Center. Ann Surg Oncol 2022;29(2): 1423–32.
46. Singh J, Thota N, Singh S, et al. Screening of over 1000 Indian patients with breast and/or ovarian cancer with a multi-gene panel: prevalence of BRCA1/2 and non-BRCA mutations. Breast Cancer Res Treat 2018;170(1):189–96.
47. Mannan AU, Singh J, Lakshmikeshava R, et al. Detection of high frequency of mutations in a breast and/or ovarian cancer cohort: implications of embracing a multi-gene panel in molecular diagnosis in India. J Hum Genet 2016;61(6): 515–22.
48. Parikh PM, Wadhwa J, Minhas S, et al. Practical consensus recommendation on when to do BRCA testing. South Asian J Cancer 2018;7(2):106–9.
49. Laskar SG, Sinha S, Krishnatry R, et al. Access to Radiation Therapy: From Local to Global and Equality to Equity. JCO Glob Oncol 2022;(8):e2100358.
50. Mehrotra R, Yadav K. Breast cancer in India: Present scenario and the challenges ahead. World J Clin Oncol 2022;13(3):209–18. https://doi.org/10.5306/wjco.v13. i3.209.
51. Indian Association of Surgical Oncology. Available at: https://www.iasoindia.in/. Accessed January 3, 2023.
52. Pramesh CS, Badwe RA, Borthakur BB, et al. Delivery of affordable and equitable cancer care in India. Lancet Oncol 2014;15(6):e223–33.
53. Jain M, Mukherjee K. Economic burden of breast cancer to the households in Punjab, India. Int J Med Public Health 2016;6(1):13.
54. Rajpal S, Kumar A, Joe W. Economic burden of cancer in India: Evidence from cross-sectional nationally representative household survey, 2014. PLoS One 2018;13(2):e0193320.
55. WHO report on cancer: setting priorities, investing wisely and providing care for all. Available at: https://www.who.int/publications-detail-redirect/9789240001299. Accessed October 27, 2022.
56. Sun L, Legood R, Dos-Santos-Silva I, et al. Global treatment costs of breast cancer by stage: A systematic review. PLoS One 2018;13(11):e0207993.
57. Vijaykumar DK, Arun S, Abraham AG, et al. Breast Cancer Care in South India: Is Practice Concordant With National Guidelines? J Glob Oncol 2019;5:1–7.
58. Rangarajan B, Shet T, Wadasadawala T, et al. Breast cancer: An overview of published Indian data. South Asian J Cancer 2016;5(3):86–92.
59. Hassan Ali S, Somashekhar SP, Arun Kumar N. Rate of Breast-Conserving Surgery vs Mastectomy in Breast Cancer: a Tertiary Care Centre Experience from South India. Indian J Surg Oncol 2019;10(1):72–6.

60. Kadam SS, Tripathi P, Jagtap R, et al. Modified Radical Mastectomy vs Breast-Conserving Surgery: Current Clinical Practice in Women with Early Stage Breast Cancer at a Corporate Tertiary Cancer Center in India. Indian J Surg Oncol 2022; 13(2):322–8.

61. Nadkarni MS, Gupta PB, Parmar VV, et al. Breast conservation surgery without pre-operative mammography–a definite feasibility. Breast Edinb Scotl 2006; 15(5):595–600.

62. Chatterjee S. Is India Overdoing Mastectomy? Indian J Surg 2021;83(2):275–7.

63. Available at: Breast_Cancer.pdf. Accessed November 10, 2022. https://tmc.gov.in/NCG/docs/PDF/Breast/Breast_Cancer.pdf.

64. Parmar V, Hawaldar R, Nair NS, et al. Sentinel node biopsy versus low axillary sampling in women with clinically node negative operable breast cancer. Breast Edinb Scotl 2013;22(6):1081–6.

65. Chatterjee S, Arunsingh M, Agrawal S, et al. Outcomes Following a Moderately Hypofractionated Adjuvant Radiation (START B Type) Schedule for Breast Cancer in an Unscreened Non-Caucasian Population. Clin Oncol R Coll Radiol G B 2016; 28(10):e165–72.

66. Yadav BS, Sharma SC, Singh R, et al. Postmastectomy radiation and survival in patients with breast cancer. J Cancer Res Ther 2007;3(4):218–24.

67. Neoadjuvant Platinum Plus Standard Chemotherapy Improves Survival in TNBC. OncLive. Available at: https://www.onclive.com/view/neoadjuvant-platinum-plus-standard-chemotherapy-improves-survival-in-tnbc. Accessed December 25, 2022.

68. Ghosh J, Gupta S, Desai S, et al. Estrogen, progesterone and HER2 receptor expression in breast tumors of patients, and their usage of HER2-targeted therapy, in a tertiary care centre in India. Indian J Cancer 2011;48(4):391.

69. Agrawal S, Banswal L, Saha A, et al. Progesterone Receptors, Pathological Complete Response and Early Outcome for Locally Advanced Breast Cancer - a Single Centre Study. (PPLB - 01). Indian J Surg Oncol 2016;7(4):397–406.

70. Nair NS, Gupta S, Ghosh J, et al. Access to Human Epidermal Growth Factor Receptor 2–Targeted Therapy at a Tertiary Care Center in India: An Evolution. J Glob Oncol 2018;4(Supplement 3):27s.

71. An Indian survey with oncologists for the use of biosimilar Trastuzumab in clinical practice. Available at: https://www.hilarispublisher.com/proceedings/an-indian-survey-with-oncologists-for-the-use-of-biosimilar-trastuzumab-in-clinical-practice-31003.html. Accessed November 3, 2022.

72. Kalinsky K, Barlow WE, Gralow JR, et al. 21-Gene Assay to Inform Chemotherapy Benefit in Node-Positive Breast Cancer. N Engl J Med 2021;385(25):2336–47.

73. Cardoso F, van't Veer LJ, Bogaerts J, et al. 70-Gene Signature as an Aid to Treatment Decisions in Early-Stage Breast Cancer. N Engl J Med 2016;375(8):717–29.

74. Sparano JA, Gray RJ, Makower DF, et al. Adjuvant Chemotherapy Guided by a 21-Gene Expression Assay in Breast Cancer. N Engl J Med 2018;379(2):111–21.

75. Parikh PM, Bhattacharyya GS, Biswas G, et al. Practical Consensus Recommendations for Optimizing Risk versus Benefit of Chemotherapy in Patients with HR Positive Her2 Negative Early Breast Cancer in India. South Asian J Cancer 2021;10(04):213–9.

76. Bhattacharyya GS, Doval DC, Desai CJ, et al. Overview of Breast Cancer and Implications of Overtreatment of Early-Stage Breast Cancer: An Indian Perspective. JCO Glob Oncol 2020;(6):789–98.

77. Attuluri AK, Serkad CPV, Gunda A, et al. Analytical validation of CanAssist-Breast: an immunohistochemistry based prognostic test for hormone receptor positive breast cancer patients. BMC Cancer 2019;19(1):249.

78. Sankaran S, Dikshit JB, Prakash Sv C, et al. CanAssist Breast Impacting Clinical Treatment Decisions in Early-Stage HR+ Breast Cancer Patients: Indian Scenario. Indian J Surg Oncol 2021;12(Suppl 1):21–9.

79. Bakre MM, Ramkumar C, Attuluri AK, et al. Clinical validation of an immunohistochemistry-based CanAssist-Breast test for distant recurrence prediction in hormone receptor-positive breast cancer patients. Cancer Med 2019; 8(4):1755–64.

80. Akhade A, Mathew A. To Give or Not to Give Adjuvant Chemotherapy in Breast Cancer? Can CanAssist Breast Assist? South Asian J Cancer 2022;11(01):001–2.

81. Arora S, Gogia DA, Deo S, et al. Neoadjuvant pertuzumab plus trastuzumab in combination with anthracycline- free chemotherapy regimen in patients with HER2 positive breast cancer-Real-world data from a single center in India. Cancer Treat Res Commun 2021;29:100483.

82. Chakraborty S, Wadasadawala T, Ahmed R, et al. Breast Cancer Demographics, Types and Management Pathways: Can Western Algorithms be Optimally used in Eastern Countries? Clin Oncol 2019;31(8):502–9.

83. Joel A, Georgy JT, Thumaty DB, et al. Neoadjuvant chemotherapy with biosimilar trastuzumab in human epidermal growth factor receptor 2 overexpressed non-metastatic breast cancer: patterns of use and clinical outcomes in India. Ecancermedicalscience 2021;15:1207.

84. Gupta S, Singh M, Vora A, et al. Practical consensus recommendations on duration of adjuvant hormonal therapy in breast cancer. South Asian J Cancer 2018; 7(2):142–5.

85. Gogia A, Deo SVS, Sharma D, et al. Discordance in Biomarker Expression in Breast Cancer After Metastasis: Single Center Experience in India. J Glob Oncol 2019;5:1–8.

86. Badwe R, Hawaldar R, Nair N, et al. Locoregional treatment versus no treatment of the primary tumour in metastatic breast cancer: an open-label randomised controlled trial. Lancet Oncol 2015;16(13):1380–8.

87. Mathew A, Joseph S, Boby J, et al. Clinical Benefit of Comprehensive Genomic Profiling for Advanced Cancers in India. JCO Glob Oncol 2022;(8):e2100421.

88. Patel A, Gupta VG, Guleria B, et al. Real-World Breast Cancer Patient Follow-Up Practices by Medical Oncologists in India-A Survey Report. South Asian J Cancer 2022;11(1):9–13.

89. Mohanti BK, Kaur J. Living experiences of Indian adult cancer survivors–a brief report. Asian Pac J Cancer Prev APJCP 2015;16(2):507–12.

90. Kaur N, Gupta A, Sharma AK, et al. Survivorship issues as determinants of quality of life after breast cancer treatment: Report from a limited resource setting. Breast Edinb Scotl 2018;41:120–6.

91. Available at: Breast_Cancer.pdf. Accessed November 3, 2022. http://cancerindia.org.in/wp-content/uploads/2017/11/Breast_Cancer.pdf.

92. Boby JM, Rajappa S, Mathew A. Financial toxicity in cancer care in India: a systematic review. Lancet Oncol 2021;22(12):e541–9.

Part II: Innovations to Improve Access and Outcomes

Breast Cancer and Lifestyle Factors: Umbrella Review

Ilir Hoxha, MD, PhD[a,b,c],*, Fitim Sadiku, MS[b], Lot Hoxha, MD[b],
Midhet Nasim, MS[b,d], Marie Anne Christine Buteau, MD[e],
Krenare Grezda, MD[b], Mary D. Chamberlin, MD[e]

KEYWORDS

- Breast cancer • Body mass index • Obesity • Overweight • Waist-to-hip ratio
- Physical activity • Smoking • Sleep

KEY POINTS

- Different lifestyle factors are known to cause cancer.
- We examined the latest evidence in the form of systematic reviews that establish a quantitative relation between the effect of different lifestyle factors and breast cancer.
- We analyzed 64 systematic reviews with meta-analysis examining the relationship between breast cancer and body mass and height, central obesity, physical activity, sleep duration and disruption, alcohol intake, and smoking.
- We found an increased risk for breast cancer due to obesity, alcohol intake, and smoking and a decreased risk due to physical activity.
- The evidence for sleep disruption and duration indicates risk for breast cancer but is limited in size, statistical significance, and quality of evidence.

INTRODUCTION

There were 2.3 million new cases of female breast cancer worldwide in 2020. Breast cancer remains the most commonly diagnosed malignancy and the first cause of cancer-specific deaths in women.[1,2] It claims the lives of more than 600 000 people worldwide each year. High-income countries such as the United States, Western and Northern Europe, and Australia/New Zealand have a higher incidence rate of this disease than low- to middle-income countries in sub-Saharan Africa and South Central Asia.[1] Interestingly, with the advent of industrialization and globalization, breast cancer incidence rates have increased also in low- to middle-income

[a] The Dartmouth Institute for Health Policy and Clinical Practice, Geisel School of Medicine at Dartmouth, Lebanon, NH, USA; [b] Evidence Synthesis Group, Prishtina, Kosovo; [c] Heimerer College, Prishtina, Kosovo; [d] Japan International Cooperation Agency, Mother and Child Health Project, Lahore, Punjab, Pakistan; [e] Department of Hematology-Oncology, Geisel School of Medicine at Dartmouth, Hanover, NH, USA
* Corresponding author.
E-mail address: ilir.s.hoxha@dartmouth.edu

Hematol Oncol Clin N Am 38 (2024) 137–170
https://doi.org/10.1016/j.hoc.2023.07.005
0889-8588/24/© 2023 Elsevier Inc. All rights reserved.

countries.[3,4] This correlation between industrialization, globalization, certain ways of living, exposure to certain factors, and increased incidence rates of breast cancer warrants a closer look as to what lifestyle factors may alter breast tissue to increase risk for breast cancer. As this malignancy constitutes a major public health issue worldwide, it is imperative to identify these factors and understand how and to what extent they contribute to the pathogenesis of breast cancer.

Breast tissue changes under the influence of immutable and exogenous factors. In some instances, these factors cause the development of malignant cells and breast cancer. Epidemiological studies such as the Surveillance, Epidemiology, and End Results Program database in the United States have continued to demonstrate that breast cancer risk increases with older age and occurs more frequently in white women compared with other racial groups.[5] Other publications, including a Danish Epidemiology Science Center cohort study, established a link between height and risk of breast cancer,[6] whereas other studies a direct proportional relationship with larger waist circumference, weight throughout adulthood, and height. In a 2010 review of 13 cohort and 14 case-control studies, from 2007 to 2010, evaluating risk and protective factors for breast cancer, breastfeeding, and physical activity were found to be protective factors against breast cancer, whereas alcohol consumption was a risk factor. The accumulated evidence suggested that breastfeeding and a healthy lifestyle were the factors most strongly associated with breast cancer prevention.[7] A 2013 systematic review and meta-analysis found a significant level of evidence that tea consumption and physical activity were significantly associated with a decreased risk of breast cancer in Chinese females.[8]

Given this knowledge of the effect of lifestyle factors, it is essential to consider and use existing evidence in the prevention but also treatment of individuals with breast cancer. The most robust evidence is in the form of high-quality systematic reviews. Given this, our objective was to identify and assess the quality of the most recent evidence that examines the effect of select lifestyle factors on risk for breast cancer.

METHODS

We performed an umbrella review of systematic reviews as per guidelines provided by Cochrane.[9] We systematically searched four key databases for identifying papers of interest, including CINAHL, PubMed, Scopus, and Web of Science. The search strategy consisted of search terms related to breast cancer and different lifestyle factors of interest, such as alcohol, smoking, physical activity, and obesity. The search strategy for each individual database is available in the Online Appendix. The search was last updated in July 2022.

Screening and the full-text review of articles were performed by two researchers. To be included, articles had to be systemic reviews with meta-analysis establishing a quantative association of risk or protective factors of interest with breast cancer in human subjects. Risk factors of interest were alcohol consumption, obesity, physical activity, smoking, sleep quality, and duration. Papers had to be published from 2000 and on and in English language. We first performed two rounds of screening of titles and abstracts, followed by full-text review. Disagreements in inclusion of articles were solved with consensus and consultation with an experienced reviewer.

Data extraction was performed in duplicate, and we extracted general information on the studies, information on effect estimates, risk measurement, study design, population, and quality of the reviews included in the study.

Quality assessment was performed using GRADE assessment for systematic reviews.[10] We examined five key domains, including the risk of bias from the quality rating of studies included in a review, inconsistency of effect estimate from the heterogeneity of included studies, indirectness, as a measure of population homogeneity among included studies, imprecision as a measure of the precision of overall effect estimate and its confidence intervals, and finally, the risk of publication bias. Studies were rated as having high, moderate, low, or very low quality of evidence. In case of fulfillment of all criteria, a review was ranked as high-quality review. In the case of nonfulfillment of one criterion, the study was downgraded to a moderate quality. In the case of nonfulfillment of two criteria, a review was downgraded to low quality. In case of nonfulfillment of more than two criteria, the study was downgraded as being of very low quality.

We performed a descriptive analysis of the data. We analyzed data by organizing them into three categories depending on the menopause status of women, that is, risk assessments that did not specify the menopausal status of women and risk assessments of women in the premenopausal or postmenopausal stage. Further on, the data presentation was organized to present the risk for breast cancer by each of the key risk categories of interest. We present a summary of data on effect estimate, setting information, specification of risk factors and their measurement, and the quality ranking of each meta-analysis included in the study. Data were processed using STATA 17BE (Stata Corp, College Station, TX, USA).

RESULTS

We identified 3147 records in all four databases (**Fig. 1**). Two hundred fifty-four in CINAHL, 1250 in PubMed, 1153 in Scopus, and 490 in Web of Science. Nine hundred eighty-two duplicates were excluded. Two thousand and one hundred and sixty five records were screened from titles and abstracts. Two thousand and thirty-two records were excluded after reviewing the titles and abstracts, which left us with 133 records that were assessed full text for eligibility. Sixty-nine studies were excluded after full-text review. Five did not report breast cancer, five did not report lifestyle factors, and 59 studies reported breast cancer and lifestyle factors that did not match to our study's aim. In the end, we included 64 articles reporting 174 meta-analyses (ie, risk estimations for breast cancer) and performed a synthesis of results with them.[8,11–15,16–30,31–50,51–73]

Most studies were published between 2010 and 2021 (**Table 1**).[8,11–15,16–30,31–50,51–73] The included systematic reviews reported data from multiple countries and continents. These reviews reported the breast cancer risk for alcohol intake, body mass and height, physical activity, sleep disruption and quality, smoking, and waist and hip measures. Fifty-five studies reported the risk of breast cancer among women without specification of the menopause status. Twenty-three studies reported risk for premenopausal, and 21 for postmenopausal women.

OVERALL BREAST CANCER

In **Table 2**, we present findings from the studies that reported the risk of breast cancer among women in general, without specification of menopause status. For alcohol intake, three risk estimations reported moderate, eleven low, and six a very low quality evidence. Eighteen out of twenty risk estimations reported a higher risk of breast cancer due to alcohol intake. Two out of three risk estimations with moderate quality of evidence reported a higher risk for breast cancer due to alcohol intake. Overall, the risk estimates ranged from OR = 0.76 (95%CI 0.60, 0.97) to RR = 1.61 (95%CI

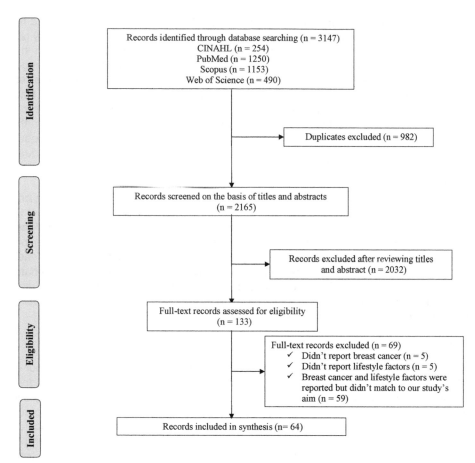

Fig. 1. Selection of studies.

1.33, 1.94). However, for moderate quality evidence, risk estimates ranged from OR = 0.85 (95%CI 0.72, 1.02) to RR = 1.08 (95%CI 1.06, 1.11).

For body mass measures, one risk estimation was evidence of high quality. Twelve were moderate, nine low, and one very low-quality evidence. Eighteen risk estimations reported a higher risk for breast cancer due to the higher value of body mass or height measures (obesity, weight gain, and so forth). Ten risk estimations with moderate- or high-quality evidence reported a higher risk for breast cancer. Overall, the risk estimates ranged from OR = 0.82 (95%CI 0.70, 0.96) to RR = 2.90 (95%CI 2.00, 4.21). For moderate or high-quality evidence, risk estimates ranged from OR = 0.87 (95% CI 0.82, 0.92) to RR = 2.90 (95%CI 2.00, 4.21). Three dose-response meta-analyses reported a higher risk for breast cancer with an increase in body mass. For waist and hip measures as measures of central obesity, two risk estimations reported very low-quality evidence. Both these risk estimations reported a higher risk of breast cancer for higher waist-to-hip measures ranging from OR = 1.27 (95%CI 1.07, 1.51) to OR = 1.80 (95%CI 1.29, 2.50).

For physical activity, one risk estimation was evidence of high quality. Nine were moderate, five low, and two very low-quality evidence. All risk estimations reported

Table 1
Included studies

Study/Year	Countries	Menopause	Risk Factor Examined
Khuder et al,[11] 2000	Canada, China, Japan, South Korea, Switzerland, United Kingdom, United States	Overall	Smoking
Ellison et al,[12] 2001	Unclear	Overall	Alcohol
Khuder et al,[13] 2001	Australia, Canada, Denmark, France, Italy, Japan, Norway, Poland, Sweden, Switzerland, United Kingdom, United States	Overall Premenopausal Postmenopausal	Smoking
Connolly et al,[14] 2002	Canada, China, Finland, Italy, Netherlands, Singapore, United States	Overall Premenopausal Postmenopausal	Waist and hip measures
Lagerros et al,[15] 2004	Canada, China, Italy, Japan, Netherlands, Norway, Sweden, Switzerland, United States	Overall Premenopausal Postmenopausal	Physical activity
Lee et al,[16] 2006	Unclear	Overall Premenopausal Postmenopausal	Smoking
Miller et al,[17] 2007	Canada, China, Germany, Japan, South Korea, Switzerland, United Kingdom, United States	Overall	Smoking
Pirie et al,[18] 2008	Canada, China, Germany, Japan, South Korea, Poland, Switzerland, United Kingdom, United States	Overall	Smoking
Renehan et al,[19] 2008	Australia, Asia-Pacific, Europe, North America	Premenopausal Postmenopausal	Body mass and height
Suzuki et al,[21] 2008	Australia, Canada, Sweden, United States	Overall	Body mass and height
Suzuki et al,[20] 2008	Canada, Sweden, United States	Overall	Alcohol
DeRoo et al,[22] 2011	Canada, Germany, Norway, Poland, Sweden, Switzerland, United States	Overall	Smoking
Li et al,[23] 2011	China	Overall	Alcohol

(continued on next page)

Table 1
(continued)

Study/Year	Countries	Menopause	Risk Factor Examined
Cheraghi et al,[24] 2012	Unclear	Premenopausal Postmenopausal	Body mass and height
Pierobon et al,[30] 2012	Unclear	Premenopausal Postmenopausal	Body mass and height
Seitz et al,[25] 2012	Asia, Europe, North America	Overall	Alcohol
Amadou et al,[26] 2013	Canada, China, Finland, France, Germany, Japan, Netherlands, Nigeria, Norway, Sweden, Taiwan, Thailand, United Kingdom, United States, Vietnam	Premenopausal	Body mass and height Waist and hip measures
Bagnardi et al,[27] 2013	Asia, Europe, North America	Overall	Alcohol
Chen et al,[39] 2013	China	Overall	Smoking
Gao et al,[8] 2013	China	Overall	Alcohol Physical activity
Gaudet et al,[28] 2013	Unclear	Overall	Smoking
Jjaz et al,[29] 2013	China, Denmark, France, Germany, Norway, United States	Overall	Sleep
Qin et al,[35] 2013	Australia, Finland, Japan, Singapore, United States	Overall	Sleep
Wu et al,[31] 2013	Canada, China, Denmark, Europe, Finland, France, Japan, Norway, Sweden, United States	Overall	Physical activity
Yang et al,[32] 2013	Denmark, France, Germany, Greece, Italy, Japan, South Korea, Netherlands, Norway, Spain, Sweden, United Kingdom, United States	Overall Premenopausal Postmenopausal	Smoking
Bagnardi et al,[38] 2014	Asia, Europe, North America	Overall	Alcohol
Chen et al,[33] 2014	China	Overall	Smoking
Namiranian et al,[34] 2014	Eastern Mediterranean Region	Overall	Body mass and height Physical activity Smoking
Xia et al,[36] 2014	Unclear	Overall	Body mass and height

Study	Countries	Menopausal status	Factor
Yang et al,[37] 2014	Australia, Finland, Japan, Singapore, United States	Overall	Sleep
Jayasekara et al,[44] 2015	Canada, Greece, Sweden, United States	Overall	Alcohol
Keum et al,[40] 2015	Japan, Norway, United States, other European countries	Premenopausal / Postmenopausal	Body mass and height
Liu et al,[46] 2015	Unclear	Overall / Premenopausal / Postmenopausal	Physical activity
Macacu et al,[41] 2015	Unclear	Overall / Premenopausal / Postmenopausal	Smoking
Chen et al,[43] 2016	Canada, Denmark, France, Italy, Japan, Netherlands, Norway, Spain, Sweden, Switzerland, United Kingdom, United States	Overall	Alcohol
Chen et al,[42] 2016	Australia, Canada, China, France, Italy, Netherlands, United States, other European countries	Premenopausal / Postmenopausal	Waist and hip measures
Kyu et al,[45] 2016	Unclear	Overall	Physical activity
Neilson et al,[53] 2016	Australia, Canada, China, Denmark, France, Germany, Greece, Italy, Japan, Netherlands, Norway, Mexico, Poland, Spain, Sweden, Switzerland, United Kingdom, United States	Premenopausal / Postmenopausal	Physical activity
Ordóñez-Mena et al,[47] 2016	Unclear	Overall	Smoking
Pizot et al,[48] 2016	Canada, China, Denmark, Finland, France, Japan, Nether ands, Norway, Sweden, United States	Overall / Premenopausal / Postmenopausal	Physical activity
Travis et al,[49] 2016	China, Netherlands, Sweden, United Kingdom, United States	Overall	Sleep
Wang et al,[50] 2016	Asian Pacific, Australia, Europe, North America	Overall / Premenopausal / Postmenopausal	Body mass and height
Chen et al,[51] 2017	Austria, China, Denmark, Japan, South Korea, Netherlands, North America, Norway, Sweden, United Kingdom	Overall / Premenopausal / Postmenopausal	Body mass and height

(continued on next page)

Table 1
(continued)

Studyf Year	Countries	Menopause	Risk Factor Examined
Hardefeldt et al,[56] 2017	Unclear	Overall	Body mass and height Physical activity
Hidayat et al,[57] 2017	Australia, Canada, China, Denmark, Finland, Israel, Japan, Netherlands, Norway, Sweden, United Kingdom, United States	Overall Premenopausal Postmenopausal	Body mass and height
Lu et al,[52] 2017	Australia, China, Finland, Japan, Singapore, United States	Overall	Sleep
Zahmatkesh et al,[54] 2017	Iran	Overall	Body mass and height
Chen et al,[59] 2018	Canada, China, Denmark, Finland, France, Netherlands, Norway, Puerto Rico, Sweden, United States, other European countries	Overall Premenopausal Postmenopausal	Physical activity
Choi et al,[55] 2018	Canada, Denmark, France, Japan, Netherlands, Norway, Sweden, United Kingdom, United States, other European countries	Overall	Alcohol
Kim et al,[58] 2018	Canada, China, Germany, Japan, Switzerland, United Kingdom, United States	Overall	Smoking
Dong et al,[61] 2019	Japan, Denmark, Norway, Sweden, Netherlands, United States, other European countries	Overall	Alcohol
Hidayat et al,[63] 2019	Asia, Europe, North America	Overall Premenopausal Postmenopausal	Physical activity
Nindrea et al,[60] 2019	Bangladesh, China, India, Japan, Saudi Arabia, South Korea, Taiwan, Thailand, Vietnam	Premenopausal	Body mass and height
Dun et al,[62] 2020	Australia, Canada, China, Denmark, France, Germany, India, Norway, Spain, Sweden, United Kingdom, United States	Overall	Sleep
Shamshirian et al,[64] 2020	Iran	Overall	Body mass and height Physical activity Smoking

Study	Countries	Menopausal status	Factors
Sun et al,[65] 2020	Canada, Denmark, France, Germany, Greece, Italy, Japan, Netherlands, Norway, Spain, Sweden, United Kingdom, United States	Overall	Alcohol
Wong et al,[72] 2020	Canada, Finland, Japan, Singapore, United Kingdom, United States	Overall	Sleep
Arafat et al,[66] 2021	Palestine	Overall	Body mass and height Sleep Smoking
Byun et al,[73] 2021	Australia, Denmark, Japan, Netherlands, Norway, Sweden, United Kingdom, United States	Premenopausal Postmenopausal	Body mass and height
Hao et al,[67] 2021	Australia, Canada, China, Japan, Netherlands, Norway, United Kingdom, United States, other European countries	Overall	Body mass and height
Larsson et al,[68] 2021	Europe	Overall	Body mass and height
Poorolajal et al,[69] 2021	Unclear	Overall	Alcohol Body mass and height Physical activity Smoking
Schwarz et al,[70] 2021	Australia, Canada, China, Denmark, Germany, Netherlands, Norway, Sweden, United Kingdom, United States	Overall Premenopausal Postmenopausal	Sleep
Wei et al,[71] 2021	Canada, China, South Korea, United States	Overall	Sleep

Table 2
Results for breast cancer overall

Study, Year	Risk Factor	Measurement of Risk	Other Characteristics	Number of Studies	Type of Outcome	Type of Effect	Effect Size	Lower CI	Upper CI	Quality of Evidence (GRADE)
Alcohol										
Ellison et al,[12] 2001	Alcohol intake	6 g a day		na	Binary	RR	1.05	1.03	1.07	Low
Ellison et al,[12] 2001	Alcohol intake	12 g a day		na	Binary	RR	1.10	1.06	1.14	Low
Ellison et al,[12] 2001	Alcohol intake	24 g a day		na	Binary	RR	1.21	1.13	1.30	Very low
Suzuki et al,[20] 2008	Alcohol intake	10 g a day	ER + PR+	5	Dose–response	RR	1.04	0.76	1.43	Very low
Suzuki et al,[20] 2008	Alcohol intake	10 g a day	ER– PR–	12	Dose–response	RR	1.04	0.98	1.09	Low
Li et al,[23] 2011	Alcohol intake	Alcohol vs no alcohol intake		4	Binary	OR	0.76	0.60	0.97	Low
Seitz et al,[25] 2012	Alcohol intake	≤12.5 g a day of ethanol; ≤1 drink/day		113	Binary	RR	1.05	1.02	1.08	Very low
Bagnardi et al,[27] 2013	Light alcohol intake	≤12.5 g or one drink a day		110	Binary	RR	1.05	1.02	1.08	Low
Gao et al,[8] 2013	Alcohol intake	Exposure to drinking		26	Binary	OR	0.85	0.72	1.02	Moderate
Bagnardi et al,[38] 2015	Heavy alcohol intake	>50 g a day		na	Binary	RR	1.61	1.33	1.94	Very low
Bagnardi et al,[38] 2015	Moderate alcohol intake	≤50 g a day		na	Binary	RR	1.23	1.19	1.28	Very low

Study	Exposure	Comparison	Subtype	N	Type	Measure				Certainty
Bagnardi et al,[38] 2015	Light alcohol intake	<=12.5 g a day		na	Binary	RR	1.04	1.01	1.07	Very low
Jayasekara et al,[44] 2016	Alcohol intake	Highest vs lowest		15	Binary	RR	1.28	1.07	1.52	Low
Chen et al,[43] 2016	Wine intake	Wine vs no wine intake		26	Binary	RR	1.36	1.20	1.54	Low
Choi et al,[55] 2018	Very light alcohol intake	≤0.5 drink a day		20	Binary	RR	1.04	1.01	1.07	Low
Choi et al,[55] 2018	Moderate alcohol intake	Wine vs no wine intake		15	Binary	RR	1.13	1.11	1.15	Low
Choi et al,[55] 2018	Light alcohol intake	≤1 drink a day		25	Binary	RR	1.09	1.06	1.12	Low
Dong et al,[61] 2020	Alcohol intake	Alcohol intake		8	Binary	RR	1.07	0.99	1.14	Moderate
Sun et al,[65] 2020	Alcohol intake	Alcohol intake		22	Binary	RR	1.17	1.11	1.24	Low
Poorolajal et al,[69] 2021	Alcohol intake	Alcohol intake vs no intake		53	Binary	RR	1.08	1.06	1.11	Moderate
Body mass and height										
Suzuki et al,[20] 2008	Body weight	Highest vs reference	ER− PR−	20	Binary	RR	1.04	0.92	1.17	Moderate
Suzuki et al,[20] 2008	Body weight	Highest vs reference	ER + PR−	11	Binary	RR	0.91	0.79	1.04	Moderate
Suzuki et al,[20] 2008	Body weight	Highest vs reference	ER− PR+	8	Binary	RR	1.19	0.96	1.47	Low
Namiranian et al,[34] 2014	Body mass index	25–30 vs <25 kg/m²		8	Binary	OR	1.71	1.09	2.68	Moderate

(continued on next page)

Table 2
(continued)

Study, Year	Risk Factor	Measurement of Risk	Other Characteristics	Number of Studies	Type of Outcome	Type of Effect	Effect Size	Lower CI	Upper CI	Quality of Evidence (GRADE)
Namiranian et al,[34] 2014	Body mass index	>30 vs <25 kg/m^2		8	Binary	OR	2.21	1.71	2.36	Moderate
Xia et al,[36] 2014	Body mass index	35 vs 21.75 kg/m^2		na	Binary	RR	1.26	1.07	1.50	Low
Xia et al,[36] 2014	Body mass index	30 vs 21.75 kg/m^2		na	Binary	RR	1.12	1.01	1.24	Low
Xia et al,[36] 2014	Body mass index	25 vs 21.75 kg/m^2		na	Binary	RR	1.02	0.98	1.06	Moderate
Wang et al,[50] 2016	Body mass index	5 kg/m^2 increase		61	Dose–response	RR	1.07	1.05	1.09	Low
Chen et al,[51] 2017	Body mass index	Highest vs normal		31	Binary	RR	1.19	1.06	1.33	Low
Hardefeldt et al,[56] 2018	Weight loss	Overall weight loss		20	Binary	OR	0.82	0.70	0.96	Low
Hidayat et al,[57] 2018	Body mass index at young age	age ≤ 30 years; 5 kg/m^2 increase		24	Dose–response	RR	0.86	0.82	0.90	Very low
Hidayat et al,[57] 2018	Body mass index gain from young age	5 kg/m^2 increase		7	Dose–response	RR	1.13	1.05	1.20	Moderate
Zahmatkesh et al,[54] 2017	Obesity	30 vs 18.5 -24.9 kg/m^2		7	Binary	OR	1.81	1.24	2.64	Low
Zahmatkesh et al,[54] 2017	Overweight	25-30 kg/m^2 vs 18.5-24.9 kg/ m^2		7	Binary	OR	1.45	1.13	1.89	Low

Study	Factor	Comparison	N	Type	Effect				Quality
Shamshirian et al,[64] 2020	Body mass index	25–29.9 vs 19–24.9	3	Binary	OR	1.07	0.82	1.32	High
Shamshirian et al,[64] 2020	Body mass index	30 vs 18–24.9	3	Binary	OR	1.21	0.90	1.52	Moderate
Arafat et al,[66] 2021	Obesity	>30 kg/m²	3	Binary	OR	2.90	2.00	4.21	Moderate
Hao et al,[67] 2021	Weight gain	5 kg/m² increase	16	Dose–response	RR	1.08	1.07	1.09	Low
Hao et al,[67] 2021	Weight gain	Highest vs lowest adult weight gain	16	Binary	RR	1.55	1.40	1.71	Moderate
Hao et al,[67] 2021	Weight gain	Highest vs lowest adult weight gain	7	Binary	RR	1.00	0.83	1.21	Moderate
Larsson et al,[68] 2021	Body mass index	Around 4.8 kg/m² increase	5	Binary	OR	0.87	0.82	0.92	Moderate
Poorolajal et al,[69] 2021	Overweight and obesity	25.0–≥30.0 vs 18.5–24.9 kg/m²	45	Binary	RR	1.11	1.08	1.15	Moderate
Physical activity									
Lagerros et al,[15] 2004	Physical activity in adolescence and young adulthood	Physical activity	25	Binary	RR	0.81	0.73	0.89	Low
Gao et al,[8] 2013	Physical activity	Physical activity	15	Binary	OR	0.73	0.63	0.85	Moderate
Wu et al,[31] 2013	Physical activity	Exposure to physical activity	31	Binary	RR	0.87	0.83	0.92	Moderate

(continued on next page)

Table 2
(continued)

Study, Year	Risk Factor	Measurement of Risk	Other Characteristics	Number of Studies	Type of Outcome	Type of Effect	Effect Size	Lower CI	Upper CI	Quality of Evidence (GRADE)
Namiranian et al,[34] 2014	Physical activity	5.5 hours/week/year		4	Binary	OR	0.32	0.27	0.38	Moderate
Liu et al,[46] 2016	Leisure time physical activity	Physical activity		33	Binary	RR	0.88	0.84	0.91	Moderate
Kyu et al,[45] 2016	Physical activity	≥8000 metabolic equivalent minutes a week		na	Binary	RR	0.86	0.83	0.90	Moderate
Kyu et al,[45] 2016	Physical activity	600–3999 metabolic equivalent minutes a week		na	Binary	RR	0.97	0.94	1.00	Moderate
Kyu et al,[45] 2016	Physical activity	4000–7999 metabolic equivalent minutes a week		na	Binary	RR	0.94	0.90	0.98	Moderate
Pizot et al,[48] 2016	Physical activity level	na		38	Binary	RR	0.88	0.85	0.90	Low
Hardefeldt et al,[56] 2018	High-intensity physical activity	Running, competitive sports		35	Binary	OR	0.73	0.65	0.81	Low
Hardefeldt et al,[56] 2018	Low-intensity physical activity	Walking, dancing, and gardening		32	Binary	OR	0.79	0.72	0.86	Low

Study	Factor	Comparison	N	Type	Measure	Estimate	Lower	Upper	Quality
Hardefeldt et al,[56] 2018	Nonspecific physical activity	Overall physical activity	129	Binary	OR	0.78	0.76	0.81	Low
Chen et al,[59] 2019	Physical activity	Physical activity	38	Binary	RR	0.85	0.82	0.89	Moderate
Hidayat et al,[63] 2020	Physical activity at a young age	5-30 years old	29	Binary	RR	0.81	0.76	0.87	Very low
Hidayat et al,[63] 2020	Lifetime physical activity	>10 years	20	Binary	RR	0.79	0.72	0.86	Very low
Shamshirian et al,[64] 2020	Daily exercise	Daily physical activity	3	Binary	OR	0.59	0.44	0.73	High
Poorolajal et al,[69] 2021	Sufficient physical activity	≥30 minutes	15	Binary	RR	0.89	0.85	0.94	Moderate
Sleep									
Ijaz et al,[29] 2013	Night shift work	≥300 shifts	8	Binary	RR	1.04	1.00	1.10	Low
Ijaz et al,[29] 2013	Night shift work	5 years	12	Binary	RR	1.05	1.01	1.10	Low
Qin et al,[35] 2014	Long sleep duration	>8 - ≥ 10 vs 6-8 hours	6	Binary	OR	0.95	0.86	1.04	Moderate
Qin et al,[35] 2014	Short sleep duration	≥4 – ≤6 h) vs 7-8 hours	6	Binary	OR	1.01	0.90	1.14	Moderate
Yang et al,[37] 2014	Sleep duration	≥9 vs <6 hhours	6	Binary	RR	0.96	0.77	1.19	Low

(continued on next page)

Table 2
(continued)

Study, Year	Risk Factor	Measurement of Risk	Other Characteristics	Number of Studies	Type of Outcome	Type of Effect	Effect Size	Lower CI	Upper CI	Quality of Evidence (GRADE)
Yang et al,[37] 2014	Sleep duration	1 hour a night increase		6	Dose–response	RR	1.00	1.00	1.01	Moderate
Travis et al,[49] 2016	Night shift work	≥30 years vs no night shift work		4	Binary	RR	1.00	0.87	1.14	Moderate
Travis et al,[49] 2016	Night shift work	Ever vs never night shift work		10	Binary	RR	0.99	0.95	1.03	Low
Travis et al,[49] 2016	Night shift work	≥20 years vs never night shift work		10	Binary	RR	1.01	0.93	1.10	Low
Lu et al,[52] 2017	Sleep duration	10 vs 6 hours		10	Binary	RR	1.11	1.03	1.19	Low
Lu et al,[52] 2017	Sleep duration	8 vs 6 hours		10	Binary	RR	1.05	1.00	1.10	Low
Lu et al,[52] 2017	Sleep duration	7 vs 6 hours		10	Binary	RR	1.02	1.00	1.04	Low
Lu et al,[52] 2017	Sleep duration	9 vs 6 hours		10	Binary	RR	1.08	1.02	1.14	Low
Lu et al,[52] 2017	Sleep duration	5 vs 6 hours		10	Binary	RR	1.00	0.99	1.00	Low
Lu et al,[52] 2017	Sleep duration	4 h vs 6 hours		10	Binary	RR	1.00	0.99	1.01	Low
Dun et al,[62] 2020	Night shift work	Ever exposure to night shift work		26	Binary	OR	1.01	0.98	1.03	Moderate
Wong et al,[72] 2021	Short sleep duration	<7 vs 7-9 hours		15	Binary	RR	0.99	0.98	1.01	Moderate
Wong et al,[72] 2021	Long sleep duration	>9 vs 6 - <8 hours		15	Binary	RR	1.01	0.98	1.04	Moderate

Study	Exposure	Category	N	Type	Effect	Estimate	Lower	Upper	Quality
Arafat et al,[66] 2021	Sleep duration	<7 hours	2	Binary	OR	2.51	0.79	7.97	Low
Schwarz et al,[70] 2021	Long-term night shift work	≥15 years	17	Binary	RR	1.13	1.01	1.27	Low
Wei et al,[71] 2021	Sleep-disordered breathing	Presence of sleep-disordered breathing	8	Binary	RR	1.36	1.08	1.71	Very low
Smoking									
Khuder et al,[11] 2000	Passive smoking	Exposure to passive smoking	11	Binary	RR	1.41	1.14	1.75	Low
Khuder et al,[13] 2001	Past smoking	Former active smoking	25	Binary	RR	1.10	1.00	1.21	Low
Khuder et al,[13] 2001	Current smoking	Current active smoking	24	Binary	RR	1.11	1.01	1.22	Low
Khuder et al,[13] 2001	Ever smoking	Ever active smoking	40	Binary	RR	1.10	1.02	1.18	Low
Lee et al,[16] 2006	Passive smoking	Exposure to passive smoking	22	Binary	RR	1.12	1.02	1.24	Very low
Miller et al,[17] 2007	Passive smoking	Exposure to passive smoking	19	Binary	RR	1.25	1.08	1.44	Low
Pirie et al,[18] 2008	Passive smoking	Exposure to passive smoking	8	Binary	RR	1.06	1.01	1.11	Moderate
DeRoo et al,[22] 2011	Smoking after first pregnancy	Smoking after first pregnancy vs women who never smoked	16	Binary	RR	1.07	0.99	1.15	Low

(continued on next page)

Table 2
(continued)

Study, Year	Risk Factor	Measurement of Risk	Other Characteristics	Number of Studies	Type of Outcome	Type of Effect	Effect Size	Lower CI	Upper CI	Quality of Evidence (GRADE)
DeRoo et al,[22] 2011	Smoking before first pregnancy	Smoking before first pregnancy vs women who never smoked		23	Binary	RR	1.10	1.07	1.14	Moderate
Chen et al,[39] 2015	Passive smoking	>15 minutes a day, at least 1 day a week		6	Binary	OR	1.60	1.08	2.37	Very low
Gaudet et al,[28] 2013	Past smoking	10 to 30 cigarettes a day		15	Binary	HR	1.09	1.04	1.15	Low
Gaudet et al,[28] 2013	Current smoking	Current vs no smoking		15	Binary	HR	1.12	1.08	1.16	Moderate
Gaudet et al,[28] 2013	Smoking initiation before first birth	Smoking initiation before first birth		9	Binary	HR	1.21	1.14	1.28	Moderate
Gaudet et al,[28] 2013	Younger age at smoking initiation	Younger age at smoking initiation		10	Binary	HR	1.12	1.06	1.19	Moderate
Yang et al,[32] 2013	Passive smoking	Exposure to passive smoking		10	Binary	RR	1.01	0.96	1.06	Moderate
Chen et al,[33] 2014	Active smoking	Active smoking		31	Binary	OR	1.04	0.89	1.20	Moderate

Study	Exposure	Comparison	N	Type	Measure	OR			Quality
Chen et al,[33] 2014	Passive smoking	Exposure to passive smoking	26	Binary	OR	1.60	1.39	1.82	Moderate
Namiranian et al,[34] 2014	Smoking	Smoking versus no smoking	10	Binary	OR	1.25	1.12	1.39	Moderate
Macacu et al,[41] 2015	Active ever smoking	Unclear	12	Dose–response	RR	1.01	1.00	1.01	Low
Macacu et al,[41] 2015	Active ever smoking	Active smoking	73	Binary	RR	1.09	1.06	1.12	Moderate
Macacu et al,[41] 2015	Passive ever smoking	Exposure to passive smoking	31	Binary	RR	1.20	1.07	1.33	Low
Ordóñez-Mena et al,[47] 2016	Current smoking	Current vs never smoking	na	Binary	HR	1.07	1.00	1.15	High
Ordóñez-Mena et al,[47] 2016	Past smoking	Former vs never smoking	na	Binary	HR	1.08	1.04	1.12	High
Kim et al,[58] 2018	Passive smoking	Exposure to passive smoking	15	Binary	RR	1.24	1.10	1.39	Very low
Shamshirian et al,[64] 2020	Passive smoking	Exposure to passive smoking	3	Binary	OR	1.68	1.34	2.03	Moderate
Shamshirian et al,[64] 2020	Active smoking	Active smoking	3	Binary	OR	1.70	0.66	2.74	Low
Arafat et al,[66] 2021	Passive smoking	Exposure to passive smoking	3	Binary	OR	1.50	1.12	2.02	Moderate
Poorolajal et al,[69] 2021	Smoking	Smoking vs no smoking	84	Binary	RR	1.08	1.06	1.10	Moderate

(continued on next page)

Table 2
(continued)

Study, Year	Risk Factor	Measurement of Risk	Other Characteristics	Number of Studies	Type of Outcome	Type of Effect	Effect Size	Lower CI	Upper CI	Quality of Evidence (GRADE)
Waist and hip measures										
Connolly et al,[14] 2002	Waist-to-hip ratio	>0.778 vs ≤0.79		9	Binary	OR	1.27	1.07	1.51	Very low
Connolly et al,[14] 2002	Waist-to-hip ratio	≥0.81 vs <0.79		16	Binary	OR	1.80	1.29	2.50	Very low

a lower risk of breast cancer. The risk estimates ranged from OR = 0.32 (95%CI 0.27, 0.38) to RR = 0.97 (95%CI 0.94, 1.00).

For risk measures related to sleep disruption and quality, seven risk estimations reported evidence of moderate quality. Thirteen reported low and one a very low quality of evidence. Five estimations reported a higher risk for sleep disruption due to night shift employment. All but one, which was moderate, were low-quality evidence. Estimates from moderate-quality studies show minor insignificant effects of sleep duration or disruption on breast cancer risk.

For smoking, two estimations reported high, 13 moderate, ten low, and three very low-quality evidence. All risk estimations from reported reviews reported a higher risk of breast cancer for different forms of smoking exposure or initiation. Overall, the risk estimates ranged from RR = 1.01 (95%CI 1.00, 1.01) to OR = 1.70 (95%CI 0.66, 2.74). However, for high or moderate-quality evidence, risk estimates ranged from RR = 1.01 (95%CI 0.96, 1.06) to OR = 1.68 (95%CI 1.34, 2.03). For subgroup of passive smoking, risk estimates (five with moderate, six with low or very low quality evidence) ranged from RR = 1.01 (95%CI 0.96, 1.06) to OR = 1.68 (95%CI 1.34, 2.03). For subgroup of active smokers, risk estimates (one high, three moderate, and three low quality evidence) ranged from RR = 1.01 (95%CI 1.00, 1.01) to OR = 1.70 (95%CI 0.66, 2.74). For subgroup of past smoking, risk estimates (one high and two low quality evidence) ranged from HR = 1.08 (95%CI 1.04, 1.12) to RR = 1.10 (95%CI 1.00, 1.21). For subgroup of ever smoking, risk estimates (two moderate and one low quality evidence) ranged from RR = 1.08 (95%CI 1.06, 1.10) to OR = 1.25 (95%CI 1.12, 1.39).

PREMENOPAUSAL BREAST CANCER

In **Table 3**, we present findings from the studies that reported the risk of breast cancer among premenopausal women. For body mass measures, eight risk estimations were moderate, five low, and one very low-quality evidence. For subgroup of body mass index (BMI), two risk estimations reported a higher and seven lower risk of breast cancer for a higher value of the BMI. However, all but two estimations reported small statistically nonsignificant effects. Three dose–response meta-analyses reported a lower risk for breast cancer with a 5 kg/m^2 increase in BMI. Two of them were statistically significant. Two other dose–response meta-analyses reported a lower and one a higher risk for breast cancer with a 5 kg/m^2 increase in BMI from young age. Both estimations reporting lower risk were statistically significant. For waist and hip measures, one risk estimation reported moderate, two low, and two very low-quality evidence. All risk estimations reported a higher risk of breast cancer.

For physical activity, one risk estimation was moderate, four low, and two very low quality evidence. All risk estimations reported a lower risk of breast cancer. The risk estimates ranged from RR = 0.79 (95%CI 0.63, 0.99) to RR = 0.87 (95%CI 0.78, 0.96). For measures related to sleep disruption and quality, there was only one risk estimation with low quality of evidence, reporting a higher risk for breast cancer for women working 15 or more years on night shift RR = 1.27 (95%CI 0.96, 1.68). For smoking, there was one risk estimation with moderate, two with low, and four with very low quality of evidence. All risk estimations reported a higher risk of breast cancer for different forms of smoking exposure or initiation. Overall, the risk estimates ranged from RR = 1.11 (95%CI 0.55, 2.24) to RR = 1.54 (95%CI 1.16, 2.05). For subgroup of passive smoking, risk estimates (three with low quality evidence) ranged from RR = 1.11 (95%CI 0.55, 2.24) to RR = 1.55 (95%CI 1.16, 2.05). For subgroup of active smokers, risk estimates (one with moderate and one with very low quality evidence) ranged from RR = 1.11 (95%CI 1.00, 1.25) to RR = 1.18 (95%CI 0.94, 1.48). For

Table 3
Results for premenopausal breast cancer

Study Year	Risk Factor	Measurement of Risk	Number of Studies	Type of Outcome	Type of Effect	Effect Size	Lower CI	Upper CI	Quality of Evidence (GRADE)
Body mass and height									
Renehan et al,[19] 2008	Body mass index	5 kg/m² increase	20	Dose–response	RR	0.92	0.88	0.97	Moderate
Cheraghi et al,[24] 2012	Overweight and obesity	≥25 vs <25 kg/m²	4	Binary	RR	0.97	0.92	1.16	Low
Cheraghi et al,[24] 2012	Overweight and obesity	≥25 vs <25 kg/m²	26	Binary	OR	0.93	0.86	1.02	Low
Pierobon et al,[30] 2012	Obesity	≥30 vs <30 kg/m²	6	Binary	OR	0.99	0.79	1.24	Low
Amadou et al,[26] 2013	Body height	10 cm increase	14	Dose–response	RR	1.03	1.02	1.05	Moderate
Amadou et al,[26] 2013	Body mass index	5 kg/m² increase	30	Dose–response	RR	0.95	0.94	0.97	Low
Keum et al,[40] 2015	Adult weight gain	5 kg increase	3	Dose–response	RR	0.99	0.95	1.03	Moderate
Wang et al,[50] 2016	Body mass index	5 kg/m² increase	24	Dose–response	RR	0.99	0.97	1.01	Moderate
Chen et al,[51] 2017	Body mass index	Highest vs normal	18	Binary	RR	0.94	0.80	1.11	Moderate
Hidayat et al,[57] 2018	Body fatness gain from young age	5 kg/m² increase	2	Dose–response	RR	1.01	0.84	1.20	Moderate
Hidayat et al,[57] 2018	Body mass index at young age	age ≤ 30 years; 5 kg/m² increase	10	Dose–response	RR	0.88	0.81	0.95	Very low
Nindrea et al,[60] 2019	Overweight	23.0–24.9 vs <23 kg/m²	15	Binary	OR	1.17	1.10	1.25	Low

Study	Exposure	Comparison	No.	Type	Measure				Quality
Nindrea et al,[60] 2019	Obesity	≥25 vs <23 kg/m²	10	Binary	OR	1.36	1.26	1.47	Moderate
Byun et al,[73] 2021	Body mass index at young age	5 kg/m² increase	6	Dose–response	RR	0.82	0.78	0.87	Moderate
Physical activity									
Lagerros et al,[15] 2004	Physical activity in adolescence and young adulthood	Physical activity	9	Binary	RR	0.85	0.70	1.02	Low
Liu et al,[46] 2015	Leisure time physical activity	Physical activity	6	Binary	RR	0.79	0.63	0.99	Low
Neilson et al,[53] 2016	Moderate-vigorous recreational physical activity	Metabolic equivalent value 3.0	43	Binary	RR	0.80	0.74	0.87	Low
Pizot et al,[48] 2016	Physical activity level	na	18	Binary	RR	0.87	0.78	0.96	Very low
Chen et al,[59] 2018	Physical activity	Physical activity	9	Binary	RR	0.80	0.75	0.86	Moderate
Hidayat et al,[63] 2019	Physical activity at a young age	5-30 years old	14	Binary	RR	0.87	0.78	0.96	Low
Hidayat et al,[63] 2019	Lifetime physical activity	>10 years	12	Binary	RR	0.81	0.66	0.99	Very low
Sleep									
Schwarz et al,[70] 2021	Long-term night-shift work	≥15 years	6	Binary	RR	1.27	0.96	1.68	Low
Smoking									
Khuder et al,[13] 2001	Past smoking	Former active smoking	9	Binary	RR	1.30	1.19	1.51	Low
Khuder et al,[13] 2001	Ever smoking	Ever active smoking	13	Binary	RR	1.21	1.08	1.36	Low

(continued on next page)

Table 3
(continued)

Study Year	Risk Factor	Measurement of Risk	Number of Studies	Type of Outcome	Type of Effect	Effect Size	Lower CI	Upper CI	Quality of Evidence (GRADE)
Khuder et al,[13] 2001	Current smoking	Current active smoking	9	Binary	RR	1.18	0.94	1.48	Very low
Lee et al,[16] 2006	Passive smoking	Exposure to passive smoking	10	Binary	RR	1.54	1.16	2.05	Very low
Yang et al,[32] 2013	Passive smoking	Exposure to passive smoking	3	Binary	RR	1.11	0.55	2.24	Very low
Macacu et al,[41] 2015	Passive ever smoking	Exposure to passive smoking	5	Binary	RR	1.16	0.62	2.16	Very low
Macacu et al,[41] 2015	Active ever smoking	Active smoking	6	Binary	RR	1.11	1.00	1.25	Moderate
Waist and hip measures									
Connolly et al,[14] 2002	Waist-to-hip ratio	≥0.81 vs <0.78	6	Binary	OR	2.07	1.15	3.73	Very low
Connolly et al,[14] 2002	Waist-to-hip ratio	>0.778 vs ≤0.75	4	Binary	OR	1.44	1.01	2.04	Very low
Amadou et al,[26] 2013	Waist-to-hip ratio	0.1 unit increase	12	Dose–response	RR	1.08	1.01	1.16	Low
Chen et al,[42] 2016	Waist circumference	10 cm increase	8	Dose–response	RR	1.05	0.99	1.10	Moderate
Chen et al,[42] 2016	Waist-to-hip ratio	0.1 unit increase	11	Dose–response	RR	1.07	0.95	1.21	Low

subgroup of past smoking, one risk estimation with a low quality evidence reported a RR = 1.30 (95%CI 1.19, 1.51). For subgroup of ever smoking, one risk estimation with low quality evidence reported a risk estimate RR = 1.21 (95%CI 1.08, 1.36).

POSTMENOPAUSAL BREAST CANCER

In **Table 4**, we present findings from the studies that reported the risk of breast cancer among postmenopausal women. For body mass, three risk estimations for breast cancer were moderate, six low, and one very low-quality evidence. Eight risk estimations reported a higher risk of breast cancer for a higher value of body mass measures (obesity, weight gain, and so forth). Three risk estimations with moderate quality evidence reported a higher risk for breast cancer. Overall, the risk estimates ranged from RR = 0.83 (95%CI 0.77, 0.89) to OR = 1.43 (95%CI 1.23, 1.65). For moderate quality evidence, risk estimates ranged from OR = 1.11 (95%CI 1.08, 1.13) to RR = 1.43 (95%CI 1.23, 1.65). Two dose–response meta-analyses reported a higher risk for breast cancer with an increase in body mass. For waist and hip measures, one risk estimation was moderate, one low, and two very low quality evidence. All these risk estimations reported a higher risk of breast cancer ranging from RR = 1.06 (95%CI 1.04, 1.09) to OR = 1.75 (95%CI 1.07, 2.87).

For physical activity, we found three risk estimations of moderate, two of low, and two of very low-quality evidence. All risk estimations reported a lower risk of breast cancer. The risk estimates ranged from RR = 0.69 (95%CI 0.59, 0.81) to RR = 0.91 (95%CI 0.82, 0.99).

For risk measures related to sleep disruption and quality, there was only one risk estimation with low quality evidence, reporting a higher risk for breast cancer for women working 15 or more years on night shift RR = 1.05 (95%CI 0.90, 1.24). For smoking, two estimations reported moderate, four low, and one very low quality evidence. Six risk estimations reported a minor, often insignificant higher risk of breast cancer for different forms of smoking exposure or initiation.

DISCUSSION

This review identifies the most recent evidence that examines the size of the effect of select lifestyle factors on risk for breast cancer. We found evidence that shows an increased risk for breast cancer due to obesity. Furthermore, there is evidence to demonstrate an increased risk for breast cancer due to alcohol intake and smoking. The evidence shows the physical activity as a protective factor for breast cancer. The evidence for night work is inconclusive. One important limitation of all this review is that most studies are from high-income countries.

Overall, umbrella reviews studying factors impacting breast cancer risk are scarce. This lack of reviews exploring risk factors related to breast cancer highlights a gap in the current state of knowledge. This ubmrella review reduces such gap. Furthermore, considering epidemiologic trends, it reminds us of the importance of analyzing factors tied to industrialization which have been linked to breast cancer risk. The added value and strength of our review is in a thorough search of relevant studies across four databases using reliable tools and standards for performing review, organization, and assessment of evidence.

In an umbrella review of the evidence associating diet and cancer risk published in 2021, alcohol consumption was found to be positively associated with the risk of multiple cancers, including postmenopausal breast cancer.[74] In another review, it was concluded that overweight/obesity increases the risk of multiple cancers, including postmenopausal breast cancer.[75] Kyrgiou and colleagues published an umbrella

Table 4
Results for postmenopausal breast cancer

Study Year	Risk Factor	Measurement of Risk	Number of Studies	Type of Outcome	Type of Effect	Effect Size	Lower CI	Upper CI	Quality of Evidence (GRADE)
Body mass and height									
Renehan et al,[19] 2008	Body mass index	5 kg/m² increase	31	Dose–response	RR	1.12	1.08	1.16	Low
Cheraghi et al,[24] 2012	Overweight and obesity	≤25 vs < 25 kg/m²	8	Binary	RR	1.14	1.09	1.19	Low
Cheraghi et al,[24] 2012	Overweight and obesity	≥ 25 vs <25 kg/m²	29	Binary	OR	1.15	1.07	1.24	Low
Pierobon et al,[30] 2012	Obesity	≥30 vs <30 kg/m²	5	Binary	OR	1.43	1.23	1.65	Moderate
Keum et al,[40] 2015	Adult weight gain	5 kg increase	7	Dose–response	RR	1.11	1.08	1.13	Moderate
Wang et al,[50] 2016	Body mass index	5 kg/m² increase	37	Dose–response	RR	1.11	1.08	1.14	Low
Chen et al,[51] 2017	Body mass index	Highest vs normal	26	Binary	RR	1.33	1.20	1.48	Low
Hidayat et al,[57] 2018	Body fatness gain from young age	5 kg/m² increase	5	Dose–response	RR	1.14	1.06	1.23	Moderate
Hidayat et al,[57] 2018	Body mass index at young age	age ≤ 30 years; 5 kg/ m² increase	17	Dose–response	RR	0.83	0.77	0.89	Very low
Byun et al,[73] 2022	Body mass index	5 kg/m² increase	12	Dose–response	RR	0.83	0.79	0.87	Low
Physical activity									
Lagerros et al,[15] 2004	Physical activity in adolescence and young adulthood	Physical activity	11	Binary	RR	0.88	0.78	0.99	Moderate

Study	Exposure	Measure	No.	Type					Evidence
Liu et al,[46] 2016	Leisure time physical activity	Physical activity	15	Binary	RR	0.89	0.84	0.93	Moderate
Neilson et al,[53] 2017	Moderate-vigorous recreational physical activity	Metabolic equivalent value 3.0	58	Binary	RR	0.79	0.74	0.84	Low
Pizot et al,[48] 2016	Physical activity level	Physical activity	32	Binary	RR	0.88	0.85	0.91	Low
Chen et al,[59] 2019	Physical activity	Physical activity	23	Binary	RR	0.91	0.82	0.99	Moderate
Hidayat et al,[63] 2020	Physical activity at a young age	5-30 years old	19	Binary	RR	0.86	0.78	0.94	Very low
Hidayat et al,[63] 2020	Lifetime physical activity	>10 years	13	Binary	RR	0.69	0.59	0.81	Very low
Sleep									
Schwarz et al,[70] 2021	Long-term night shift work	≥15 years	7	Binary	RR	1.05	0.90	1.24	Low
Smoking									
Khuder et al,[13] 2001	Past smoking	Former active smoking	8	Binary	RR	1.10	1.03	1.18	Moderate
Khuder et al,[13] 2001	Ever smoking	Ever active smoking	12	Binary	RR	1.07	1.02	1.19	Low
Khuder et al,[13] 2001	Current smoking	Current active smoking	8	Binary	RR	1.05	0.96	1.15	Low
Lee et al,[16] 2006	Passive smoking	Exposure to passive smoking	10	Binary	RR	0.98	0.86	1.12	Very low
Yang et al,[32] 2013	Passive smoking	Exposure to passive smoking	4	Binary	RR	1.01	0.85	1.20	Low
Macacu et al,[41] 2015	Passive ever smoking	Exposure to passive smoking	6	Binary	RR	1.04	0.90	1.21	Low

(continued on next page)

Table 4
(continued)

Study Year	Risk Factor	Measurement of Risk	Number of Studies	Type of Outcome	Type of Effect	Effect Size	Lower CI	Upper CI	Quality of Evidence (GRADE)
Macacu et al,[41] 2015	Active ever smoking	Active smoking	10	Binary	RR	1.10	1.07	1.13	Moderate
Waist and hip measures									
Connolly et al,[14] 2002	Waist-to-hip ratio	>0.80 vs ≤ 0.79	5	Binary	OR	1.21	0.99	1.48	Very low
Connolly et al,[14] 2002	Waist-to-hip ratio	≥ 0.83 vs <0.79	6	Binary	OR	1.75	1.07	2.87	Very low
Chen et al,[42] 2016	Waist-to-hip ratio	0.1 unit increase	15	Dose–response	RR	1.07	1.01	1.14	Low
Chen et al,[42] 2016	Waist circumference	10 cm increase	14	Dose–response	RR	1.06	1.04	1.09	Moderate

review of systematic reviews and meta-analyses evaluating the association between adiposity and the risk of developing or dying from cancer. They found that the risk of postmenopausal breast cancer among women who have never used hormone replacement therapy increased by 11% for each 5 kg weight gain in adulthood (RR = 1.11, 95%CI 1.09, 1.13).[76] Rezende and colleagues[77] explored the association between physical activity and cancer incidence and mortality in their umbrella review and found a protective association with breast cancer. Moreover, a review of 14 meta-analyses, concluded that high sedentary behavior levels increase the risk for multiple cancers, including breast with a relative risk of 1.08 (95%CI,1.04, 1.11).[78] Our review provides most recent and updated evidence on this domain.

It would not be enough just to know that these lifestyle factors are likely causes of breast cancer. The evidence for factors with higher quality of evidence, should inform medical practice, and find use for developing assessment and behavioral change tools that support lifestyle changes that prevent breast cancer. Or when it occurs, they can help reduce the effect of the risk factors that caused it. For example, identifying measurable biomarkers in blood or tissue to determine how different risk factors may exacerbate or ameliorate risk on a personalized level is needed to better control for genetic and other factors. This could even extend to identifying targetable biomarkers which could be modified by certain interventions.

SUMMARY

Lifestyle factors play a major role in the risk of breast cancer. We found evidence for an increased risk for breast cancer due to obesity, alcohol intake, and smoking and a decreased risk due to physical activity. The evidence for sleep disruption and duration indicates risk for breast cancer, but it is limited in size, statistical significance, and quality of evidence. The work for further investigation and generation of high-quality evidence should continue. At the same time, existing knowledge should inform the way medicine is practiced and encourage the development of tools and methods that use this knowledge to shape lifestyle behavior and change.

AUTHOR CONTRIBUTIONS

The study was conceived and designed by I Hoxha. The data were screened by F Sadiku, L Hoxha, M Nasim and extracted by I Hoxha, F Sadiku, L Hoxha, K Grezda. Quality assessment was performed by I Hoxha and F Sadiku. I Hoxha has analyzed the data. The article was prepared by I Hoxha, F Sadiku, MAC Buteau and was critically reviewed by all authors.

DISCLOSURE

No external funding was received for this study. I Hoxha has stock and other ownership interests at LifestylediagnostiX. M.D. Chamberlin has a past consulting or advisory role with Genomic Health International and received research funding from Archer, Inc over 5 years ago. No other potential conflicts of interest were reported.

CLINICS CARE POINTS

- Lifestyle factors play a significant role in the risk of breast cancer.
- The evidence shows an increased risk for breast cancer due to obesity, alcohol intake, and smoking and a decreased risk due to physical activity.

- The evidence for sleep disruption and duration indicates risk for breast cancer but is limited in size, statistical significance, and quality of evidence.
- The evidence on the effect of lifestyle factors should inform how medicine is practiced and encourage the development of tools and methods that use this knowledge to shape lifestyle behavior and change.
- The support for lifestyle changes should occur before and after breast cancer.

SUPPLEMENTARY DATA

Supplementary data related to this article can be found online at https://doi.org/10.1016/j.hoc.2023.07.005.

REFERENCES

1. Sung H, Ferlay J, Siegel RL, et al. Global cancer statistics 2020: GLOBOCAN estimates of incidence and mortality worldwide for 36 cancers in 185 countries. CA Cancer J Clin 2021;71(3):209–49 [published Online First: 20210204].
2. Hoxha I, Islami DA, Uwizeye G, et al. Forty-five years of research and progress in breast cancer: progress for some, disparities for most. JCO Global Oncology 2022;8.
3. Tfayli A, Temraz S, Abou Mrad R, et al. Breast cancer in low- and middle-income countries: an emerging and challenging epidemic. J Oncol 2010;2010:490631 [published Online First: 20101215].
4. De Moulin D. A short history of breast cancer. Dordrecht, Netherlands: Springer Science & Business Media; 2012.
5. Siegel RL, Miller KD, Fuchs HE, et al. Cancer Statistics, 2021. CA Cancer J Clin 2021;71(1):7–33 [published Online First: 20210112].
6. Ahlgren M, Melbye M, Wohlfahrt J, et al. Growth patterns and the risk of breast cancer in women. N Engl J Med 2004;351(16):1619–26.
7. Inumaru LE, Silveira EA, Naves MM. [Risk and protective factors for breast cancer: a systematic review]. Cad Saúde Pública 2011;27(7):1259–70.
8. Gao Y, Huang YB, Liu XO, et al. Tea consumption, alcohol drinking and physical activity associations with breast cancer risk among Chinese females: a systematic review and meta-analysis. Asian Pac J Cancer Prev 2013;14(12):7543–50.
9. Higgins JP, Thomas J, Chandler J, et al. Cochrane handbook for systematic reviews of interventions. Chichester, UK: John Wiley & Sons; 2019.
10. Guyatt GH, Oxman AD, Vist GE, et al. GRADE: an emerging consensus on rating quality of evidence and strength of recommendations. BMJ 2008;336(7650):924–6.
11. Khuder SA, Simon VJ Jr. Is there an association between passive smoking and breast cancer? Eur J Epidemiol 2000;16(12):1117–21.
12. Ellison RC, Zhang Y, McLennan CE, et al. Exploring the relation of alcohol consumption to risk of breast cancer. Am J Epidemiol 2001;154(8):740–7.
13. Khuder SA, Mutgi AB, Nugent S. Smoking and breast cancer: a meta-analysis. Rev Environ Health 2001;16(4):253–61.
14. Connolly BS, Barnett C, Vogt KN, et al. A meta-analysis of published literature on waist-to-hip ratio and risk of breast cancer. Nutr Cancer 2002;44(2):127–38.
15. Lagerros YT, Hsieh SF, Hsieh CC. Physical activity in adolescence and young adulthood and breast cancer risk: a quantitative review. Eur J Cancer Prev 2004;13(1):5–12.

16. Lee PN, Hamling J. Environmental tobacco smoke exposure and risk of breast cancer in nonsmoking women: a review with meta-analyses. Inhal Toxicol 2006; 18(14):1053–70.

17. Miller MD, Marty MA, Broadwin R, et al. The association between exposure to environmental tobacco smoke and breast cancer: a review by the California Environmental Protection Agency. Prev Med 2007;44(2):93–106 [published Online First: 20061005].

18. Pirie K, Beral V, Peto R, et al. Passive smoking and breast cancer in never smokers: prospective study and meta-analysis. Int J Epidemiol 2008;37(5): 1069–79 [published Online First: 20080610].

19. Renehan AG, Tyson M, Egger M, et al. Body-mass index and incidence of cancer: a systematic review and meta-analysis of prospective observational studies. Lancet 2008;371(9612):569–78.

20. Suzuki R, Orsini N, Mignone L, et al. Alcohol intake and risk of breast cancer defined by estrogen and progesterone receptor status–a meta-analysis of epidemiological studies. Int J Cancer 2008;122(8):1832–41.

21. Suzuki R, Orsini N, Saji S, et al. Body weight and incidence of breast cancer defined by estrogen and progesterone receptor status–a meta-analysis. Int J Cancer 2009;124(3):698–712.

22. DeRoo LA, Cummings P, Mueller BA. Smoking before the first pregnancy and the risk of breast cancer: a meta-analysis. Am J Epidemiol 2011;174(4):390–402 [published Online First: 20110630].

23. Li Y, Yang H, Cao J. Association between alcohol consumption and cancers in the Chinese population–a systematic review and meta-analysis. PLoS One 2011;6(4): e18776 [published Online First: 20110415].

24. Cheraghi Z, Poorolajal J, Hashem T, et al. Effect of body mass index on breast cancer during premenopausal and postmenopausal periods: a meta-analysis. PLoS One 2012;7(12):e51446 [published Online First: 20121207].

25. Seitz HK, Pelucchi C, Bagnardi V, et al. Epidemiology and pathophysiology of alcohol and breast cancer: update 2012. Alcohol Alcohol 2012;47(3):204–12 [published Online First: 20120329].

26. Amadou A, Ferrari P, Muwonge R, et al. Overweight, obesity and risk of premenopausal breast cancer according to ethnicity: a systematic review and dose-response meta-analysis. Obes Rev 2013;14(8):665–78 [published Online First: 20130425].

27. Bagnardi V, Rota M, Botteri E, et al. Light alcohol drinking and cancer: a meta-analysis. Ann Oncol 2013;24(2):301–8 [published Online First: 20120821].

28. Gaudet MM, Gapstur SM, Sun J, et al. Active smoking and breast cancer risk: original cohort data and meta-analysis. J Natl Cancer Inst 2013;105(8):515–25 [published Online First: 20130228].

29. Ijaz S, Verbeek J, Seidler A, et al. Night-shift work and breast cancer–a systematic review and meta-analysis. Scand J Work Environ Health 2013;39(5):431–47 [published Online First: 20130626].

30. Pierobon M, Frankenfeld CL. Obesity as a risk factor for triple-negative breast cancers: a systematic review and meta-analysis. Breast Cancer Res Treat 2013;137(1): 307–14 [published Online First: 20121120].

31. Wu Y, Zhang D, Kang S. Physical activity and risk of breast cancer: a meta-analysis of prospective studies. Breast Cancer Res Treat 2013;137(3):869–82 [published Online First: 20121230].

32. Yang Y, Zhang F, Skrip L, et al. Lack of an association between passive smoking and incidence of female breast cancer in non-smokers: evidence from 10

prospective cohort studies. PLoS One 2013;8(10):e77029 [published Online First: 20131018].

33. Chen C, Huang YB, Liu XO, et al. Active and passive smoking with breast cancer risk for Chinese females: a systematic review and meta-analysis. Chin J Cancer 2014;33(6):306–16 [published Online First: 20140505].

34. Namiranian N, Moradi-Lakeh M, Razavi-Ratki SK, et al. Risk factors of breast cancer in the eastern mediterranean region: a systematic review and meta-analysis. Asian Pac J Cancer Prev 2014;15(21):9535–41.

35. Qin Y, Zhou Y, Zhang X, et al. Sleep duration and breast cancer risk: a meta-analysis of observational studies. Int J Cancer 2014;134(5):1166–73 [published Online First: 20130914].

36. Xia X, Chen W, Li J, et al. Body mass index and risk of breast cancer: a nonlinear dose-response meta-analysis of prospective studies. Sci Rep 2014;4:7480 [published Online First: 20141215].

37. Yang WS, Deng Q, Fan WY, et al. Light exposure at night, sleep duration, melatonin, and breast cancer: a dose-response analysis of observational studies. Eur J Cancer Prev 2014;23(4):269–76.

38. Bagnardi V, Rota M, Botteri E, et al. Alcohol consumption and site-specific cancer risk: a comprehensive dose-response meta-analysis. Br J Cancer 2015;112(3):580–93 [published Online First: 20141125].

39. Chen Z, Shao J, Gao X, et al. Effect of passive smoking on female breast cancer in China: a meta-analysis. Asia Pac J Public Health 2015;27(2):NP58–64 [published Online First: 20130409].

40. Keum N, Greenwood DC, Lee DH, et al. Adult weight gain and adiposity-related cancers: a dose-response meta-analysis of prospective observational studies. J Natl Cancer Inst 2015;107(2). https://doi.org/10.1093/jnci/djv088 [published Online First: 20150310].

41. Macacu A, Autier P, Boniol M, et al. Active and passive smoking and risk of breast cancer: a meta-analysis. Breast Cancer Res Treat 2015;154(2):213–24 [published Online First: 20151106].

42. Chen GC, Chen SJ, Zhang R, et al. Central obesity and risks of pre- and postmenopausal breast cancer: a dose-response meta-analysis of prospective studies. Obes Rev 2016;17(11):1167–77 [published Online First: 20160719].

43. Chen JY, Zhu HC, Guo Q, et al. Dose-dependent associations between wine drinking and breast cancer risk - meta-analysis findings. Asian Pac J Cancer Prev 2016;17(3):1221–33.

44. Jayasekara H, MacInnis RJ, Room R, et al. Long-term alcohol consumption and breast, upper aero-digestive tract and colorectal cancer risk: a systematic review and meta-analysis. Alcohol Alcohol 2016;51(3):315–30 [published Online First: 20150922].

45. Kyu HH, Bachman VF, Alexander LT, et al. Physical activity and risk of breast cancer, colon cancer, diabetes, ischemic heart disease, and ischemic stroke events: systematic review and dose-response meta-analysis for the Global Burden of Disease Study 2013. BMJ 2016;354:i3857 [published Online First: 20160809].

46. Liu L, Shi Y, Li T, et al. Leisure time physical activity and cancer risk: evaluation of the WHO's recommendation based on 126 high-quality epidemiological studies. Br J Sports Med 2016;50(6):372 8 [published Online First: 20151023].

47. Ordonez-Mena JM, Schottker B, Mons U, et al. Quantification of the smoking-associated cancer risk with rate advancement periods: meta-analysis of individual participant data from cohorts of the CHANCES consortium. BMC Med 2016;14:62 [published Online First: 20160405].

48. Pizot C, Boniol M, Mullie P, et al. Physical activity, hormone replacement therapy and breast cancer risk: a meta-analysis of prospective studies. Eur J Cancer 2016;52:138–54 [published Online First: 20151211].

49. Travis RC, Balkwill A, Fensom GK, et al. Night Shift Work and Breast Cancer Incidence: Three Prospective Studies and Meta-analysis of Published Studies. J Natl Cancer Inst 2016;108(12). https://doi.org/10.1093/jnci/djw169 [published Online First: 20161006].

50. Wang J, Yang DL, Chen ZZ, et al. Associations of body mass index with cancer incidence among populations, genders, and menopausal status: A systematic review and meta-analysis. Cancer Epidemiol 2016;42:1–8 [published Online First: 20160303].

51. Chen Y, Liu L, Zhou Q, et al. Body mass index had different effects on premenopausal and postmenopausal breast cancer risks: a dose-response meta-analysis with 3,318,796 subjects from 31 cohort studies. BMC Publ Health 2017; 17(1):936 [published Online First: 20171208].

52. Lu C, Sun H, Huang J, et al. Long-Term Sleep Duration as a Risk Factor for Breast Cancer: Evidence from a Systematic Review and Dose-Response Meta-Analysis. BioMed Res Int 2017;2017:4845059 [published Online First: 20171010].

53. Neilson HK, Farris MS, Stone CR, et al. Moderate-vigorous recreational physical activity and breast cancer risk, stratified by menopause status: a systematic review and meta-analysis. Menopause 2017;24(3):322–44.

54. Zahmatkesh BH, Alavi N, Keramat A, et al. Body mass index and risk of breast cancer: a systematic review and meta-analysis in Iran. International Journal of Cancer Management 2017;10(4). https://doi.org/10.5812/ijcm.5921.

55. Choi YJ, Myung SK, Lee JH. Light alcohol drinking and risk of cancer: a meta-analysis of cohort studies. Cancer Res Treat 2018;50(2):474–87 [published Online First: 20170522].

56. Hardefeldt PJ, Penninkilampi R, Edirimanne S, et al. Physical activity and weight loss reduce the risk of breast cancer: a meta-analysis of 139 prospective and retrospective studies. Clin Breast Cancer 2018;18(4):e601–12 [published Online First: 20171017].

57. Hidayat K, Yang CM, Shi BM. Body fatness at a young age, body fatness gain and risk of breast cancer: systematic review and meta-analysis of cohort studies. Obes Rev 2018;19(2):254–68 [published Online First: 20171112].

58. Kim AS, Ko HJ, Kwon JH, et al. Exposure to secondhand smoke and risk of cancer in never smokers: a meta-analysis of epidemiologic studies. Int J Environ Res Publ Health 2018;15(9). https://doi.org/10.3390/ijerph15091981 [published Online First: 20180911].

59. Chen X, Wang Q, Zhang Y, et al. Physical Activity and Risk of Breast Cancer: A Meta-Analysis of 38 Cohort Studies in 45 Study Reports. Value Health 2019;22(1): 104–28 [published Online First: 20181214].

60. Nindrea RD, Aryandono T, Lazuardi L, et al. Association of overweight and obesity with breast cancer during premenopausal period in asia: a meta-analysis. Int J Prev Med 2019;10:192 [published Online First: 20191106].

61. Dong JY, Qin LQ. Education level and breast cancer incidence: a meta-analysis of cohort studies. Menopause 2020;27(1):113–8.

62. Dun A, Zhao X, Jin X, et al. Association between night-shift work and cancer risk: updated systematic review and meta-analysis. Front Oncol 2020;10:1006 [published Online First: 20200623].

63. Hidayat K, Zhou HJ, Shi BM. Influence of physical activity at a young age and lifetime physical activity on the risks of 3 obesity-related cancers: systematic review and meta-analysis of observational studies. Nutr Rev 2020;78(1):1–18.

64. Shamshirian A, Heydari K, Shams Z, et al. Breast cancer risk factors in Iran: a systematic review & meta-analysis. Horm Mol Biol Clin Investig 2020;41(4). https://doi.org/10.1515/hmbci-2020-0021 [published Online First: 20201021].

65. Sun Q, Xie W, Wang Y, et al. Alcohol consumption by beverage type and risk of breast cancer: a dose-response meta-analysis of prospective cohort studies. Alcohol Alcohol 2020;55(3):246–53.

66. Arafat HM, Omar J, Muhamad R, et al. Breast cancer risk from modifiable and non-modifiable risk factors among Palestinian women: a systematic review and meta-analysis. Asian Pac J Cancer Prev 2021;22(7):1987–95 [published Online First: 20210701].

67. Hao Y, Jiang M, Miao Y, et al. Effect of long-term weight gain on the risk of breast cancer across women's whole adulthood as well as hormone-changed menopause stages: A systematic review and dose-response meta-analysis. Obes Res Clin Pract 2021;15(5):439–48 [published Online First: 20210826].

68. Larsson SC, Burgess S. Causal role of high body mass index in multiple chronic diseases: a systematic review and meta-analysis of Mendelian randomization studies. BMC Med 2021;19(1). https://doi.org/10.1186/s12916-021-02188-x.

69. Poorolajal J, Heidarimoghis F, Karami M, et al. Factors for the primary prevention of breast cancer: a meta-analysis of prospective cohort studies. J Res Health Sci 2021;21(3):e00520 [published Online First: 20210720].

70. Schwarz C, Pedraza-Flechas AM, Pastor-Barriuso R, et al. Long-term nightshift work and breast cancer risk: an updated systematic review and meta-analysis with special attention to menopausal status and to recent nightshift work. Cancers 2021;13(23):5952 [published Online First: 20211126].

71. Wei L, Han N, Sun S, et al. Sleep-disordered breathing and risk of the breast cancer: a meta-analysis of cohort studies. Int J Clin Pract 2021;75(11):e14793 [published Online First: 20210917].

72. Wong ATY, Heath AK, Tong TYN, et al. Sleep duration and breast cancer incidence: results from the Million Women Study and meta-analysis of published prospective studies. Sleep 2021;44(2). https://doi.org/10.1093/sleep/zsaa166.

73. Byun D, Hong S, Ryu S, et al. Early-life body mass index and risks of breast, endometrial, and ovarian cancers: a dose-response meta-analysis of prospective studies. Br J Cancer 2022;126(4):664–72 [published Online First: 20211112].

74. Papadimitriou N, Markozannes G, Kanellopoulou A, et al. An umbrella review of the evidence associating diet and cancer risk at 11 anatomical sites. Nat Commun 2021;12(1):4579 [published Online First: 20210728].

75. Key TJ, Schatzkin A, Willett WC, et al. Diet, nutrition and the prevention of cancer. Public Health Nutr 2004;7(1A):187–200.

76. Kyrgiou M, Kalliala I, Markozannes G, et al. Adiposity and cancer at major anatomical sites: umbrella review of the literature. BMJ 2017;356:j477 [published Online First: 20170228].

77. Rezende LFM, Sa TH, Markozannes G, et al. Physical activity and cancer: an umbrella review of the literature including 22 major anatomical sites and 770 000 cancer cases. Br J Sports Med 2018;52(13):826–33 [published Online First: 20171116].

78. Hermelink R, Leitzmann MF, Markozannes G, et al. Sedentary behavior and cancer-an umbrella review and meta-analysis. Eur J Epidemiol 2022;37(5):447–60 [published Online First: 20220525].

Lung Cancer and Lifestyle Factors: Umbrella Review

Jeta Bunjaku, MD, PhD[a], Arber Lama, MD, PhD[a],
Tawanda Pesanayi, MS[a], Jeton Shatri, MD PhD[b,c],
Mary Chamberlin, MD[d], Ilir Hoxha, MD, PhD[a,e,*]

KEYWORDS

- Lung cancer • Alcohol • Tea • Coffee • Lifestyle factors

KEY POINTS

- Lifestyle factors are known to cause lung cancer.
- We review the latest evidence examining the effect of various lifestyle factors such as alcohol, coffee and tea intake on lung cancer risk.
- We analyzed 15 systematic reviews and 30 meta-analyses examining the relationship between lung cancer and alcohol, coffee, and tea intake.
- We found an increased risk for lung cancer due to alcohol and coffee intake and a decreased risk due to tea intake.
- The evidence is low quality or, in the case of coffee consumption, confounded by other factors.

INTRODUCTION

Globally, lung cancer continues to be the neoplastic disease with the highest morbidity rates, accounting for 11.4% of all neoplasms.[1] Lung cancer ranks second after breast cancer in incidence rates for both sexes. The appearance of symptoms in the late stages of the disease often results in a relatively late diagnosis when the disease has progressed or even metastasized.[2] Due to such diagnostic delays, the 5-year survival rate of people suffering from lung cancer is only 19%,[3] making disease treatment and prevention very difficult.

The increase in lung cancer incidence makes it increasingly important to understand the avoidable risk factors for lung cancer.[4] After water, tea is the most popular beverage

[a] Evidence Synthesis Group, Ali Vitia Street PN, 10000 Prishtina, Kosovo; [b] Clinic of Radiology, University Clinical Center of Kosovo, 10000 Prishtina, Kosovo; [c] Department of Anatomy, University of Prishtina, 10000 Prishtina, Kosovo; [d] Dartmouth Cancer Center at Dartmouth-Hitchcock Medical Center Lebanon, NH 03756, USA; [e] The Dartmouth Institute for Health Policy and Clinical Practice, Geisel School of Medicine at Dartmouth, Lebanon NH 03766, USA
* Corresponding author.
E-mail address: ilir.s.hoxha@dartmouth.edu

Hematol Oncol Clin N Am 38 (2024) 171–184
https://doi.org/10.1016/j.hoc.2023.05.018
0889-8588/24/© 2023 Elsevier Inc. All rights reserved.

consumed worldwide,[5,6] for its health benefits, especially as a protective effect on various cancers, have garnered much attention[7,8]. In-vitro studies and in vivo experiments have shown that active tea ingredients such as polyphenols,[9] can inhibit cell proliferation and tumor progression.[10,11] For green tea, health benefits[12] including anti-inflammatory,[13] antibacterial,[14] neuroprotective,[15] cholesterol-lowering effects[16] have been reported. Tang and colleagues in a 2009 meta-analysis found that green tea consumption has a protective effect on lung cancer, though this same effect was not observed with black tea.[17]

Coffee is another very popular beverage worldwide. It contains anti-oxidative and anti-inflammatory chemical compounds,[18] as well as flavonoids that reduce the risk of lung cancer. Chlorogenic acid (CGA), an important biochemical substance found in coffee, is thought to play an important role in reducing tumor expansion and metastasis. According to Kudwongsa and colleagues, coffee consumption can have a protective role in the risk of lung cancer,[19] though other studies have observed that this benefit may largely be confounded by smoking.[20–22]

The health effects of alcohol vary depending on the amount of consumption and an individual's lifestyle routine. Recently, one study suggested positive health outcomes from alcohol, including reduced mortality risk, by reducing risk for cardiovascular disease and type-2 diabetes, for short or long-term light to moderate alcohol consumers.[23] Meta-analyses reveal varying results for alcohol consumption and its effect on lung cancer, though.[24–27] Bagnardi and colleagues, with an increase of 25 g of alcohol per day found stronger risk for cancers of the oral cavity and pharynx, esophagus, and larynx, and weaker risk for cancers of the stomach, colon and rectum, liver, breast and ovary.[24] But like Thun and colleagues they found no association between lung cancer mortality and any level of alcohol consumption.[24,25] In the study carried out by Korte and colleagues a smoking-adjusted association between alcohol and lung cancer risk is present for at the very high consumption populations. The lower level observed associations are likely to be explained by confounding.[26] Analysis carried by Freudenheim and colleagues reveals small risk for lung cancer with the consumption of > or = 30 g alcohol a day.[27] An analysis conducted by Chao found that the high consumption of beer and liquors may be associated with increased lung cancer risk, and wine consumption may reduce lung cancer risk.[28] Further, according to the International Agency for Research on Cancer, though, alcohol is ranked as a group 1 carcinogen, and alcohol consumption increases the risk of lung cancer,[29] amidst being a substantial risk factor for many cancers worldwide.[30]

Based on such conflicting evidence, we aimed to clarify the association between beverages such as tea, coffee, and alcohol consumption and the risk of the lung cancer, using an umbrella review of systematic reviews with meta-analyses.

METHODS

The umbrella review of systematic reviews was performed according to Cochrane guidelines.[31] Our search was performed across five databases, including CINAH, Cochrane, PubMed, Scopus, and Web of Science. We used search terms related to lung cancer and lifestyle factors of interest, such as alcohol, coffee, and tea, to construct a search strategy for finding relevant records. We limited the search to publication year (2000 and on), systematic reviews with meta-analysis, and human subjects reporting reviews. The search strategy is available in the Online Appendix. The search was last updated in July 2022.

Screening and the full-text review of articles were performed by two reviewers. We included English-written systemic reviews with meta-analysis establishing a qualitative association of risk or protective factors with lung cancer in human subjects. Risk factors of interest were alcohol, coffee, and tea intake. Two rounds of screening of titles and abstracts were performed, and the full-text review was performed afterward. Disagreements, such as whether to include or not a article, were solved with consensus and the involvement of an experienced reviewer.

Data extraction was done by two reviewers in parallel and reviewed by an experienced reviewer. We extracted information on the study's characteristics and general information, effect estimates, risk factors measurement, design, and population.

GRADE assessment for systematic reviews was used to assess the quality of systematic reviews.[32] Five key domains, as foreseen by GRADE, were assessed: the risk of bias related to the quality of studies, inconsistency of effect estimates, indirectness, imprecision, and the risk of publication bias. A four level (high, moderate, low, and very low quality) rating was used. Reviews were ranked as high quality if they fulfilled all criteria of GRADE. The meta-analyses were downgraded to lower levels of quality with each additional unfulfilled criterion.

A descriptive analysis of the data was used for all analyses performed. We present a summary of each of the key risk categories of interest, including the effect estimate, setting, risk factors and their measurement, and quality ranking for each meta-analyses. STATA 17BE (Stata Corp., College Station, TX, USA) was used for all analyses.

RESULTS

A total of 1950 records were identified. (**Fig. 1**) One hundred ninety-four publications were found in CINAHL, 198 in Cochrane, 749 in PubMed, 538 in Scopus, and 271 in Web of Science; an additional 18 articles were identified via a manual search of references. One thousand and four hundred and eighty one records were screened, after four hundred eighty-seven duplicates were excluded. Nine hundred eighty-one records were excluded after the screening of the titles and abstracts. The remaining 500 records were reviewed in full-text, and four hundred and eighty-five studies were subsequently excluded due to not reporting lung cancer or lifestyle factors of interest, or were reporting lung cancer treatment or other non-relevant studies. We finally included 15 records reporting 30 meta-analyses (ie, risk estimations).[17,20,22,24,26–28,33–40]

Ten studies were published from 2010 and on, and five before that period (**Table 1**).[17,20,22,24,26–28,33–40] These studies reported data from multiple countries. Eight studies reported the risk of alcohol on lung cancer, three studies reported the role of coffee intake, and four reported the role of tea intake in lung cancer. **Table 2** and **Fig. 2** present findings from all meta-analyses found.

Alcohol Intake

For alcohol intake, we found a total of 12 binary outcomes and four dose-response meta-analyses. The number of studies included in the meta-analyses ranged from 3 to 21, and the cumulative sample sizes of studies included in each meta-analysis ranged from over 14,000 to close to 2,500,000. The number of cases ranged from a few hundred to over 8000. One meta-analysis reported high, one moderate, 12 low, and two very low-quality evidence. Eleven meta-analyses reported a higher risk of lung cancer as a result of alcohol intake, but none of these meta-analyses were of high or moderate quality evidence; these risk estimates ranged from OR = 0.65 (95%CI 0.53, 0.77) to RR = 1.99 (95%CI 1.66, 2.39). For high or moderate quality evidence, risk estimates ranged from OR = 0.65 (95%CI 0.53, 0.77) to RR = 0.98 (95%CI

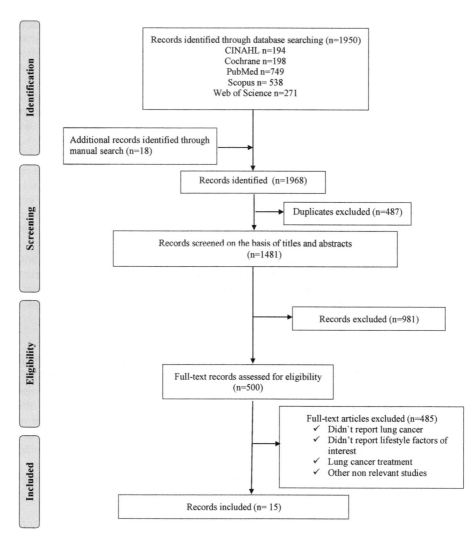

Fig. 1. Flowchart of the review

0.91, 1.07). Interestingly, four dose-response meta-analyses of various levels of alcohol intake reported a higher risk of lung cancer for alcohol intake, with statistically significant effects reported for three of them, though all of these meta-analyses were of low-quality evidence.

Coffee Intake

For coffee intake, we found a total of four binary outcomes and one dose-response meta-analyses. The number of studies included in the meta-analyses ranged from 9 to 21, and the cumulative sample sizes of studies included in each meta-analysis ranged from over 51,000 to over 600,000. The number of cases ranged from close to four thousand to close two twenty thousand. Three meta-analyses reported moderate, one low, and another of very low-quality evidence. Two meta-analyses of low or very low quality, and three meta-analyses of moderate quality, reported a higher risk of

Table 1
Included studies

Study Year	Countries	Risk Factor Category
Bagnardi et al,[24] 2001	Unclear	Alcohol
Korte et al,[26] 2002	Canada, Denmark, Finland, Ireland, Norway, Sweden, United Kingdom, United States	Alcohol
Freudenheim et al,[27] 2005	Canada, Finland, Netherlands, United States	Alcohol
Chao[28] 2007	Canada, Czech Republic, Denmark, Europe, Spain, United States, Uruguay	Alcohol
Tang et al,[17] 2009	Canada, China, Czech, Finland, Japan, Netherlands, Sweden, Uruguay, United States	Tea
Tang et al,[20] 2010	Canada, Czech Republic, Japan, Norway, Sweden, United States, Uruguay	Coffee
Uehara et al,[39] 2010	Japan	Alcohol
Bagnardi et al,[33] 2011	Canada, China, Italy, Japan, Netherland, Poland, United States, Other European countries	Alcohol
Li et al,[38] 2011	China	Alcohol
Wang et al,[40] 2014	Canada, China, Czech, Finland, India, Japan, Netherlands, Sweden, Taiwan China, Uruguay, United Kingdom, United States	Tea
Galarraga et al,[36] 2016	Canada, China, Czech Republic, France, India, Japan, Korea, Norway, Pakistan, Sweden, Uruguay, United States	Coffee
Xie et al,[22] 2016	Canada, Czech, France, Hong Kong, India, Japan, Korea, Pakistan, Sweden, United States, Uruguay	Coffee
Choi et al,[34] 2018	Canada, Denmark, Japan, United States	Alcohol
Guo et al,[37] 2019	Canada, China, Finland, India, Italy, Japan, Netherlands, Poland, Sweden, United Kingdom, Uruguay, United States	Tea
Filippini et al,[35] 2020	China, Czech Republic, Japan, United States	Tea

Table 2
Results for lung cancer

Study Year	Risk Factor	Measurement of Risk	Number of Studies	Total Sample	Total Cases	Type of Outcome	Type of Effect	Effect Size	Lower CI	Upper CI	Quality of Evidence (GRADE)
Alcohol											
Bagnardi et al,[24] 2001	Alcohol intake	25 g a day increaes of alcohol intake	6	Unclear	2314	Dose-response	RR	1.02	1.00	1.04	Low
Bagnardi et al,[24] 2001	Alcohol intake	100 g a day increaes of alcohol intake	6	Unclear	2314	Dose-response	RR	1.08	1.00	1.18	Low
Bagnardi et al,[24] 2001	Alcohol intake	50 g a day increaes of alcohol intake	6	Unclear	2314	Dose-response	RR	1.04	1.00	1.08	Low
Korte et al,[26] 2002	Beer intake	Beer intake vs no intake	3	22,169	482	Binary	RR	1.17	0.99	1.39	Low
Korte et al,[26] 2002	Alcohol intake	Acohol intake vs no intake	12	147,256	1311	Binary	RR	1.99	1.66	2.39	Very low
Freudenheim et al,[27] 2005	Alcohol intake	≥30 g a day vs 0 g a day of alcohol intake	9	468,074	3137	Binary	RR	1.18	0.99	1.39	Low
Chao[28] 2007	Beer intake	Average beer intake of one drink or greater a day vs no intake	21	464,075	8510	Binary	RR	1.23	1.06	1.41	Low
Chao[28] 2007	Wine intake	Average wine intake of less than one drink a day vs no intake	14	464,075	8510	Binary	RR	0.78	0.60	1.02	Low
Chao[28] 2007	Liquor intake	Average liquor intake of one drink or greater a day vs no intake	15	464,075	8510	Binary	RR	1.33	1.10	1.62	Low
Uehara et al, 2010	Alcohol intake	Highest vs lowest alcohol intake	4	80,232	1209	Binary	OR	0.65	0.53	0.77	High
Bagnardi et al,[33] 2011	Alcohol intake	Alcohol intake vs no alcohol intake	10	605,474	1913	Binary	RR	1.21	0.95	1.55	Very low

Study	Factor	Exposure	Ref	N	Cases	Type	Measure	Estimate	Lower	Upper	Quality
Bagnardi et al,[33] 2011	Alcohol intake	10 g a day increase of acohol intake	8	605,086	1771	Dose-response	RR	1.01	0.92	1.10	Low
Li et al,[38] 2011	Alcohol intake	Highest vs lowest alcohol intake	6	14,731	1104	Binary	OR	1.39	0.93	2.07	Low
Choi et al,[34] 2018	Moderate alcohol intake	1–2 drinks a day	8	1,957,494	Unclear	Binary	RR	0.98	0.91	1.07	Moderate
Choi et al,[34] 2018	Very light alcohol intake	≤0.5 drink a day	3	892,669	Unclear	Binary	RR	0.89	0.84	0.93	Low
Choi et al,[34] 2018	Light alcohol intake	<1 drink a day	10	2,458,402	Unclear	Binary	RR	0.91	0.90	0.94	Low
Coffee											
Tang et al,[20] 2010	Coffee intake	Highest vs lowest coffee intake	13	106,911	5347	Binary	RR	1.27	1.04	1.54	Low
Tang et al,[20] 2010	Coffee intake	2 cups a day increase of coffee intake	9	59,713	3862	Dose-response	RR	1.14	1.04	1.26	Moderate
Galarraga et al,[36] 2016	Coffee intake	Ever vs never coffee intake	21	623,645	19,892	Binary	RR	1.09	1.00	1.19	Very low
Xie et al,[22] 2016	Coffee intake	Coffee intake vs no intake	14	55,155	10,982	Binary	OR	1.17	1.03	1.33	Moderate
Xie et al,[22] 2016	Coffee intake	Highest vs lowest coffee intake	17	102,516	12,276	Binary	OR	1.31	1.11	1.55	Moderate
Tea											
Tang et al,[17] 2009	Green tea intake	Highest vs lowest green tea intake	12	102,042	5495	Binary	RR	0.78	0.61	1.00	Low

(continued on next page)

Table 2
(continued)

Study Year	Risk Factor	Measurement of Risk	Number of Studies	Total Sample	Total Cases	Type of Outcome	Type of Effect	Effect Size	Lower CI	Upper CI	Quality of Evidence (GRADE)
Tang et al,[17] 2009	Black tea intake	Highest vs lowest black tea intake	14	194,282	6936	Binary	RR	0.86	0.70	1.05	Low
Wang et al,[40] 2014	Black tea intake		13	191,124	6888	Binary	RR	0.82	0.71	0.94	Low
Wang et al,[40] 2014	Green tea intake		16	109,999	23,549	Binary	RR	0.75	0.62	0.91	Low
Wang et al,[40] 2014	Tea intake		38	396,664	59,041	Binary	RR	0.78	0.70	0.87	Very low
Guo et al,[37] 2019	Tea intake	Tea intake vs no intake	42	718,854	19,433	Binary	RR	0.80	0.73	0.87	Low
Guo et al,[37] 2019	Green tea intake	Green tea intake vs no intake	14	111,640	5750	Binary	RR	0.75	0.61	0.92	Low
Guo et al,[37] 2019	Black tea intake	Black tea intake vs no intake	9	159,909	4797	Binary	RR	0.80	0.70	0.91	Low
Filippini et al,[35] 2020	Green tea intake	Highest vs lowest greet tea intake	17	269,565	9180	Binary	RR	0.88	0.76	1.02	Low

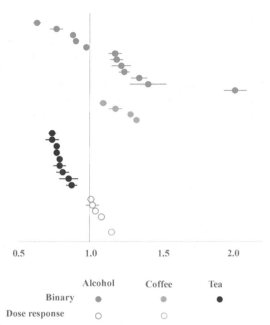

	Alcohol	Coffee	Tea
Binary	●	●	●
Dose response	○	○	

Fig. 2. Risk for lung cancer with effect estimates for alcohol, coffee and team intake

lung cancer as a result of coffee intake. Risk estimates for meta-analyses of low to very low-quality evidence ranged from OR = 1.09 (95%CI 1.00, 1.19) to OR = 1.27 (95%CI 1.04, 1.54), and for moderate quality evidence, ranged from OR = 1.17 (95%CI 1.03, 1.33) to OR = 1.31 (95%CI 1.11, 1.55). One dose-response meta-analysis of moderate quality evidence reported a statistically significant higher risk of lung cancer for coffee intake OR = 1.14 (95%CI 1.04, 1.26), too. All three studies reporting five meta-analysis considered the effect of smoking in interpretation[20,36] or analyses of results.[22,36] While Tang and colleagues only put some caution in the interpretation of results without performing specific analyses to show the confounding effect of smoking,[20] Galarraga and colleagues found that when smoking is controlled for, coffee intake does not show a risk for lung cancer. The dose–response analysis in never-smokers, resulted in an RR = 0.95 (95% CI, 0.83, 1.09).[36] Xie and colleagues to control for confounding by smoking, analyzed studies by omitting studies with no adjustment for smoking. In such case, the overall effect reduced but did not change substantially. The overall effect was RR = 1.15 (95% CI, 1.01, 1.32) for coffee drinkers as compared to nondrinkers and RR 1.29 (95% CI, 1.08, 1.54) for the highest category versus the lowest category of cofee drinkers.[22]

Tea Intake

For tea intake, we found a total of 9 binary outcome meta-analyses. The number of studies included the in meta-analyses ranged from 9 to 42 studies, and the cumulative sample sizes of studies included in each meta-analysis ranged from over 100,000 to over 700,000. The number of cases ranged from nearly 5000 to close to 60,000. All meta-analyses reported a lower risk for lung cancer as a result of tea intake, though 8 of these analyses were of low and 1 was of very low quality of evidence. Overall, the risk estimates ranged from RR = 0.75 (95%CI 0.61, 0.92) to RR = 0.88 (95%CI 0.76, 1.02).

DISCUSSION SECTION

This umbrella review (systematic review of systematic reviews) examines the association between beverages such as tea, coffee, and alcohol consumption and the risk of the lung cancer. We found that overall evidence suggests there is a risk of lung cancer from alcohol consumption, though, the evidence is largely of low quality. For coffee intake, too, evidence suggests an increased risk of lung cancer from coffee consumption, though evidence was of very low-moderate quality. We also found evidence to support tea drinking's protective effect against lung cancer, but evidence was also of low quality according to GRADE.

An umbrella review published in 2021 found that alcohol consumption was positively associated with the risk of multiple, including lung, cancers,[41] supporting our findings presented in the current article, despite evidence largely being of low quality. Though ethanol itself is not carcinogenic, its first metabolite (acetaldehyde) has been shown to be a local carcinogen in humans.[42] Acetaldehyde damages DNA and may block DNA synthesis and repair, leading to structural changes to chromosomes.[43,44]

Similar to our findings, an umbrella review of the evidence associating tea and cancer risk published in 2020 showed tea's protective effect by decreasing the risk of multiple cancers, including lung cancer.[45] This may be due to tea containing many bioactive components, such as catechins, flavonols, lignans, and phenolic acids, that protect against cancer. Its polyphenolic antioxidants, too, work by inhibiting nitrosation, cell proliferation, and tumor progression, and induce carcinoma cell apoptosis.[9] In fact, Ju and colleagues found that epigallocatechin gallate (EGCG) is the most abundant tea catechin and plays the most important role in inhibiting cancer progression.[46]

A relationship between coffee drinking and lung cancer risk is justified in that coffee contains agents which may cause cancer under experimental conditions, such as acrylamide,[47] which is formed during the roasting of coffee beans. Coffee contains o lot of bioactive compounds with antioxidant, anti-inflammatory, and anticancer effects. However, the coffee intake effect on lung cancer can be confounded by tobacco smoking.[36] Shafiei and colleagues found no significant association between total caffeine and caffeinated coffee intake and the risk for ovarian cancer risk, but an inverse association of decaffeinated coffee intake with the risk of ovarian cancer.[48] Je and colleagues, comparing high-versus low-consumption found no significant effect of coffee consumption on colorectal cancer risk. However, there was a slight suggestion of an inverse association between coffee consumption and colon cancer in women and in studies that controlled for smoking and alcohol.[49] Similarly, Sartini and collegues found no significant association between coffee intake and colorectal cancer. However, a protective effect was detected in European men and in Asian women.[50] In another study, decaffeinated coffee again showed a protective effect for colorectal cancer. In subgroup analysis, for colon cancer, coffee reduced risk and there was no association for rectal cancer.[50]

Yu and colleagues examining 59 studies, looking at multiple cancers found that an increase in coffee consumption was associated reduced risk of cancers. Subgroup analyses, revealed that, coffee intake reduced the risk for bladder, breast, buccal, and pharyngeal, colorectal, endometrial, esophageal, hepatocellular, leukemic, pancreatic, and prostate cancers. No association with lung cancer with coffee intake was determined.[51]

Though the strength of this review lies in the extensive search of literature across key databases, closely following the standards for umbrella reviews laid by Cochrane, the quality of evidence was low for alcohol, coffee, and tea consumption, and likely confounded by smoking for coffee consumption. Future studies with large, diverse samples should thoroughly explore the relationship between these beverages and risk of lung cancer, while adjusting for confounding factors.

SUMMARY

The evidence on the role of lifestyle factors in the risk of lung cancer is indicative of their role as risk or protective factors. We found evidence for an increased risk for lung cancer due to alcohol and coffee intake, amidst a protective role for tea intake, though evidence quality is low; evidence on the risk of coffee intake may further be confounded by smoking. Further research is needed to provide high-quality evidence in elucidating the effects of these common habitual lifestyle behaviors and the risk for lung cancer.

AUTHOR CONTRIBUTIONS

The study was conceived and designed by J. Bunjaku and I. Hoxha. The data were screened by J Bunjaku, A. Lama, T. Pesanayi, and extracted by J. Bunjaku, A. Lama, T. Pesanayi, and I. Hoxha. Quality assessment was performed by J. Bunjaku and I. Hoxha. I Hoxha has analyzed the data. The article was prepared by J Bunjaku, A Lama, and I Hoxha and was critically reviewed by all authors.

DISCLOSURE

No external funding was received for this study. Ilir Hoxha has stock and other owner-ship interests at LifestylediagnostiX. Mary D. Chamberlin has a past consulting or advisory role with Genomic Health International and received research funding from ARCHER, United States (Inst). No other potential conflicts of interest were reported.

SUPPLEMENTARY DATA

Supplementary data related to this article can be found online at https://doi.org/10.1016/j.hoc.2023.05.018.

REFERENCES

1. Sung H, Ferlay J, Siegel RL, et al. Global Cancer Statistics 2020: GLOBOCAN Estimates of Incidence and Mortality Worldwide for 36 Cancers in 185 Countries. CA Cancer J Clin 2021;71(3):209–49.
2. Shankar A, Dubey A, Saini D, et al. Environmental and occupational determinants of lung cancer. Transl Lung Cancer Res 2019;8(Suppl 1):S31–49.
3. Vieira AR, Abar L, Vingeliene S, et al. Fruits, vegetables and lung cancer risk: a systematic review and meta-analysis. Ann Oncol 2016;27(1):81–96.
4. Chen C, Hu Q, Wang J, et al. Habitual consumption of alcohol with meals and lung cancer: a Mendelian randomization study. Ann Transl Med 2021;9(3):263.
5. Bushman JL. Green tea and cancer in humans: a review of the literature. Nutr Cancer 1998;31(3):151–9.
6. Weisburger JH. Tea and health: a historical perspective. Cancer Lett 1997;114(1–2):315–7.
7. Yang CS, Ju J, Lu G, et al. Cancer prevention by tea and tea polyphenols. Asia Pac J Clin Nutr 2008;17(Suppl 1):245–8.
8. Shankar S, Marsh L, Srivastava RK. EGCG inhibits growth of human pancreatic tumors orthotopically implanted in Balb C nude mice through modulation of FKHRL1/FOXO3a and neuropilin. Mol Cell Biochem 2013;372(1–2):83–94.

9. Yang CS, Wang X, Lu G, et al. Cancer prevention by tea: animal studies, molecular mechanisms and human relevance. Nat Rev Cancer 2009;9(6):429–39.

10. Ahmad N, Mukhtar H. Green tea polyphenols and cancer: biologic mechanisms and practical implications. Nutr Rev 1999;57(3):78–83.

11. Cabrera C, Gimenez R, Lopez MC. Determination of tea components with antioxidant activity. J Agric Food Chem 2003;51(15):4427–35.

12. Xing L, Zhang H, Qi R, et al. Recent Advances in the Understanding of the Health Benefits and Molecular Mechanisms Associated with Green Tea Polyphenols. J Agric Food Chem 2019;67(4):1029–43.

13. Dona M, Dell'Aica I, Calabrese F, et al. Neutrophil restraint by green tea: inhibition of inflammation, associated angiogenesis, and pulmonary fibrosis. J Immunol 2003;170(8):4335–41.

14. Sudano Roccaro A, Blanco AR, Giuliano F, et al. Epigallocatechin-gallate enhances the activity of tetracycline in staphylococci by inhibiting its efflux from bacterial cells. Antimicrob Agents Chemother 2004;48(6):1968–73.

15. Weinreb O, Mandel S, Amit T, et al. Neurological mechanisms of green tea polyphenols in Alzheimer's and Parkinson's diseases. J Nutr Biochem 2004;15(9):506–16.

16. Raederstorff DG, Schlachter MF, Elste V, et al. Effect of EGCG on lipid absorption and plasma lipid levels in rats. J Nutr Biochem 2003;14(6):326–32.

17. Tang N, Wu Y, Zhou B, et al. Green tea, black tea consumption and risk of lung cancer: a meta-analysis. Lung Cancer 2009;65(3):274–83.

18. Ludwig IA, Clifford MN, Lean ME, et al. Coffee: biochemistry and potential impact on health. Food Funct 2014;5(8):1695–717.

19. Kudwongsa W, Promthet S, Suwanrungruang K, et al. Coffee Consumption and Lung Cancer Risk: A Prospective Cohort Study in Khon Kaen Thailand. Asian Pac J Cancer Prev 2020;21(8):2367–71.

20. Tang N, Wu Y, Ma J, et al. Coffee consumption and risk of lung cancer: a meta-analysis. Lung Cancer 2010;67(1):17–22.

21. Seow WJ, Koh WP, Jin A, et al. Associations between tea and coffee beverage consumption and the risk of lung cancer in the Singaporean Chinese population. Eur J Nutr 2020;59(7):3083–91.

22. Xie Y, Qin J, Nan G, et al. Coffee consumption and the risk of lung cancer: an updated meta-analysis of epidemiological studies. Eur J Clin Nutr 2016;70(2):199–206.

23. Hendriks HFJ. Alcohol and Human Health: What Is the Evidence? Annu Rev Food Sci Technol 2020;11:1–21.

24. Bagnardi V, Blangiardo M, La Vecchia C, et al. A meta-analysis of alcohol drinking and cancer risk. Br J Cancer 2001;85(11):1700–5.

25. Thun MJ, Hannan LM, DeLancey JO. Alcohol consumption not associated with lung cancer mortality in lifelong nonsmokers. Cancer Epidemiol Biomarkers Prev 2009;18(8):2269–72.

26. Korte JE, Brennan P, Henley SJ, et al. Dose-specific meta-analysis and sensitivity analysis of the relation between alcohol consumption and lung cancer risk. Am J Epidemiol 2002;155(6):496–506.

27. Freudenheim JL, Ritz J, Smith-Warner SA, et al. Alcohol consumption and risk of lung cancer: a pooled analysis of cohort studies. Am J Clin Nutr 2005;82(3):657–67.

28. Chao C. Associations between beer, wine, and liquor consumption and lung cancer risk: a meta-analysis. Cancer Epidemiol Biomarkers Prev 2007;16(11):2436–47.

29. Fehringer G, Brenner DR, Zhang ZF, et al. Alcohol and lung cancer risk among never smokers: A pooled analysis from the international lung cancer consortium and the SYNERGY study. Int J Cancer 2017;140(9):1976–84.

30. Boffetta P, Hashibe M. Alcohol and cancer. Lancet Oncol 2006;7(2):149–56.

31. Higgins JP, Thomas J, Chandler J, et al. Cochrane handbook for systematic reviews of interventions. Chichester, UK: John Wiley & Sons; 2019.

32. Guyatt GH, Oxman AD, Vist GE, et al. GRADE: an emerging consensus on rating quality of evidence and strength of recommendations. BMJ 2008;336(7650):924–6.

33. Bagnardi V, Rota M, Botteri E, et al. Alcohol consumption and lung cancer risk in never smokers: a meta-analysis. Ann Oncol 2011;22(12):2631–9.

34. Choi YJ, Myung SK, Lee JH. Light Alcohol Drinking and Risk of Cancer: A Meta-Analysis of Cohort Studies. Cancer Res Treat 2018;50(2):474–87.

35. Filippini T, Malavolti M, Borrelli F, et al. Green tea (Camellia sinensis) for the prevention of cancer. Cochrane Database Syst Rev 2020;2020(3). https://doi.org/10.1002/14651858.CD005004.pub3.

36. Galarraga V, Boffetta P. Coffee Drinking and Risk of Lung Cancer-A Meta-Analysis. Cancer Epidemiol Biomarkers Prev 2016;25(6):951–7.

37. Guo ZJ, Jiang M, Luo WT, et al. Association of Lung Cancer and Tea-Drinking Habits of Different Subgroup Populations: Meta-Analysis of Case-Control Studies and Cohort Studies. Iran J Public Health 2019;48(9):1566–76.

38. Li Y, Yang HA, Cao J. Association between Alcohol Consumption and Cancers in the Chinese Population-A Systematic Review and Meta-Analysis. PLoS One 2011;6(4). https://doi.org/10.1371/journal.pone.0018776.

39. Uehara Y, Kiyohara C. Alcohol consumption and lung cancer risk among Japanese: a meta-analysis. Fukuoka Igaku Zasshi 2010;101(5):101–8.

40. Wang L, Zhang X, Liu J, et al. Tea consumption and lung cancer risk: a meta-analysis of case-control and cohort studies. Nutrition 2014;30(10):1122–7.

41. Papadimitriou N, Markozannes G, Kanellopoulou A, et al. An umbrella review of the evidence associating diet and cancer risk at 11 anatomical sites. Nat Commun 2021;12(1):4579.

42. Salaspuro MP. Alcohol consumption and cancer of the gastrointestinal tract. Best Pract Res Clin Gastroenterol 2003;17(4):679–94.

43. Seitz HK, Stickel F. Molecular mechanisms of alcohol-mediated carcinogenesis. Nat Rev Cancer 2007;7(8):599–612.

44. Garaycoechea JI, Crossan GP, Langevin F, et al. Alcohol and endogenous aldehydes damage chromosomes and mutate stem cells. Nature 2018;553(7687):171–7.

45. Kim TL, Jeong GH, Yang JW, et al. Tea Consumption and Risk of Cancer: An Umbrella Review and Meta-Analysis of Observational Studies. Adv Nutr 2020;11(6):1437–52.

46. Ju J, Lu G, Lambert JD, et al. Inhibition of carcinogenesis by tea constituents. Semin Cancer Biol 2007;17(5):395–402.

47. Beland FA, Mellick PW, Olson GR, et al. Carcinogenicity of acrylamide in B6C3F(1) mice and F344/N rats from a 2-year drinking water exposure. Food Chem Toxicol 2013;51:149–59.

48. Shafiei F, Salari-Moghaddam A, Milajerdi A, et al. Coffee and caffeine intake and risk of ovarian cancer: a systematic review and meta-analysis. International Journal of Gynecologic Cancer 2019;29(3):579–84.

49. Je Y, Liu W, Giovannucci E. Coffee consumption and risk of colorectal cancer: A systematic review and meta-analysis of prospective cohort studies. Int J Cancer 2009;124(7):1662–8.
50. Sartini M, Bragazzi NL, Spagnolo AM, et al. Coffee Consumption and Risk of Colorectal Cancer: A Systematic Review and Meta-Analysis of Prospective Studies. Nutrients 2019;11(3):694.
51. Yu X, Bao Z, Zou J, et al. Coffee consumption and risk of cancers: a meta-analysis of cohort studies. BMC Cancer 2011;11(1):96.

Education and Training Models for Remote Learning

Victoria E. Forbes, MD, MS[a],*, Mary D. Chamberlin, MD[b],
Vincent Dusabejambo, MBBS[c], Tim Walker, MBBS, FRACP, MPHTM[d],
Steve P. Bensen, MD[e], Norrisa Haynes, MD, MPH, MSHP[f],
Kathryn Nunes, BA[g], Veauthyelau Saint-Joy, MD[h],
Frederick L. Makrauer, MD[i]

KEYWORDS

- Remote learning • Haiti • Rwanda • United States • LMICs • Global health
- Global oncology • Partnerships

KEY POINTS

- Insufficient local provider capacity, technology restrcitions population displacement, diminishing material resources, and persistent socioeconomic inequity make it imperative for the medical profession to hasten its pursuit of affordable, humane, community-based healthcare for all.
- In order to prevent disease, improve health, and achieve equity in health, we must find meaningful ways to gain and share knowledge globally in a bidirectional and sustainable manner.
- Remote and hybrid learning models expand the scope of global health training and can provide equitable and effective global health education.
- Remote learning allows learners to connect in ways that were not possible before, overcoming logistical barriers, economic hardships with travel, and travel restrictions.
- We present 3 different applications of available technology, which serve as valuable methods for delivering meaningful education to healthcare providers.

[a] University of Connecticut Health Center, 263 Farmington Avenue, Farmington, CT 06030, USA; [b] Dartmouth-Hitchcock Medical Center, One Medical Center Drive Lebanon, NH 03756, USA; [c] University of Rwanda College of Medicine and Health Sciences, KG 11 Avenue, Kigali, Rwanda; [d] Calvary Mater Newcastle, 20 Edith Street, Waratah NSW 2298, Australia; [e] Dartmouth-Hitchcock Medical Center, One Medical Center Drive Lebanon, NH 03756, USA; [f] Yale School of Medicine, 333 Cedar Street, New Haven, CT 06510, USA; [g] Sidney Kimmel Medical College, 1025 Walnut Street, #100, Philadelphia, PA 19107, USA; [h] Centre Hospitalier de la Basse-Terre, 97100 Avenue, Gaston Feuillard, Basse-Terre 97109, Guadeloupe, France; [i] Division of Gastroenterology, Hepatology and Endoscopy, Brigham and Women's Hospital, 75 Francis Street, Boston, MA 02115, USA
* Corresponding author. University of Connecticut Health Center, Carole and Ray Neag Comprehensive Cancer Center, 263 Farmington Avenue, Farmington, CT 06030.
E-mail address: vforbes@uchc.edu

Hematol Oncol Clin N Am 38 (2024) 185–197
https://doi.org/10.1016/j.hoc.2023.06.008
0889-8588/24/© 2023 Elsevier Inc. All rights reserved.

hemonc.theclinics.com

INTRODUCTION

Global health education should seek to incorporate novel methods to teach learners and establish and maintain durable global partnerships in rising economies. The learning models described here have effectively delivered grassroots global health education to all levels of current and future healthcare professionals including medical technologists, nurses, physicians, physician assistants, nurse practitioners, public health professionals, and trainees, as well as government and institutional administrators. Emphasis should be placed on bidirectional learning modules and equitable partnerships because we aim to improve the outcomes of patients across the globe.

SECTION 1: GI RISING AND INTERNATIONAL EDUCATION AND COLLABORATION
Title: Raising the Bar for Health-care in Rwanda: A Template for Partnership in Gastroenterological Training and Health-care Innovation in Africa

Introduction

Rwanda is a small, land-locked country of more than 13 million people located in sub-Saharan East Africa with limited healthcare capacity (clinical and technological) to effectively manage a heavy burden of early onset, advanced, and often preventable disease. Prominent examples include hepatocellular carcinoma, comprising 9% of all cancer in sub-Saharan Africa (SSA), multiple types of adenocarcinoma in SSA including gastric (11%), pancreatic and biliary, colorectal (1%–3%), and human papillomavirus-related anorectal squamous cell carcinoma.[1,2] In addition, late-stage malignancy (adenocarcinoma, mucosa associated lymphoid tissue lymphoma), associated with untreated and widely endemic *Helicobacter pylori* infection, may present with malnutrition, bleeding, and gastric outlet obstruction.

The government of Rwanda made it an immediate priority to address the postgenocide extremely limited supply of expertise and tools necessary for prevention, early detection, and treatment of cancer. With the implementation of universal health insurance and international financial support, the country has already made substantial improvement in maternal and neonatal health care, and control of HIV and viral hepatitis.[3,4] Despite these clear early successes, progress in reducing cancer morbidity and mortality has not kept pace due to cultural, political, and financial challenges that delay or impede patient access to care.[5]

In response, in 2020 Rwanda created a 10-year National Strategy for Health Professional Development to establish its own, locally-trained group of highly skilled subspecialists to oversee the earlier diagnosis and care of advanced disease and guide future public health policy. By building its own in-country subspecialist capacity, support staff and technology, Rwanda could then achieve grassroots sustainability while limiting the "opportunity cost" of international training, achieving earlier diagnosis of preventable cancer, and reducing the loss of young physicians (its "intellectual treasure") attracted to greater economic opportunity during their training abroad.

REBUILDING HEALTHCARE IN POSTGENOCIDE RWANDA

After the Rwandan genocide in 1994 caused sudden and devastating loss or displacement of 80% of healthcare professionals, medical education and access to infrastructure, advanced diagnostic tools, and therapy became extremely limited. Dr Vincent Dusabejambo, a respected local internist, educator, and community leader, led the effort to restore and strengthen gastroenterology services by recruiting Dr Tim Walker, an Australian Gastroenterologist in 2003 to serve as the University of Rwanda's Academic Head of Internal Medicine. They were later joined by Drs Steven Bensen, from

Dartmouth-Geisel, and Frederick Makrauer from Brigham and Women's Hospital and Harvard Medical School. The group has grown steadily to more than 45 volunteer university gastroenterology faculty from the United States (Maryland, Wisconsin, Michigan, and USC), Australia, Netherlands, and Canada (Manitoba) and has expanded in scope to include Oncology and Hematopathology faculty from Dartmouth and the University of Connecticut. The result has been a rapidly expanded capacity to provide patient care and to educate and train local internists to diagnose and treat the most prevalent and urgent clinical disorders.

Dr Dusabejambo's initiative received vital external healthcare funding in the amount of USD $100 million through the "President's Emergency Plan for AIDS Relief" (PEPFAR). With additional funding and expertise provided by the Clinton Health Access Initiative, PEPFAR provided the momentum necessary for Dr Agnes Binagwaho to form Rwanda's "Human Resources for Health" (HRH).[6] She recruited a consortium of US academic leaders to "partner" (Dr Paul Farmer's concept of "twinning" or "Zanmi Lasante") in a 7-year effort to restore the country's depleted medical workforce. Seven US medical schools provided a cadre of almost 100 health professionals per year to join the effort in rebuilding healthcare capacity.[7,8] By 2017, "The Global Fund" (for the care of AIDS, tuberculosis, and malaria) was also contributing USD $2 to 3 billion per year to Rwanda and SSA.[9] Relying heavily on the model of grassroots partnership with international physicians,[10,11] in May 4, 2022, the Ministry of Health announced the approval of funding for 13 sustainable, advanced training programs in Rwanda for Rwandan physicians including medical fellowships in Gastroenterology and Hepatology, Oncology, Cardiology, Nephrology, and Endocrinology.[12]

From the beginning, a key to rebuilding infrastructure has been the formation of a *durable partnership* for successful collaboration between Rwandan and the above international academic institutions. A 5-year effort began to establish Memorandum of Understandings (MOU) that would prioritize Rwanda's needs, not the will of outsiders. Four *founding principles* were identified to guide stakeholders: (1) respect for community-based healthcare delivery, (2) clear objectives anchored in Rwanda's needs and administered through local governance, (3) primacy of intellectual over material resources, and (4) sustainability. In 2016, Dr Stephen Rulisa, Dean of the University of Rwanda School of Medicine, recruited Drs Frederick Makrauer and Richard Johannes from Brigham and Women's Hospital and Harvard Medical School to join Drs Dusabejambo, Walker, and Bensen, bringing additional expertise in curriculum and faculty development, teaching skills, and clinical research for designing a web-based, "bottom-up" (community-based) model with a strictly *beneficiary-focus*, and clear, sustainable objectives consistent with the country's healthcare model.[13] It was agreed that the necessary training must occur predominantly in Rwanda and the region to accommodate local work demands and funding realities.

By 2016, Dr Dusabejambo had founded the *Rwanda Society for Endoscopy*, providing the framework for developing and coordinating the country's gastrointestinal (GI) patient care and endoscopy services. Furthermore, he drafted an educational curriculum in a web-based format for all training sites to serve as the foundation for a planned future GI fellowship. Outside reviewers were recruited from Yale and Pittsburgh to monitor program quality. Drs Johannes and Makrauer, with guidance from Dr Traci Wolbrink of "OpenPediatrics" at Boston Childrens' Hospital and Christian Ulstrup, an electronics engineer, converted weekly communications to an online vehicle, "Zoom" with failsafe systems to overcome frequent weather-related interruptions in 3G function. Dr Rulisa emphasized the value of "bidirectional exchange" of Fellows between Rwanda and international partners that included "hands-on" experience in teaching and clinical care. The benefits of such mutual training, based on a recent US survey of GI program directors and fellows, would be to increase all fellows' cultural competence and respect for healthcare equity, and their expertise in program design and operation, evidence-based decision-making, and performance assessment.[14,15] Funding was carefully allocated by HRH based on PEPFAR's "Technical Working Group's Rapid Site-Level Health Workforce Assessment Tool."

In 2017, Drs Dusabejambo, Walker, Bensen, and Makrauer, in partnership with *all* Rwandan stakeholders at the professional, university, and government levels including Dr Patrick Ndimubanzi, the HRH Secretariat, formed the "International Working Group" (IWG), which has met by Zoom regularly to oversee GI clinical operations and program development.[16] The newly formed IWG realized that, despite strong government, political, and financial support (generated in part by fellows' clinical service and existing international funding), Rwanda would still require a temporary external source of experienced medical faculty and proper equipment for several years as a foundation for sustainable advanced patient care, education, and in-country training programs. For example, by 2019 Dartmouth, Harvard and selected international private practitioners had donated scholarships and diagnostic equipment (including endoscopy instruments, "Fibroscan" to determine severity of liver disease, and "Endosim" a self-teaching training device to develop endoscopy) amounting to USD $250,000. IWG has proven to be a strong and effective vehicle for supporting the unique future GI Fellowship Program's mission, principles, curriculum, governance, and funding. In 2022, a joint MOU was approved, demonstrating the power of "twinning," and a US-based 501-C3 NGO, "GI Rising," was incorporated to coordinate recruitment of qualified volunteer faculty and raise further funds for bidirectional visiting faculty,trainee scholarships, and essential equipment. Dartmouth-Hitchcock Medical Center (New Hampshire) and Brigham Women's Hospital (Boston) then rapidly formed partnerships among Africa, Australia (University of Newcastle), Netherlands, and the Universities of Maryland, Michigan, Wisconsin, and California-Davis, in addition to with US private practitioners.[17]

THE EARLY IMPACT OF A STRONG GRASSROOTS PARTNERSHIP AND JUDICIOUS USE OF MODERN TECHNOLOGY ON THE QUALITY OF COMMUNITY-BASED HEALTH CARE IN A RISING ECONOMY

In September2022, Rwanda's government launched the country's first medical specialty training programin gastroenterology and hepatology, designated to be a model for the country and thought by the authors to be Africa's only third fully accredited program of its kind and its very first to be fully sustainable. Fellows and medical residents, with regular mentoring from a steadily expanding group of screened visiting teaching faculty, have already improved patient access to GI specialty care (**Table 1**) and increased clinical research activity with the design and completion of their own pilot observational research studies to begin quantifying the country's burden serious GI diseases and guide future healthcare policy (**Table 2**).

RECENT GI PUBLICATIONS AND PRESENTATIONS BY RWANDAN GI FELLOWS

Ingabire, P. Bensen, S, Dusabejambo, V., Hannon, N., Makrauer, F., Aberra, H, Shikama F. 5th Annual Rwanda Endoscopy Week: Successful Endoscopic Practice in a Resource-Limited Setting *Submitted for AGA DDW Poster Session, May 2023.*

Shikama, F., Bensen, S., Giraneza, R., Ndayisaba, P., Hategekimana, E., Rutaganda, E., Tuyizere, A., Nkakyekorera, T., Seminega, B., Ngabonziza, F., Kamali, P., Dusabejambo, V., van Leeuwen, D., Munyaneza, M., Makrauer, F., Calderwood, A. Upper Gastrointestinal Cancers in Rwanda: Epidemiologic, Clinical and

Table 1
Five-year trend: Rwanda/GI Rising joint clinical activity (2017–2022)

	2017 (Rutanga, 2017)	2022 (Ingabire, 2022)
# Treatment Centers	4	8
# Consultations	50	1021
# Procedures (all types)	241	897
ERCP/with EUS	1/0	16/7
Gastric cancer (% ofEGDs)	4	4
Colon cancer (% of colonoscopies)	1.5	1

Notes: (1) Procedural activity has greatly expanded in both the number of treatment sites and diagnostic studies performed. Fellows began performing procedures (under faculty supervision) in 2022. Training for banding of esophageal varices for physicians began in 2017.(2) Absolute numbers of gastric and colon cancers are small, but their prevalence compared with the Western world is quite high.

Histopathological Features in Patients Presenting to a Tertiary Referral Hospital *Open Journal of Gastroenterology 2022;12: 286–298.*

SUMMARY

Although initially Rwanda's venture Into postgraduate medical education seemed far from assured, in retrospect the gains made in educational delivery, as well as the clinical and academic accomplishments of Rwandan doctors through these programs, clearly mark important progress. An institutional framework was established early on with strong bidirectional relationships, shared mission, and local leadership. A single, local, highly respected internist and dedicated educator, after founding The Rwanda Society for Endoscopy in 2016, and today recognized as a training site by the World Gastroenterology Organization, formed a durable bond with 3 visiting gastroenterologists that inspired the birth of GI Rising, Incand a highly effective MOU to establish a durable international partnership between Rwanda and cooperating international medical schools. GI Rising, Inc. is providing bidirectional educational scholarships, highly qualified and dedicated volunteer visiting teaching faculty, and vital equipment, which is stimulating community-based, equitable GI care, and grassroots healthcare planning for the entire country. In September2022, the effectiveness of the joint Rwanda/GI Rising MOU was validated with the establishment of the "University of Rwanda Fellowship in Gastroenterology and Hepatology" and the enrollment of its first 4 fellows, all Rwandan citizens, under the leadership of Dr Hanna Aberra, MD, PhD, an leader in liver disease treatment in Africa and the Program's first Director. Rwanda's first medical fellowship program will graduate the country's very own GI specialists and future leaders in August2024, bringing better understanding to bear on Rwanda's most pressing GI diseases and offering Africa a promising model for restoring and maintaining the capacity for grassroots specialty care in rising economies.

SECTION 2: THE GLOBAL ONCOLOGY AND DISPARITIES OF CARE PROGRAM
Title: Hematology-Oncology Fellowship Curriculum Goes Global: Creating the Next Generation of Global Hematologist-Oncologists Through Remote Learning

The global burden of cancer and cancer-related mortality are increasing. By the year 2030, there will be an estimated 13 million total deaths from cancer worldwide with three-quarters of these deaths occurring in low-income and middle-income countries.[18] These countries are ill equipped to cope with the escalating burden of the disease.

Comprehensive patient care requires an understanding of medical guidelines and available resources as well as the intersectional context of the patient's identity and experiences. Many Hematology and Oncology Fellows in the United States lack exposure to disparities of care and global oncology at large. Hematology and Oncology training programs must teach topics addressing various disparities of care to prepare trainees to provide informed care. Central in such preparation is for trainees to gain understanding of cancer on a global scale and recognize disparities of care in domestic and international settings.

To begin to address the knowledge gap and establish, maintain, and improve international cancer education and collaborations, an elective was created for Dartmouth Hematology and Oncology fellows in 2015 in which fellows rotated in Rwanda with our partners. In 2019, we created an online course in global oncology for 9 Hematology and Oncology fellows at Dartmouth with participants from around the world. The course first used the Project ECHO (Extension for Community Healthcare Outcomes) model of teaching. Project ECHO was developed by Dr Sanjeev Arora at the University of New Mexico Health Sciences and uses telehealth and case-based learning to connect providers wherever they live. For our course, Zoom was used as a teleconferencing platform to facilitate a flow of knowledge between the fellows and clinicians abroad. The program became an ideal model for remote learning as the coronavirus disease 2019 (COVID-19) pandemic transpired. As the course evolved and broadened in scope, we detached from the ECHO model in order to include additional time for presentations by experts in the field and discussion by participants. Hematology and Oncology fellows from the University of Connecticut joined. Monthly hour-long sessions were held from September to June.

The expanded course was named the "Global Oncology and Disparities of Care" program, an innovative, interdisciplinary, remote learning program that brings health professionals together in a common space. Participants hailed from locations across the globe as shown in **Fig. 1**. They ranged from medical trainees to global health and public health experts, researchers, and clinicians. The core learners included the Hematology and Oncology fellows from Dartmouth and the University of Connecticut. Rwanda's first Gastroenterology fellows, Internal mMedicine residents from the University of Connecticut and Dartmouth, and other learners joined. This upcoming year, we anticipate fellows from several other Hematology and Oncology fellowships to participate.

A global network of multidisciplinary faculty in radiation oncology, palliative, gynecologic oncology, research, education, public health, and many hematology and oncology subspecialties presented focusing on the internationalization of the curriculum. The sessions were facilitated by the program director and senior fellows interested in global oncology. The presenters were global experts in the field and often identified by the connections we have fostered in the global health community. The geographic range, number, and disciplines of our participants continue to grow. A range of topics presented is outlined in **Table 2**.

The 2021 to 2022 course survey data demonstrated an increase in participation number during the years and revealed a need and desire for this content from participants.[19] Postcourse surveys showed that the Global Oncology and Disparities of Care program participants felt prepared to recognize and discuss global risk factors, resource constraints, and disparities in care in domestic and international settings. Participants perceived the program as providing several opportunities for growth and development. They reported the strongest skill development around

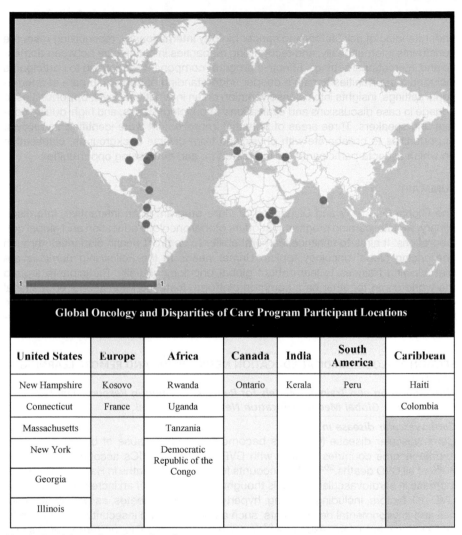

Fig. 1. Participant locations thus far.

United States	Europe	Africa	Canada	India	South America	Caribbean
New Hampshire	Kosovo	Rwanda	Ontario	Kerala	Peru	Haiti
Connecticut	France	Uganda				Colombia
Massachusetts		Tanzania				
New York		Democratic Republic of the Congo				
Georgia						
Illinois						

Caption above table: **Global Oncology and Disparities of Care Program Participant Locations**

Table 2
A sample of topics presented

Topics Presented	
Esophageal and gastrointestinal cancers in Rwanda	HIV-related malignancies
Hepatocellular Carcinoma and Cholangiocarcinoma	COVID-19 and Cancer
Gastric Cancer	Social Networking for Global Oncology
ASCO International	University of Global Health Equity in Rwanda
Global Medical Education Network in Haiti	Palliative Care in India and Haiti
Breast Cancer in Kosovo and India	Radiation Oncology in Latin America
Breast Cancer and Lifestyle Factors	Access to Essential Cancer Medicines
Hemoglobinopathies Sickle Cell Anemia in Canada	Management of Cervical Cancer in LMICs and a Case Study in Rwanda

understanding of risk factors and cancer biology internationally, recognizing resource constraints internationally, and recognizing disparities in health care between domestic and international settings. Effective program components according to participants included: opportunities to gain a deeper understanding of barriers to care at international settings, insights into disease variation on an international level, opportunities to engage in case discussions and evaluations of oncology cases, and high-quality content and speakers. Three areas of potential improvement were identified as follows: opportunities to collaborate with physicians from diverse backgrounds, clarification on which aspects participants are interested in, and networking opportunities.

SUMMARY

The Global Oncology and Disparities of Care program is an interactive, interdisciplinary, remote learning program that offers global oncology education and global collaborations. It aims to enhance learners' ability to confront health disparities through challenging global oncology topics. Unmet needs in the Fellowship curricula are met allowing trainees to learn about global oncology virtually. Participants around the world come together on a common platform, fostering international educational exchange and collaborations. An educational program to address disparities of care both domestically and internationally is an important addition to hematology-oncology training programs.

SECTION 3: GLOBAL MEDICAL EDUCATION NETWORK INC AND REMOTE LEARNING IN HAITI
Title: Education and Training Models for Remote Learning in Resource Limited Communities: Global Medical Education Network Inc Model

Cardiovascular disease in Haiti
Cardiovascular disease (CVD) has become the leading cause of death in low and middle-income countries (LMICs) with CVD deaths in LMICs accounting for nearly 80% of all CVD deaths.[20,21] CVD accounts for 29% of all deaths in Haiti.[22] The relative increase in cardiovascular deaths is thought to be a result of an increase in traditional CVD risk factors, including smoking, hypertension, and diabetes, as well as other social and environmental determinants, such as poverty, food insecurity, dietary habits, and environmental lead exposure.[23] In an analysis of the Global Burden of Disease Study, Haiti had significantly higher years of life lost, a metric of premature death, due to heart disease than other Caribbean countries.[24] Additionally, Haiti has one of the highest incidences of peripartum cardiomyopathy in the world at approximately 1 in 300 deliveries.[25] Haiti also has a relatively high prevalence of rheumatic heart disease, hypertension, and stroke.[25]

SCARCITY OF SUBSPECIALISTS AND TRAINING OPPORTUNITIES

For a population of more than 11 million people, there is a significant lack of cardiovascular healthcare infrastructure.[25] Currently, there are no formal Cardiology training programs in Haiti.[25] There are only 16 Cardiologists, all of whom received their training outside of the country.[25] Additionally, there are no catheterization laboratories in Haiti and therefore acute coronary syndromes are typically medically managed.[25] There is limited access to cardiac surgery through nongovernmental organizations.[25] Most hospitals have access to electrocardiogram machines, but due to a lack of trained professionals, few hospitals routinely use cardiac ultrasound despite its high diagnostic value.[25]

GLOBAL MEDICAL EDUCATION NETWORK INC AND ITS ORIGINS

Global Medical Education Network Inc (GMEN) began as a collaborative program among chief residents at Hôpital Universitaire de Mirebalais (HUM) and cardiology trainees in the United States and France, specifically from the University of Pennsylvania and Centre Hospitalier d'Antibes Juan-les-Pins. GMEN started with 2 chief residents and 16 Internal Medicine (IM) residents at HUM. GMEN's program—International Cardiology Curriculum Accessible by Remote Distance Learning (ICARDs-Haiti)—was established with the goal of improving access to cardiovascular education for clinicians in Haiti and providing novel training experiences for American and French trainees. What started as small group meetings to discuss interesting cardiology cases and treatment plans developed into a transcontinental collaboration.

The ICARDS-Haiti program was implemented in Haiti in 2019. Through the implementation of a culturally competent remote classroom, ICARDs-Haiti has demonstrated noteworthy participant improvement in subjective and objective assessment scores. Several topics included in the program were heart failure, echocardiography, valvular disease, and hypertension. Based on the end of the year evaluation, 94% of participants rated the curriculum as educational and relevant to their medical practice. One hundred percent of participants reported the curriculum as good to excellent. ICARDS-Haiti is one example of GMEN's successful implementation of a virtual education program.

GMEN has since expanded its efforts beyond HUM to include all IM residency programs in the country. In collaboration with the Center for Haitian Studies, GMEN has created Continuing Medical Education content for general practitioners in Haiti. There are currently more than 600 physicians enrolled in GMEN's educational programming. GMEN's mission is to improve the quality of patient care by providing high-quality, evidence-based medical education to clinicians and patients around the world.

GLOBAL MEDICAL EDUCATION NETWORK INC'S IMPLEMENTATION STRATEGY

GMEN's approach to medical education is rooted in the modified analysis, design, development, implementation, and evaluation (ADDIE) model (**Fig. 2**). This model involves local healthcare professionals in every aspect of the implementation and analysis process. It includes 5 stages: analysis, design, development, implementation, and

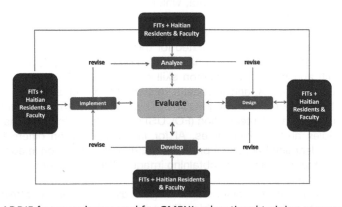

Fig. 2. The ADDIE framework was used for GMEN's educational training programs. EC, early career; FIT, fellows-in-training.

evaluation.[26] GMEN's approach to medical education is unique, involving local healthcare providers in every stage of the process.[26] This ensures that the educational programs are tailored to the specific needs of the community and are effective in improving patient care.

This approach to medical education is unique in that it leverages technology to provide cost-effective and accessible medical education to physicians in LMICs. Much of the structure of GMEN aligns with the core principles of Community Based Participatory Research (CBPR). CBPR was created to combine addressing health disparities and promoting community empowerment with scientific principles and rigor.[27] It focuses on continuous inquiry, evaluation, and action implementation "*with* instead of *on*" marginalized individuals.[25] For GMEN, community members have been essential in generating intervention and implementation ideas and leveraging community stakeholders such as local healthcare providers. Local community members also help generate research questions, develop methodologies, and cowrite scholarly publications. Aside from objective assessments demonstrating knowledge acquisition, the program was found to have a positive influence on patient care and physician-patient communication through semistructured interviews and focus groups. Improved patient care and better communication directly benefits the community. Additionally, because the implementation strategies are created in a collaborative way, they are more likely to be sustainable. Through the use of the ADDIE model and incorporation of CBPR strategies, GMEN hopes to personalize cardiovascular training to meet the needs of specific communities and thereby democratize access to specialized medical education.

FUTURE DIRECTIONS

In collaboration with academic institutions, GMEN plans to expand cardiovascular teaching to include diagnostic capacity building by incorporating focused cardiac ultrasound (FOCUS). FOCUS has proven successful in LMICs as a means of task-shifting, whereby noncardiologists are trained to perform ultrasound scans and diagnose cardiovascular conditions. The goal is to implement the FOCUS training in August 2023 with buy-in from the Ministry of Health and additional local hospital leadership. By building FOCUS capacity in public hospitals, healthcare providers in Haiti can improve the characterization and diagnostic accuracy of heart failure, as well as improve patient management and clinical outcomes. In the end, it may also lead to improved accuracy in prevalence data, which is currently likely underestimated due to the reliance on private institutions for data collection. Of note, given the lack of technology in many public hospitals in Haiti, necessary ultrasound equipment with artificial intelligence (AI) capability will be donated for this pilot study.

The current geopolitical instability has created barriers for supporting medical providers in Haiti and providing in-person skill development. To address these challenges, GMEN will use AI and telehealth to train IM residents in Haiti to diagnose and characterize heart failure using FOCUS. This innovative approach aims to implement an evidence-based intervention (FOCUS) using telehealth and AI as implementation strategies and teaching aides. AI for image acquisition differs from online module-based learning because it provides real-time feedback on image acquisition while novice ultrasound users are obtaining images. This allows for real-time directive feedback on hand positioning and image quality.

Overall, GMEN's effort to build cardiovascular diagnostic and treatment capacity through education is commendable. By providing training to noncardiologists, healthcare providers in Haiti can improve their ability to diagnose and manage cardiovascular conditions, which may ultimately lead to improved patient outcomes. GMEN's efforts are scalable and it is the hope of the organization to eventually expand to other LMICs. GMEN's use of technology to deliver education serves as a valuable tool for overcoming geopolitical instability, economic hardship, global pandemics and logistical barriers to medical training, and patient care delivery.

CLINICS CARE POINTS

- Program development in emerging economies requires careful formation of partnerships and a clear mission defined by the host country.
- A firm commitment to local governance and sustainability is essential for success.
- The most important resources are intellectual capital, *not* bricks and mortar. In program development, well-meaning health professionals must never underestimate the influence of "opportunity costs" and differences in values, culture, and history.

SUMMARY

Global health education must evolve to meet the barriers we face in the world from disparities to pandemics. Training programs should recognize the need for future medical professionals to receive education in global health issues in order to respond to global health inequities. Virtual teaching models are a valuable tool with the power to connect trainees and clinicians from around the world. The learning models described above effectively deliver global health education to healthcare professionals. Emphasis should be placed on bidirectional learning modules and equitable partnerships as we aim to improve the outcomes of patients across the globe.

ACKNOWLEDGMENTS

The authors are thankful to our colleagues listed below who provided their time, effort, and expertise to make the work described in this article possible. They are dedicated to global health and educating the next generations of health professionals. Eric Rutaganda, MBBS, MPH, University of Rwanda College of Medicine and Health Sciences, rutagander@gmail.com. Dirk J van Leeuwen, MD, PhD, Dartmouth Geisel School of Medicine, dirk.j.vanleeuwen@gmail.com. Kenechukwu Chudy-Onwugaje, MBBS, MPH, University of Michigan School of Medicine, kenechudy@gmail.com. Rebecca Laird, MD, MPH, Dartmouth Geisel School of Medicine, Rebecca.E.Laird@dartmouth.edu. Erik von Rosenvinge, MD, University of Maryland School of Medicine, evonrose@som.umaryland.edu.

FUNDING

We would like to recognize our funding sources, the Department of Medicine at Dartmouth-Hitchcock and the Geisel School of Medicine Scholarship Enhancement in Academic Medicine Award 2020. Dr. Makrauer has received funding from Gift of Private Patient and Gift of 'Bridge Growth Partners, NYC.'

REFERENCES

1. Sung H, Ferlay J, Siegel RL, et al. Global Cancer Statistics 2020: GLOBOCAN Estimates of Incidence and Mortality Worldwide for 36 Cancers in 185 Countries. CA Cancer J Clin 2021;71(3):209–49.

2. Wang H, Dwyer-Lindgren L, Lofgren KT, et al. Age-specific and sex-specific mortality in 187 countries, 1970-2010: a systematic analysis for the Global Burden of Disease Study 2010. Lancet 2012;380(9859):2071–94.
3. Fauci AS, Eisinger RW. PEPFAR - 15 Years and Counting the Lives Saved. N Engl J Med 2018;378(4):314–6.
4. Wang H, Dwyer-Lindgren L, Lofgren KT, et al. Age-specific and sex-specific mortality in 187 countries, 1970-2010: a systematic analysis for the Global Burden of Disease Study 2010. Lancet 2012;380(9859):2071–94.
5. Nyandekwe M, Nzayirambaho M, Kakoma JB. Universal health insurance in Rwanda: major challenges and solutions for financial sustainability case study of Rwanda community-based health insurance part I. Pan Afr Med J 2020;37:55.
6. Binagwaho A, Kyamanywa P, Farmer PE, et al. The Human Resources for Health Program in Rwanda - A New Partnership. N Engl J Med 2013;369:2054–9.
7. Cancedda C, Cotton P, Shema J, et al. Health Professional Training and Capacity Strengthening Through International Academic Partnerships: The First Five Years of the Human Resources for Health Program in Rwanda. Int J Health Policy Manag 2018;7(11):1024–39.
8. Delisle H. The Human Resources for Health Program in Rwanda - Reflections on Achievements and Challenges Comment on "Health Professional Training and Capacity Strengthening Through International Academic Partnerships: The First Five Years of the Human Resources for Health Program in Rwanda. Int J Health Policy Manag 2018;8(2):128–31.
9. The Global Fund – Overview of the 2023-2025 Allocations, 13 January 2023, Fig. 3, p.3.
10. National Academies of Sciences, Engineering, and Medicine; Health and Medicine Division; Board on Global Health; Committee on the Evaluation of Strengthening Human Resources for Health Capacity in the Republic of Rwanda Under the President's Emergency Plan for AIDS Relief (PEPFAR). Evaluation of PEPFAR's Contribution (2012-2017) to Rwanda's Human Resources for Health Program. Washington (DC): National Academies Press (US); 2020.
11. Rwanda Standards of Postgraduate Medical Education, Rwanda Medical and Dental Council, 2019. Available at: https://www.rmdc.rw/IMG/pdf/posgraduate_standards.pdf.
12. Niyingabira J. The Ministry of health launches 13 medical training programs, Rwanda BioMedical Centre. Published on May 20th, 2022. Available at: https://rbc.gov.rw/index.php?id=100&tx_news_pi1%5Bnews%5D=640&tx_news_pi1%5Bday%5D=20&tx_news_pi1%5Bmonth%5D=5&tx_news_pi1%5Byear%5D=2022&cHash=d322466b34896dae2bcf0fd5f7545d85.
13. Rulisa, S. Advances in Global Health' Address at Yale U, 2014 YouTube.
14. Jirapinyo P, Hunt RS, Tabak YP, et al. Global Health Education in Gastroenterology Fellowship: A National Survey. Dig Dis Sci 2016;61(12):3443–50.
15. Dusabejambo V., Rulisa S., Johannes R., et al., Creating A Gastroenterology Fellowship in Rwanda - The Role of Relationship-Building on Successful Program Development, BWH Education Research Day, Poster, 2017. Semifinalist Award of Distinction.
16. Bensen S, Makrauer F. Giving Rise to GI in Rwanda. ACG Magazine 2018;2(2): 26–36.
17. Talib Z, Narayan L, Harrod T. Postgraduate Medical Education in Sub-Saharan Africa: A Scoping Review Spanning 26 Years and Lessons Learned. J Grad Med Educ 2019;11(4 Suppl):34–46.

18. Bray F, Jemal A, Grey N, et al. Global cancer transitions according to the Human Development Index (2008-2030): a population-based study. Lancet Oncol 2012; 13(8):790–801.
19. Forbes V., Buteau A.C., Hoxha I., et al., Global oncology and cancer disparities education. *J Clin Oncol*, 2022, 40(16_suppl), 11006-11006.
20. World Health Organization. Cardiovascular Diseases. World Health Organization 2021;11. https://www.who.int/news-room/fact-sheets/detail/cardiovascular-diseases-(cvds).
21. Kwan GF, Jean-Baptiste W, Cleophat P, et al. Descriptive epidemiology and short-term outcomes of heart failure hospitalisation in rural Haiti. Heart 2016;102(2): 140–6.
22. Institute for Health Metrics and Evaluation. https://www.healthdata.org/haiti.
23. Lookens J, Tymejczyk O, Rouzier V, et al. The Haiti cardiovascular disease cohort: study protocol for a population-based longitudinal cohort. BMC Public Health 2020;20(1):1633.
24. Fene F, Ríos-Blancas MJ, Lachaud J, et al. Life expectancy, death, and disability in Haiti, 1990-2017: a systematic analysis from the Global Burden of Disease Study 2017. Rev Panam Salud Publica 2020;44:e136.
25. Haynes NA, Saint-Joy V, Swain J, et al. Implementation of a virtual international cardiology curriculum to address the deficit of cardiovascular education in Haiti: a pilot study. BMJ Open 2021;11(6):e048690.
26. Eberly LA, Rusingiza E, Park PH, et al. 10-Year Heart Failure Outcomes From Nurse-Driven Clinics in Rural Sub-Saharan Africa. J Am Coll Cardiol 2019; 73(8):977–80.
27. Haynes N, Kaur A, Swain J, et al. Community-Based Participatory Research to Improve Cardiovascular Health Among US Racial and Ethnic Minority Groups. Curr Epidemiol Rep 2022;9(3):212–21.

Breast Cancer Disparities and Innovations
A Focus on Kosovo

Mary D. Chamberlin, MD[a], Dafina Ademi Islami, MD[b],*,
Richard J. Barth Jr, MD[c], Shqiptar Demaci, MD[d]

KEYWORDS

- Breast cancer disparities • Breast conservation • Surgical innovations
- Low- and middle-income countries (LMICs)

KEY POINTS

- Advances in systemic therapy and surgical techniques provide breast conservation as a growing option for surgical management of breast cancer around the world.
- Too many women are still over-treated by mastectomy with adverse impacts on quality of life and preventing earlier detection.
- Technological advances in international communication, access to drugs and surgical innovations can lead to international collaborations that may leapfrog over previous care patterns and lead to improvements in outcomes for women with breast cancer.
- A focus on our experience with our colleagues at Dartmouth and Kosovo illustrates a potential path forward.

INTRODUCTION

Breast cancer is the most frequent cancer among women, affecting 2.3 million globally and causing more than 685,000 deaths each year.[1] Though the age-standardized incidence of breast cancer is highest in high-income countries, 45 percent of breast cancer cases and 55 percent of breast cancer deaths occur in low- and middle-income countries.[1] While a country's age-standardized breast cancer incidence is positively correlated with income or gross domestic product (GDP), the mortality-to-incidence

[a] Department of Medicine /Hematology-Oncology, Dartmouth College of Medicine and Dartmouth Cancer Center at Dartmouth-Hitchcock Medical Center, Lebanon, NH, USA; [b] Oncology Clinic, University Clinical Center of Kosovo, Prishtina, Kosovo; [c] Department of Surgery, Section of General Surgery, Dartmouth College of Medicine and Dartmouth Cancer Center at Dartmouth-Hitchcock Medical Center, Lebanon, NH, USA; [d] Department of Thoracic Surgery, University Clinical Center of Kosovo, Prishtina, Kosovo
* Corresponding author.
E-mail address: dafinaademi@hotmail.com

Hematol Oncol Clin N Am 38 (2024) 199–207
https://doi.org/10.1016/j.hoc.2023.06.002
0889-8588/24/© 2023 Elsevier Inc. All rights reserved.

ratio is negatively correlated with GDP, indicating that breast cancer survival is significantly lower in low- and middle-income countries.

Regarding the prevalence and incidence of breast cancer across age groups, 23 percent of breast cancer cases diagnosed occur in women aged 15-49 in low- and middle-income countries (LMIC), whereas only 10 percent of cases occur in this age group in high-income countries (HIC). This is at least partially explained by the high rate of mammogram detected early breast cancers in HIC in women over 40 which substantially increases the denominator with cancers in older women and lowers the percentage of cancers in women under 40. However, even with the lack of early-detection measures in LMIC, age-standardized rates show that breast cancer is still more prevalent in younger women due to the populations' skewed age distribution.[2] As an example, the median age of breast cancer in Lebanon is 52 years compared to a median age of 63 years in the US.[1] Lack of population-based screening programs, diagnostic capabilities, and cancer registries in many areas creates a significant bias in the available data so accurate conclusions are challenging. Many studies have shown that breast cancer in LMIC is more likely to be triple negative, higher grade and higher stage, a trend also seen in the US in women who are not participating in screening, such as women under 40 or women with poor access to care.[3–6] It is well known that screening mammogram programs improve outcomes, reduce morbidity[7] and improve survival, but in countries without screening mammogram programs, further research must examine what may be done to incentivize early detection and facilitate improvements in quality of life after breast cancer treatment. Programs to raise awareness about signs of breast cancer and treatment options other than mastectomy dependent on earlier detection are in critical need.

HISTORY

In Kosovo, breast cancer remains the most widespread cancer among women. According to the hospital registry of the Oncology Clinic within the University Clinical Center of Kosovo (UCCK), the incidence of breast cancer at UCCK in 2016 was 293 new cases. In 2017, the incidence increased to 329, marking a 11% increase in new cases identified. In 2021 there were more than 400 new breast cancer cases at UCCK and over 500 in all of Kosovo (**Table 1**). The breast cancer incidence rate according to Kosovo Statistic Agency is the highest among all cancer types in Kosovo. The variations in incidence rates across different settings are related to certain risk factors such as data quality, breast-cancer awareness level, diagnostic tools, and the availability of screening though there is a sustained lack of availability of recorded incidence and mortality data in most countries of the world, with less than 20% of 178 countries presently reporting high-quality mortality data to the WHO.[8]

Table 1
Kosovo agency of statistics

Year	Breast Cancer Cases (Males and Females)
2016	380
2017	481
2018	444
2019	505
2020	471
2021	571

Estimates from the US-based Cancer Intervention and Surveillance Network (CIS-NET) show that, of the total reduction in the rate of death due to breast cancer between 1990 and 2000, between 28 and 65 percent of the reduction can be attributed to screening, while the remaining proportion of the total reduction in deaths can be attributed to adjuvant treatment.[9] Similarly, in Norway the availability of screening mammography contributed to a decrease in mortality rates from breast cancer and a third of the total reduction was attributed to screening itself. The remaining two-thirds of the total decrease was attributed to factors such as increased awareness, improved therapies, and advancements in diagnostics tools which occurred in parallel with the implementation of mammographic screening.[10]

The best approach for the earlier detection of breast cancer in LMIC's is not known although data is emerging on clinical breast exam (CBE) and opportunistic screening programs, long-term mortality data with CBE compared to screening mammography is not available.[11,12] While Kosovo does not have a national breast cancer-screening program, there have been a few initiatives to introduce mammography screening services between 2014 and 2019. A mobile mammography project called Ma-Mo 1 was implemented in 2014, which led to Ma-Mo 2 and formed the impetus for the establishment of the National Referral Centre for Breast Imaging within the University Clinical Center of Kosovo. This Center allows for the expansion of screening services with mammography being offered in specific regional hospitals in Kosovo while transmitting the patient images to the Center in Prishtina. The data revealed that more than 80% of females in Kosovo who are 40 years of age or older, had never had a screening mammogram. Upon the finalization of the second phase of the program, the professionals who implemented the program conducted an internal assessment of capacities available for the continuation of the third phase: Ma-Mo 3. Ma-Mo3 is oriented towards the assessment of the feasibility of the existing centers for the provision of mammography services and evaluating the possibility of tele-mammography, or reading mammograms remotely via internet through the National Telemedicine Center from radiologists at the Breast Diagnostics in Radiology Clinic.[13] Their assessment revealed a limited availability of data to scale the screening program and establish the national breast-imaging program due to insufficient number of mammographs (8.3 per 1 million inhabitants).There was also limited data on the condition of the mammography equipment that would be utilized in the program due to shortages in professionally trained staff and technicians.

Available statistics (personal correspondence) indicate that Ma-Mo 1 impacted municiplaities to increase supplies in family medicine centers and regional hospitals such that there are 15 static mammography machines and one mobile mammography machine currently available in Kosovo. Three of the static machines and the one mobile machine are digital, while the rest are analog. For both types of machines, there is no data available regarding their utilization rates, examination capacity, quality of imaging, or the degree of application of mammography standards. Furthermore, there is no data available on the professional preparedness of technical and radiology staff and whether their performance is in line with the regulations outlined in the Mammography Quality Standards Act.

According to health statistics published by the Kosovo Agency of Statics in 2017, there has recently been an increasing trend in the number of new cases of malignant breast neoplasms, see **Table 1**.[14] However, these data points correspond to cases drawn from the entire population of Kosovo, not just the municipality or district of Prishtina. Given that the population of Prishtina makes up a small part of Kosovo's total population (estimated to be 1,778,100 in 2017), only a fraction of the number of new cases reported above occur in Prishtina residents each year. It is also important to consider that given the current absence of a national screening program, the above figures likely underestimate the true incidence of breast cancer in Kosovo.

INNOVATIONS

Due to the current limited capacity to provide digital mammography-based screening to all women, and the lack of modern surgical oncology methods, mastectomy is still the predominant form of surgical treatment. As such there is little incentive to detect breast cancer earlier and significant fear of treatment continues to contribute to late presentations.[15]

In countries like the US where screening mammography is widespread, approximately half of the women with invasive cancer and nearly all women with ductal carcinoma in situ (DCIS) will have tumors detected before they become clinically palpable.[7,16]

For nonpalpable lesions, localization of the tumor prior to breast-conserving surgery is needed using wire-localization in which a wire is preoperatively placed near the tumor under radiographic guidance. Prospective studies have shown that wire-localized excision frequently results in positive margins requiring re-excisions between 22 and 34% of the time.[17-19] Re-excisions are emotionally difficult for patients, increase the risk of complications and poor cosmesis, and are expensive.[20,21] Quality of life for women can therefore be greatly improved by technologies that decrease the rate of positive margins and re-excisions. Furthermore, in low and middle-income countries without screening mammograms, breast cancers are universally detected when locally advanced and easily palpable. Radiographic capabilities are also important. A preliminary analysis indicates that there is only one ultrasound machine in the Pristina municipality which is located in the main Family Medicine Center (FMC) in Pristina. It was suggested that there is only one ultrasound machine available due to the limited number of radiologists currently employed in FMCs and that as the Ministry of Health hires additional radiology staff, they plan to invest in additional ultrasound equipment. Within the municipality of Pristina, the main FMC also has one mammography machine and FMC #5 also has one mammography machine. There are two currently MRI machines in tertiary care and one is getting installed in Peja a secondary care regional hospital.

In high-income countries, breast MRI is increasingly utilized for surgical staging. Our hypothesis is that awareness of and training in surgical innovations and new techniques will improve shared decision making and surgical oncologists will offer more women partial mastectomies. Surgeons report low positive margin rates (personal correspondence, thoracic surgical conference, Kosovo 11/30/22) but breast-conserving surgery is rare, even when there is access to radiation, chemotherapy and endocrine therapy. Some cancers are removed with "quadrantectomy" but most with mastectomy, and there is little data on the quality of life after surgery.

Technologies resulting in better imaging may be one route to improving surgical options and outcomes. MRI of the breast has been shown to be more sensitive than mammography or ultrasound for the detection of invasive cancer and DCIS.[22-24] Breast cancer size, as determined by histopathology, is also more accurately defined by MRI than by mammography or ultrasound.[25-27] Indications for breast MRI are expanding and can be used to improve breast cancer surgery and may detect cancers earlier than mammography.[28] Despite this increased accuracy, the use of preoperative MRI obtained with patients in the prone position has not led to decreased positive margin rates.[29] This outcome is not surprising; the shape of the breast during prone MRI is radically different from the supine position in the operating room (OR). The problem is even greater for patients with palpable cancers, where the positive margin rate is closer to 30%[30] In contrast, supine MRI replicates the surgical position and has the potential to increase the precision of breast-conserving surgery (BCS).[31,32] Sakakibara and colleagues[31] randomized patients with small foci of DCIS to wire localization or supine MRI-guided BCS and found that both the positive margin rate and resected tissue volume were lower in patients undergoing supine MRI-guided excision.

Surgical oncology investigators have developed an innovative method of MRI-guided BCS that incorporates preoperative supine MRI to define tumor extent.[33] This technique provides the surgeon with 3D views of the tumor shape and position within the breast as it appears during surgery. Supine MRI images can also be used to create a patient–specific bra-like form, the Breast Cancer Locator (BCL), which can be placed on the breast prior to surgery and allows the surgeon to place bracketing wires around the supine MRI determined tumor extent. When 3D views of the tumor in the breast are used in combination with the BCL, margin-negative resections were achieved in 33 patients treated on pilot studies[34,35]

In Prishtina, thoracic surgeons do the breast cancer surgery and of 4 interviewed after a presentation on supine MRI and 3D imaging[33] plus other 2 references, each reports 60-100 breast surgeries per year, 30-50% mastectomies, with referrals to medical oncology for neoadjuvant chemotherapy ranging from "never," 5%, 20%, to "often." (personal correspondence, 11/30/22). Although breast MRI is available to all surgeons, only 50 percent of surgeons currently utilize breast MRI, and 100% responded "yes" to participating in clinical trials with innovative technologies, offering breast-conserving surgery more often if technologies were available, and to whether women would engage in early detection if breast-conserving surgery was more widely available. (personal correspondence, Kosovo 11/30/22).

DISCUSSION

As a middle-income country in Eastern Europe, Kosovo has seen an increase in breast cancer imaging technologies and access to chemotherapy yet breast-conserving surgery is rare.

In contrast, impressive gains in breast cancer research and treatment have been made over the past 45 years in HIC and many women are now cured with a simple lumpectomy, minimal if any lymph node surgery, less if any radiation, and systemic therapy.[15] Improvements in endocrine therapy combinations, her2 targeted agents and access to oral chemotherapies are providing improvements in survival and quality of life with less surgery and radiation. Research in LMICs is critically needed as well as technological implementation and staff education o determine if survival may be at least the same if not improved with less surgery and radiation, and better access to systemic therapies.

Disparities in breast cancer outcomes are present throughout the globe. The African Breast Cancer Disparities in Outcomes (ABC-DO) is a rare example of a multi-country prospective cohort study aimed at examining the determinants of breast cancer outcomes in low- and middle-income countries.[11] These investigators found that mastectomies outnumbered breast-conserving surgery in all participating countries and that at least 30% of deaths were preventable through downstaging and improvements in treatment. While the survival of patients with breast cancer has increased in most of European countries, the highest death rates from breast cancer remain in Eastern Europe.

An interesting study in Sudan[12] trained village volunteers to screen villagers for breast cancer in 2010-12 and the data demonstrates the challenges of breast cancer care in limited resource settings. 10,300 women in 29 villages were screened. 138 had a positive clinical breast exam and were referred to a district hospital for further evaluation. No travel assistance was provided. 20 did not show for further evaluation. 118 did show for evaluation and 101 had benign disease. 17 were diagnosed with breast cancer, 8 had DCIS and received "treatment" with a good prognosis, but additional details were not reported. Nine women were diagnosed with invasive disease, 2 were Stage 4 at diagnosis, 3 refused some or all of the treatments initially recommended. Of those 3 who refused treatment, 1 refused surgery but was treated with chemotherapy and endocrine therapy and was doing well 3 years later. One initially refused treatment then returned a year later with metastasis. 1 refused treatment after diagnosis and was expected to return with metastasis at some point. 1 had stage I disease with a "wide local excision, radiation and tamoxifen." All but 1 had a mastectomy, and all had chemotherapy with or without tamoxifen depending on estrogen receptor status. This study demonstrates how the fear of treatment and the lack of options for treatment further creates late presentations and poor outcomes. If surgical options could be improved as much around the world as they have been in high-income countries, with increased breast conservation, women would be more likely to engage in awareness campaigns, opportunistic screening programs which may improve outcomes.

SUMMARY

As surgeons learn more advanced breast cancer surgical techniques, in combination with advances in systemic treatments, they may simultaneously improve quality of life and incentivize earlier presentations for women that spares unnecessary treatments without a compromise in survival.

Development of multi-disciplinary tumor boards in low- and middle-income country cancer centers is another way to advance technology to improve outcomes.[36] The breast tumor board should incorporate: thoracic surgeons, oncologists, radiotherapists, radiologists, and pathologists. In order to have a sustainable, highly professional tumor board is a need for several components. In Kosovo in particular this process of multi-disciplinary discussion should be mandatory for patient care and incorporated into national protocols in accordance with international guidelines adapting to local capacities. Partnership and collaboration with international oncology centers could enhance training and discussion of difficult cases.

Multi-disciplinary discussions tend to cause an increase in the use of neoadjuvant chemotherapy and breast-conserving surgery. Improving communication and reducing positive margin rates of breast-conserving surgery will increase the incentive for women to present earlier to their health care team, and improve outcomes. Systemic therapies for breast cancer are rapidly changing the surgical landscape for options for women with breast cancer. It is critical that cancer providers of all disciplines engage in regular discussion and research to offer options that will improve outcomes, the quality of life and result in earlier detection.

CLINICS CARE POINTS

- Research on improving breast conservation rates in the treatment of breast cancer in LMICs is needed.
- Improvements in systemic therapies have allowed for surgical sparing approaches in high-income countries with equivalent outcomes and these concepts can be applied to LMICs to improve quality of life with similar overall survival.

- Surgical innovations and multi-disciplinary international tumor boards may help reduce mastectomy rates by increasing the use of neoadjuvant chemotherapy and endocrine therapy as well as partial mastectomy approaches, which will provide incentives for women to seek medical attention for breast masses earlier in countries without screening mammogram programs.

DISCLOSURE

Dr R.J. Barth is affiliated with CairnSurgical, Inc. All other authors have no financial interests to disclose.

REFERENCES

1. Tfayli A, Temraz S, Abou Mrad R, et al. Breast cancer in low- and middle-income countries: an emerging and challenging epidemic. J Oncol 2010;2010:490631.
2. Harford JB. Breast-cancer early detection in low-income and middle-income countries: do what you can versus one size fits all. Lancet Oncologist 2011; 12(3):306–12.
3. Cathcart-Rake EJ, Ruddy KJ, Bleyer A, et al. Breast cancer in adolescent and young adult women under the age of 40 years. JCO Oncol Pract 2021;17(6): 305–13.
4. Hu X, Myers KS, Oluyemi ET, et al. Presentation and characteristics of breast cancer in young women under age 40. Breast Cancer Res Treat 2021;186(1):209–17.
5. Niraula S, Biswanger N, Hu P, et al. Incidence, characteristics, and outcomes of interval breast cancers compared with screening-detected breast cancers. JAMA Netw Open 2020;3(9):e2018179.
6. Starikov A, Askin G, Blackburn A, et al. Mode of detection matters: differences in screen-detected versus symptomatic breast cancers. Clin Imaging 2021;80:11–5.
7. Barth RJ Jr, Gibson GR, Carney PA, et al. Detection of breast cancer on screening mammography allows patients to be treated with less-toxic therapy. AJR Am J Roentgenol 2005;184(1):324–9.
8. Pineros M, Znaor A, Mery L, et al. A global cancer surveillance framework within noncommunicable disease surveillance: making the case for population-based cancer registries. Epidemiol Rev 2017;39(1):161–9.
9. Berry DA, Cronin KA, Plevritis SK, et al. Effect of screening and adjuvant therapy on mortality from breast cancer. N Engl J Med 2005;353(17):1784–92.
10. Kalager M, Zelen M, Langmark F, Adami HO. Effect of screening mammography on breast-cancer mortality in Norway. N Engl J Med 2010 Se;363(13):1203–10.
11. McCormack V, McKenzie F, Foerster M, et al. Breast cancer survival and survival gap apportionment in sub-Saharan Africa (ABC-DO): a prospective cohort study. Lancet Glob Health 2020;8(9):e1203–12.
12. Abuidris DO, Elsheikh A, Ali M, et al. Breast-cancer screening with trained volunteers in a rural area of Sudan: a pilot study. Lancet Oncol 2013;14(4):363–70.
13. Bicaku A. Mobile mammography. Available at: https://omk-rksorg/revista-mjeku. 2021. Accessed September 6, 2021.
14. European Institute of Women's Health (2017) Policy Brief: Women and Breast Cancer in the EU—a life course approach. Available at: https://eurohealth.ie/women-and-breast-cancer-in-the-eu-a-life-course-approach/.
15. Hoxha I, Islami DA, Uwizeye G, et al. Forty-five years of research and progress in breast cancer: progress for some, disparities for most. JCO Glob Oncol 2022;8: e2100424.

16. Wong JS, Kaelin CM, Troyan SL, et al. Prospective study of wide excision alone for ductal carcinoma in situ of the breast. J Clin Oncol 2006;24(7):1031–6.
17. Lovrics PJ, Goldsmith CH, Hodgson N, et al. A multicentered, randomized, controlled trial comparing radioguided seed localization to standard wire localization for nonpalpable, invasive and in situ breast carcinomas. Ann Surg Oncol 2011;18(12):3407–14.
18. Schnabel F, Boolbol SK, Gittleman M, et al. A randomized prospective study of lumpectomy margin assessment with use of MarginProbe in patients with nonpalpable breast malignancies. Ann Surg Oncol 2014;21(5):1589–95.
19. Chagpar AB, Killelea BK, Tsangaris TN, et al. A randomized, controlled trial of cavity shave margins in breast cancer. N Engl J Med 6 2015;373(6):503–10.
20. Heil J, Breitkreuz K, Golatta M, et al. Do reexcisions impair aesthetic outcome in breast conservation surgery? Exploratory analysis of a prospective cohort study. Ann Surg Oncol 2012;19(2):541–7.
21. Abe SE, Hill JS, Han Y, et al. Margin re-excision and local recurrence in invasive breast cancer: a cost analysis using a decision tree model. J Surg Oncol 2015;112(4):443–8.
22. Berg WA, Gutierrez L, NessAiver MS, et al. Diagnostic accuracy of mammography, clinical examination, US, and MR imaging in preoperative assessment of breast cancer. Radiology 2004;233(3):830–49.
23. Menell JH, Morris EA, Dershaw DD, et al. Determination of the presence and extent of pure ductal carcinoma in situ by mammography and magnetic resonance imaging. Breast J 2005;11(6):382–90.
24. Hwang ES, Kinkel K, Esserman LJ, et al. Magnetic resonance imaging in patients diagnosed with ductal carcinoma-in-situ: value in the diagnosis of residual disease, occult invasion, and multicentricity. Ann Surg Oncol 2003;10(4):381–8.
25. Kristoffersen Wiberg M, Aspelin P, Sylvan M, et al. Comparison of lesion size estimated by dynamic MR imaging, mammography and histopathology in breast neoplasms. Eur Radiol 2003;13(6):1207–12.
26. Boetes C, Mus RD, Holland R, et al. Breast tumors: comparative accuracy of MR imaging relative to mammography and US for demonstrating extent. Radiology 1995;197(3):743–7.
27. Davis PL, Staiger MJ, Harris KB, et al. Breast cancer measurements with magnetic resonance imaging, ultrasonography, and mammography. Breast Cancer Res Treat 1996;37(1):1–9.
28. Mann RM, Cho N, Moy L. Breast MRI: state of the art. Radiology 2019;292(3):520–36.
29. Turnbull L, Brown S, Harvey I, et al. Comparative effectiveness of MRI in breast cancer (COMICE) trial: a randomised controlled trial. Lancet 2010;375(9714):563–71.
30. Atkins J, Al Mushawah F, Appleton CM, et al. Positive margin rates following breast-conserving surgery for stage I-III breast cancer: palpable versus nonpalpable tumors. J Surg Res 2012;177(1):109–15.
31. Sakakibara M, Yokomizo J, Shiina N, et al. MRI-guided quadrantectomy in patients with ductal carcinoma in situ detected preoperatively by mammographic calcifications. J Am Coll Surg 2014;219(2):295–302.
32. Sakakibara Mea. J Am Coll Surg 2008;207:62–8.
33. Pallone MJ, Poplack SP, Avutu HB, et al. Supine breast MRI and 3D optical scanning: a novel approach to improve tumor localization for breast conserving surgery. Ann Surg Oncol 2014;21(7):2203–8.

34. Barth RJ Jr, Krishnaswamy V, Paulsen KD, et al. A patient-specific 3D-printed form accurately transfers supine MRI-derived tumor localization information to guide breast-conserving surgery. Ann Surg Oncol 2017;24(10):2950–6.
35. Barth RJ Jr, Krishnaswamy V, Rooney TB, et al. A pilot multi-institutional study to evaluate the accuracy of a supine MRI based guidance system, the Breast Cancer Locator, in patients with palpable breast cancer. Surg Oncol 2022;44:101843.
36. Brandao M, Guisseve A, Bata G, et al. Survival impact and cost-effectiveness of a multidisciplinary tumor board for breast cancer in mozambique, sub-saharan Africa. Oncol 2021;26(6):e996–1008.

Providing Diagnostic Pathology Services in Low and Middle-Income Countries

Deo Ruhangaza, MD[a], Linda S. Kennedy, MEd[b],
Gregory J. Tsongalis, PhD[c,d],*

KEYWORDS

- Diagnostic pathology • LMICs • CML • Cervical cancer • Breast cancer

KEY POINTS

- Providing laboratory services in low and middle-income countries (LMICs) requires a strategy to overcome diverse infrastructure barriers.
- LMICs are in dire need of robust, low-cost testing for a variety of cancer types.
- Education should be a significant part of laboratory testing initiatives in LMICs.

INTRODUCTION

Developing and delivering diagnostic pathology services in low and middle-income countries (LMICs) often requires compromise in laboratory infrastructure without compromising the quality of patient test results. In addition to the all too familiar communicable infectious diseases, LMICs are also faced with the growing challenges of providing diagnostic and clinical care services for growing numbers of patients with cancer.[1] It is often said that 70% of clinical decision-making is based on a laboratory test but if those tests do not exist or are of poor quality then patient management suffers. In LMICs, the high mortality and morbidity rates associated with these diseases can be attributed largely to the lack of affordable and accessible diagnostic testing, preventative measures, early diagnosis/screening, and treatments. In order to begin to alleviate this burden of disease, we must develop more robust infrastructures and diagnostic technologies. Here, we will discuss examples of infrastructure and diagnostic testing applications that have been implemented during the past several years.

[a] Department of Pathology, Butaro Hospital and University of Global Health Equity, Rwanda; [b] Strategic Initiatives & Global Oncology at the Dartmouth Cancer Center, Dartmouth Health, Lebanon, NH, USA; [c] Pathology and Laboratory Medicine, Dartmouth Health and the Dartmouth Cancer Center, Lebanon, NH, USA; [d] Geisel School of Medicine, Hanover, NH, USA
* Corresponding author. Department of Pathology and Laboratory Medicine, Dartmouth Hitchcock Medical Center, 1 Medical Center Drive, Lebanon, NH 03756.
E-mail address: Gregory.j.tsongalis@hitchcock.org

Hematol Oncol Clin N Am 38 (2024) 209–216
https://doi.org/10.1016/j.hoc.2023.05.015
0889-8588/24/© 2023 Elsevier Inc. All rights reserved.

A significant barrier to implementing robust and sustainable diagnostic services in LMICs may be related to insufficient awareness by health-care policy makers of the central role of pathology in cancer control.[2] This can lead to inadequate resource allocation for pathology infrastructure, inadequate development of a pipeline for well-trained staff, lack of needed reagents and consumables, and insufficient quality control practices.[3]

Providing modern health-care services in LMICs often requires development of significant infrastructure to support and sustain the efforts. Potential barriers including conflict with cultural norms, fear, language differences, distance to follow-up care, inadequate electricity and water, environmental factors, lack of health screening, poverty, and conflicting health-care policies must be addressed. Overcoming barriers requires earning the trust of local people and collaboration with authorities to ensure patients, providers, and policy makers understand the benefits of high-quality pathology services.

Individuals may not be comfortable being examined by providers of different gender or someone who does not speak their language. In addition to the study team, involving local staff and individuals from the same regions of the country can help mitigate these issues and create a bond of trust. As with any illness, patients are fearful of a diagnosis and what the outcomes may be. Patients may be concerned about stigma and providers taking time for an open conversation about treatment options may alleviate some fears with education and referral to local support groups.

From a laboratory perspective, all testing equipment and consumables must be robust with proven ability to perform at acceptable levels in various environmental conditions including the potential of limited access to electricity or laboratory grade water. Turnaround times must ensure patients can receive results in a timely manner preventing loss to follow-up if they leave the testing area. Costs of testing should be affordable to regional standards or provided for free to maximize the patients tested. More testing will increase providers' ability to make effective diagnoses. In addition, testing should be easy to perform and convenient to participate in. Depending on the population, it can be effective to take testing to nonclinical locations.

Although LMICs continue to be most heavily burdened by infectious diseases, the availability of effective therapeutic drugs has lessened the infectious disease burden, which has allowed an increase in the incidences of human cancers partially due to extended life spans. Lack of diagnostics in resource-limited settings remains a major obstacle to treating all cancers reliably. Even the least complicated of modern pathology's advanced tools and reagents are largely inaccessible in LMICs because they are expensive to stock and finicky to operate. It is critical that high complexity testing common to high-income countries (HIC) be tailored for use in LMICs.

High mortality and higher morbidity rates impose an enormous burden on LMICs. Resources available throughout health-care systems in LMICs have been characterized by the WHO into 3 categories of infrastructure: moderate-to-advanced laboratory infrastructure, minimal laboratory infrastructure, and no laboratory infrastructure. In the moderate-to-advanced laboratory infrastructure category, health care is provided in hospitals with dependable electricity, clean water, cold storage, highly trained personnel, and a dedicated laboratory space. For those regions with minimal or no infrastructure, there is a lack of reliable electricity, cold storage, trained personnel, clean water, and a sterile environment.[4] Leaders of diagnostic pathology services with broad accessibility and high impact must assume very limited health-care infrastructure in LMICs so that performance characteristics of any given test can be maintained. Below we highlight 3 examples of diagnostic implementations to improve patient health.

DIAGNOSIS AND TREATMENT OF CHRONIC MYELOID LEUKEMIA IN RURAL RWANDA

In an effort to improve pathology services in Rwanda, the Ministry of Health in collaboration with the University of Rwanda initiated a pathology training program in 2013. This 4-year residency program trains general anatomical pathologists.[5] Despite a considerable increase of pathologists and pathology services in the country, challenges on availability of reagents, especially for immunohistochemistry (IHC) tests, lack of subspecialized pathologists and complete lack of molecular pathology tests remain major limiting factors. As a pilot test to introduce molecular testing and improve the availability of molecular diagnostic tests, molecular diagnostics for chronic myeloid leukemia (CML) was introduced at the Butaro Hospital Cancer Center. CML is a myeloproliferative disorder characterized by a t(9,22) resulting in the BCR-ABL1 fusion gene product that dysregulates tyrosine kinase activity. The capacity to test for BCR-ABL1 and the availability of tyrosine kinase inhibitors (TKIs) used to treat CML is still a challenge in LMICs. To address this problem in Rwanda, support became available from the Partners in Health (a nonprofit organization), the Ministry of Health, and the Gleevec International Patient Assistance Program with partnership between Novartis and the Max Foundation.[6] The ability to perform confirmatory diagnostic and molecular testing for CML (BCR-ABL1) and the introduction of the first-line TKI (Gleevec) in Rwanda was made possible. Since 2015, 2 rural hospitals in Rwanda (Rwinkwavu and Butaro district hospitals) were equipped with the GeneXpert BCR-ABL Ultra technology (Cepheid, Sunnyvale, CA). This system uses a single-use, automated cartridge for the quantitative quantitative real time reverse transcriptase polymerase chain reaction (qRT-PCR) test for BCR-ABL1 major breakpoint (p210) transcripts that provides results within a few hours.[7] Technical labor is minimal because the cartridge performs extraction, amplification, and detection once the sample is added. Before introduction of this technology, air-dried peripheral blood smears from clinically suspected patients were sent to an external partner laboratory institution (Brigham and Womens Hospital in Boston, MA, USA) for testing. Because BCR-ABL1 detection is a diagnostic test for CML, once the diagnosis is established, patients (including those from neighboring countries) can be treated with the first-line TKI, imatinib. Treatment is provided free of charge due to the partnerships described above. The outcomes of this program from a 10-year retrospective review (2009–2018) showed that 124 patients were treated, and 91% of them achieved a complete hematologic response after 49 days.[8] Patients were younger with a median age of 34 years and 11% of patients developed imatinib resistance during treatment. This program saved many patients with CML in the country and showed that it is possible to diagnose and treat CML in a resource limited setting when public–private partnership is involved. The challenges that remain for our CML testing program include the detection of molecular resistance and the availability of second-line drugs.

THE XPERT BREAST CANCER STRAT4 ASSAY AS A POSSIBLE ALTERNATIVE FOR IMMUNOHISTOCHEMISTRY IN RWANDA

Breast cancer remains the most common type of cancer diagnosed at the Butaro rural cancer center in Rwanda. Determining breast cancer biomarker status for the estrogen receptor (ER), progesterone receptor (PR), human epidermal growth factor receptor 2/neu (HER2), and the Ki-67 proliferative marker is crucial for treatment guidance and prognostic information.[9] Testing for breast cancer biomarkers is currently being done on formalin-fixed, paraffin-embedded (FFPE) tissue blocks using manual IHC techniques in 4 public laboratories in Rwanda, including the Butaro hospital cancer center laboratory. Challenges in doing manual IHC include frequent backlog for IHC reagents due to a limited or reliable number of local suppliers, limited technical skills in interpretation of results and technical troubleshooting. These challenges significantly affect the quality of IHC results, which are critical to the management of the patient.

Due to these challenges and the often unavailability of IHC testing in LMICs, we explored implementation of a molecular diagnostic technique at the Butaro Hospital in rural Rwanda. The Xpert Breast Cancer STRAT4 assay (Cepheid, Sunnyvale, CA, USA) is a cartridge-based molecular near point-of-care technology that measures mRNA expression levels in the tumor sample rather than staining for the protein. As an alternative to IHC for ER, PR, and HER2 testing on FFPE tissues, this approach offers the advantage of a more user-friendly technique without the need for microscopic expertise to interpret staining patterns and the cartridge-based test can be performed by those without significant molecular training. The assay uses the Cepheid GeneXpert system, which is widely available for tuberculosis and other infectious disease diagnostics in Rwanda and other low-resource settings so no additional equipment purchases are necessary. A previous study conducted at an outside institution using 150 FFPE tissues processed in Rwanda assessed the breast cancer biomarkers using Xpert Breast Cancer STRAT4 assay and compared the findings with those of standard IHC.[10] STRAT4 agreement with ER IHC was 93.3% and 97.8% for HER2 IHC. A larger study is currently being conducted at the Butaro Hospital laboratory to further assess the concordance between the 2 testing methods.

IMPLEMENTATION OF CERVICAL CANCER SCREENING IN HONDURAS

In HIC, pathology laboratories are equipped with advanced technology, carefully specified infrastructure, and technicians with graduate degrees. Investigators attempting to leverage advanced technologies in LMICs can achieve significant scientific findings but only if they can successfully transplant advanced technology for real-time operation in conditions without the benefits or infrastructure of a HIC laboratory. Here we will share lessons learned from implementation of the polymerase chain reaction (PCR), a common molecular technique, for cervical screening in Honduras by Dartmouth Cancer Center (formerly known as Norris Cotton Cancer Center) investigators. Use of PCR for the detection of cancer-causing high-risk human papilloma virus (hrHPV) is standard of care in the United States for the prevention of cervical cancer. The WHO recommends worldwide implementation of PCR by 2030. HrHPV is a precursor to cervical cancer, and knowing a woman's hrHPV status allows clinicians to make proactive plans for early detection and curative treatment.

Honduras, located in Central America, is an LMIC where more than half of the population (10.2 million in 2021) lives in poverty. The cancer burden is high and many patients first present at a clinic with late-stage disease. Cervical cancer is one of the most common cancers with 491 deaths recorded in 2021.[11] In 2012, Dartmouth investigators began a true partnership, where each party brings resources the other needs, with La Liga Contra el Cancer (LCC), a full-service cancer center in San Pedro Sula, Honduras. Daily, LCC oncologists saw the tragedy of women presenting with cervical cancer that could have been prevented or treated if seen earlier. Other than poverty, the lack of trained cytopathologists was the most intractable problem in attempts to prevent cervical cancer resulting in just 10% of women of screening age being screened annually. During five years, we operationalized hrHPV screening onsite in a rural mountain area for 350 women several times and in an urban factory for 2000 women in a week.[12] Follow-up PCR analysis of samples was completed onsite at LCC's in-house pathology laboratory.

We first began by suggesting to the PCR manufacturer that testing the difference between the efficacy of their device in a modern laboratory setting versus its effectiveness in the field would open options for clinical and research use in LMICs. In this case, it was literally a world of difference between the Dartmouth laboratory and our proposed site in the mountains of Honduras. We were provided an SLAN 96 Real Time PCR instrument (Quan Dx, San Jose, CA, USA) to transport to Honduras for these studies. We started with the premise that Honduras was our index site, a proxy for the many LMICs that are similar: a mix of urban and rural poor, usually hot and dusty with bumpy roads, and intermittent electrical service. We developed workflows and laboratory processes that did not replicate the rarified atmosphere found in our laboratory at the dartmouth cancer center (DCC) but rather were modified to function in a less than ideal environment. Our goal was functional usage in the local reality including heat, dust, and bumps. The process of discovering how to implement hrHPV screening by PCR was iterative and in-country partners and alliances were essential.

The PCR instrument was the nucleus for hrHPV screening. Our device was similar in size to a kitchen microwave and came with directions for its care and use including extensive packing, narrow temperature range for optimal performance, and top-notch electrical connections. Being a solid-state device with no moving parts, we agreed it could probably travel by pickup truck on bumpy, dirt roads. A plastic bag was used to prevent dust and the heat was unavoidable. Sample testing before the PCR instrument leaving the DCC laboratory and then onsite in Honduras confirmed concordant results—the device performed as well after travel as before.

The PCR instrument tests samples of DNA using lyophilized reagents in a 96-well strip tube format. Lyophilized reagents were a key component to the success of the PCR as reagents are normally refrigerated to ensure optimal performance but these reagents did not require any refrigeration (Quan Dx, San Jose, CA, USA).[12,13] DNA was extracted from 94 samples plus 2 controls and combined in the strip tubes with the lyophilized reagents. The run-time for the PCR reaction was 2 hours, allowing for multiple runs per day. Because the automated DNA extraction equipment was cost prohibitive, we developed a rapid, inexpensive crude extraction method. Initially, we extracted DNA from cervical swab samples using a boiling water bath suitable for only several samples at a time. Toward our goal of a scalable system, we needed a way to scale-up the boiling water method for extraction with retail equipment available for sale in almost any LMIC. An extra-large pot-style home rice cooker with a perforated stainless steel insert using steam instead of boiling water provided excellent results.[14]

These methods of mitigating barriers by considering alternative sources or products yielded excellent results in multiple situations. From making advanced technologies workable, to solving low-tech problems, we succeeded by concentrating on a specific goal rather than trying to replicate the advantages of a HIC laboratory. Case in point, typically clinicians with serial appointments at a clinic, package a single Pap test swab for processing. In our rural screening program, all 350 women were tested by PCR and Pap. In this example, the pain point was how to deactivate the virus on 350 swabs and dry them for packaging without letting them cross contaminate one another. A simple solution was to use a pencil to poke holes in a scrap of Styrofoam and put each swab, handle down, into a hole, wait several hours for them to dry and proceed with packaging. In another example, lacking 12 clinical examination tables with stirrups, local men fabricated tables with detachable wooden stirrups that were later repurposed as desks in the local school.

In this "true partnership," local oncologists, medical students, community leaders, rural clinicians, factory management, and a host of others were critical to our development of scientific questions and understanding of the practical issues. An early decision was to make all frontline study personnel local Hondurans, which had benefits ranging from career development and access to local resources, to inspiring confidence among study participants, and ensuring their proper understanding of risks in the consent process. Checking for broken, missing, or unavailable infrastructure, including intermittent electricity, damaged roadways and bridges, little or low-quality water, and unreliable or nonexistent Internet are part of the study planning process. Connecting with "people who know people" can solve problems quickly. In Honduras, the rural communities had unpredictable electrical shutdowns but a query facilitated by the right person ensured that our location would have a solid connection during onsite study days.

To identify and mitigate barriers to study participation, we relied on frank conversations with local leaders to understand potential sticking points that included lack of transportation, lack of literacy, and no awareness of cancer prevention through screening. By having women call women to explain the opportunity, which included a free bus and hot lunch, we doubled our projected enrollment. Later, when we planned to screen men, we still had women call women, and quickly reached our maximum enrollment of 350, even in an environment where it is "known" that men "never" seek medical attention. This level of buy-in continued after the screening when 90% to 95% of participants referred to LCC for clinical follow-up were compliant with the recommendation.

Although it is tempting to focus on technology, these studies require human cooperation and joint effort. It is worth noting that in the rural studies, a gracious reception for study participants including a shady place to wait, a home-cooked meal, involvement of local leaders, and time to socialize, were considerations that participants appreciated. In that setting, participants were onsite for 3 to 4 hours. In the urban factory, time is money, and senior managers were eager to facilitate testing only if it took minimal time away from the sewing machines. Accordingly, everything was streamlined, and each participant was in the screening area for 7 minutes. Building capacity by working closely with local people pays dividends immediately in the ability to access populations and resources previously unavailable to HIC investigators. Long-term, the dividends are magnified when a cohort is revisited and the local leaders can mobilize their forces to repeat a study, taking their places on the team, and having pride in developing knowledge to reduce the cancer burden in LMICs. Our study in Honduras has led to lifelong relationships with colleagues and individuals clearly influenced by these efforts. We collectively have created the groundwork for sustained hrHPV screening and efforts that will lead to future screening events, and a pathway to reduction in cervical cancer mortality among Honduran women.[15]

SUMMARY

Our experience working and promoting women's health in an LMIC highlights several critical features necessary to allow for successful clinical implementation, translational research, and sustainability. Key to these successes has been the grass-roots relationships between policy-makers, investigators, local clinicians and local individuals. Working in a true partnership model of community led action research allows for inclusion of all parties in the design and implementation of clinical trials that benefit all involved. Most available molecular diagnostics require advanced infrastructure and, therefore, are largely inaccessible to populations in resource-limited areas. In addition, many settings within developed countries such as the United States could also qualify as "low infrastructure sites" (eg, rural laboratories, many nonacademic and smaller hospital laboratories, clinics of various sorts, and so forth) for which simple and rapid molecular diagnostic testing would also be beneficial. We think that implementing diagnostics in LMICs will facilitate the development of new and more robust molecular diagnostic technologies that will be improve global health.

CLINICS CARE POINTS

- Development of laboratory testing capabilities in LMICs requires a robust infrastructure and trusting relationships.
- Novel approaches to the use of existing technologies can improve testing capabilities in LMICs.
- In LMICs, near patient testing including clinics and remote health screening programs will have the largest impact on patient care.
- There are numerous opportunities to further develop testing capabilities in LMICs for various cancer types including both blood and solid tumors.

DISCLOSURE

The authors declare no disclosures with respect to this article.

FUNDING

The authors wish to acknowledge the support of the Pathology Shared Resource in the Center for Clinical Genomics and Advanced Technology of the Dartmouth Hitchcock Health System and the Dartmouth Cancer Center with NCI Cancer Center Support Grant 5P30 CA023108-37.

REFERENCES

1. Jiwnani S, Penumadu P, Ashok A, et al. Lung cancer manamegement in low and middle income countries. Thorac Surg Clin 2022;32:383–95.
2. Sayed S, Cherniac W, Lawler M, et al. Improving pathology and laboratory medicine in low-income and middle-income countries: roadmap to solutions. Lancet 2018;391:1939–52.
3. Sankarayaranana R. Screening for cancer in low and middle income countries. Annals of Global Health 2014;80:412–7.
4. Urdea M, Penny LA, Olmsted SS, et al. Requirements for high impact diagnostics in the developing world. Nature 2006;S1:73–9.
5. Nelson AM, Hale M, Isidore M, et al. Training the next generation of african pathologists. Clin Lab Med 2018;38(1):37–51.
6. Garcia-Gonzalez P, Boultbee P, Epstein D. Novel humanitarian aid program: the glivec international patient assistance program-lessons learned from providing access to breakthrough targeted oncology treatment in low- and middle-income countries. J Global Oncol 2015;1:37–45.
7. Enjeti A, Granter N, Ashraf A, et al. A longitudinal evaluation of performance of automated BCR-ABL1 quantitation using cartridge-based detection system. Pathology 2015;47:570–4.

8. Morgan J, DeBoer RJ, Bigirimana JB, et al. A ten-year experience of treating chronic myeloid leukemia in rural Rwanda: outcomes and insights for a changing landscape. JCO Glob Oncol 2022. https://doi.org/10.1200/GO.22.00131.

9. Bevers TB, Helvie M, Bonaccio E, et al. Breast cancer screening and diagnosis, version 3. 2018, NCCN clinical practice guidelines in oncology. J Natl Compr Cancer Netw 2018;16:1362–89.

10. Mugabe M, Ho KE, Ruhangaza D, et al. Use of the Xpert Breast Cancer STRAT4 for biomarker evaluation in tissue processed in a developing country. Am J Clin Pathol 2021;156:766–76.

11. Available at: https://www.who.int/teams/noncommunicable-diseases/surveillance/data/cervical-cancer-profiles. (last accessed April 3, 2023).

12. Turner SA, Deharvengt SJ, Lyons KD, et al. Implementation of multicolor melt curve analysis for high-risk human papilloma virus detection in low- and middle-income countries: a pilot study for expanded cervical cancer screening in Honduras. J Glob Oncol 2018;4:1–8.

13. Atkinson A, Studwell C, Bejarano S, et al. Rural distribution of human papilloma virus in low- and middle-income countries. Exp Mol Pathol 2018;104(2):146–50.

14. Atkinson AE, Mandujano CAM, Bejarano S, et al. Screening for human papillomavirus in a low- and middle-income country. J Glob Oncol 2019;5:JGO1800233.

15. Petersen LM, Fenton JM, Kennedy LS, et al. HPV, vaccines, and cervical cancer in a low- and middle-income country. Curr Probl Cancer 2020;44(6):100605.

Smart Solutions to Address the Global Gap in Radiation Oncology Through Trainee Engagement and Partnerships with Industry

Cecília Félix Penido Mendes de Sousa, MD[a], Jared Pasetsky, MD[b],
Gustavo Nader Marta, MD, PhD[a], Megan Kassick, MD, MPH[c],
Fabio Ynoe Moraes, MD, MBA, PhD[d,1,*], Luqman K. Dad, MD, MBA[b,1]

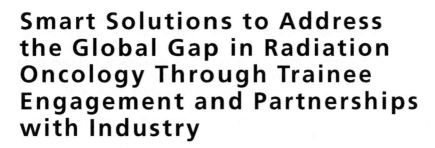

KEYWORDS

- Global oncology • Radiation oncology • Medical education
- Public–private sector partnerships • Public health

KEY POINTS

- There is a global shortage of radiation therapy supply.
- Trainee engagement initiatives are urgently needed to decrease global gaps.
- Industry partnerships have the potential to address some of the existing barriers.

INTRODUCTION

Radiotherapy (RT) is an important treatment modality in cancer management. Approximately 50% to 60% of all cancer patients globally require RT at some point during their treatment.[1,2] RT is often used in various malignancies as a primary or adjuvant treatment in curative-directed therapy as well as a palliative treatment to alleviate symptoms. Recently, treatment advances such as with intensity-modulated radiation therapy (IMRT), image-guided radiation therapy (IGRT), stereotactic radiosurgery

[a] Hospital Sírio-Libanês - Rua Dona Adma Jafet, São Paulo-SP, Bela Vista, 01308-050 Brazil;
[b] Columbia University Irving Medical Center - 630 West 168th Street, New York, NY 10032, USA;
[c] Department of Radiation Oncology, University of Pennsylvania - 3400 Civic Boulevard, Philadelphia, PA 19104-6021, USA; [d] Division of Radiation Oncology, Department of Oncology, Kingston General Hospital, Queen's University, 25 King Street West, Burr Wing, Kingston, Ontario K7L 5P9, Canada
[1] Equally contributed as senior author.
* Corresponding author. Department of Radiation Oncology, Columbia University, 622 W 168th Street, CHONY North B-Level, New York, NY 10032.
E-mail address: fymoraes@gmail.com

Hematol Oncol Clin N Am 38 (2024) 217–228
https://doi.org/10.1016/j.hoc.2023.06.009
0889-8588/24/© 2023 Elsevier Inc. All rights reserved.

(SRS), stereotactic body RT (SBRT), and proton therapy, have provided more precise and effective radiation delivery. These innovations, coupled with the integration of diagnostic imaging, have enabled RT to be given with greater accuracy to improve tumor coverage while sparing normal tissue.[3] Adaptive RT,[4] a feedback control strategy to adapt treatment planning and delivery based on patient-specific anatomical or biological variations,[5] and artificial intelligence[6] hold promise to further advance RT.

Expanding access to these technological advancements is critical, and may be enhanced through educational initiatives and global partnerships. Continuous training and education of health care providers in RT's evolving principles and techniques are necessary to ensure that providers are well-equipped to provide the best care to their patients. Collaboration between health care providers, researchers, industry, and policymakers can facilitate the development of new research projects and access to new technologies while creating updated evidence-based guidelines to ensure RT is delivered optimally and appropriately. These partnerships can also help identify barriers to accessing RT, such as access to machines, inadequate infrastructure, and lack of research funding, among others, thereby providing information to help optimize the allocation of resources nationally.

Despite its importance, access to RT remains a significant challenge in many low- and middle-income countries (LMICs), where cancer mortality rates are disproportionately higher.[7,8] Reasons for this are multifactorial and include scarcity of RT centers and shortage of trained health care personnel, among others.[3] In Latin America and the Caribbean in 2018, 30% (12/40) of countries do not have any RT centers, and only 7.5% (3/40) of countries met the International Atomic Energy Agency (IAEA) recommendation of 1 megavoltage machine (MVM) per 250,000 inhabitants.[9] In Africa, 54% (29/54) of countries do not have any RT facilities[9]; none met the IAEA recommendation regarding the population distribution per MVM.[9] Reasons for these gaps in RT are multifactorial, including workforce shortages, political instabilities, cultural barriers, inefficient partnerships, and a lack of universal health care access, funding, and cancer registries.[10] Further, a recent survey found that low salaries, work overload, lack of prestige, scarcity of resources, and centralization of centers are reasons medical graduates do not want to pursue a career in RT in Latin America.[11] Trainees who do decide to pursue a career in RT must also deal with low compensation during training (usually requiring extra shifts), insufficient supervision, high clinical demands, isolation, and the feeling of practicing suboptimal treatments, leading to frustration and a further lack of interest in pursuing RT.[11]

The multifactorial nature of these current gaps requires a complex approach to solve this problem. A trained workforce is an essential component of cancer care. Even with a trained workforce to meet the demands of a given country, without access to technology as well as funding allocated to research activities, cancer needs of that population will likely not be met. Promoting advances in trainee engagement, improving partnerships with industry, and attracting qualified professionals and educators through a structured action plan have the potential to decrease the global gap in radiation oncology by improving education, access, and delivery of RT. This article aims to describe trainee engagement and industry partnerships as two potential solutions that can help address global gaps in radiation oncology.

THE NEED FOR IMPROVED TRAINEE ENGAGEMENT

Currently, no global registry of radiation oncologists' availability and distribution exists.[10] The lack of a unified registry limits an accurate assessment of the available resources and existing gaps, hindering the implementation of an effective action plan. In addition, recommendations on staffing for RT vary considerably by country, which prevents standardized assessments of resource shortages. For example, in Europe, there are recommendations for 150 to 400 (mean 250) patients per radiation oncologist,[12] significantly higher than some LMICs like in Brazil, where the recommendation is one physician per 600 new cases/year.[13]

Despite the limitation on accurately evaluating the health care provider shortage worldwide, it is already well known that there is a global limitation in RT access.[3] The RT network faces shortages in facilities, equipment, and staff even in high-income countries (HICs) such as Australia, the UK, and Canada.[3] Furthermore, even if staffing is within recommendations for a given country, this does not mean it is appropriately distributed nationwide.[3] People living in sparsely populated regions, such as in some Canadian and Australian regions, usually have to travel long distances for treatment because the low population density does not justify the high investments needed for RT.[3] In large countries such as Brazil, RT centers tend to be centralized, and there are entire states (Roraima and Amapá) without any facility.[14] In addition, these underserved regions struggle not only with the lack of health care professionals but also with the lack of specialized training. In Brazil, 80% of RT residencies are located in the Southeast region, mostly (55%) in São Paulo State.[14]

Closing the global gap requires an absolute increase in training capacity and improvement in training quality. Health care professionals should be proficient in the various RT modalities and evidence-based medicine because it allows them to make decisions that ultimately translate into better outcomes while evaluating cost-effectiveness. However, there are still many barriers to training and continuing education. For example, RT programs exist in only 56.5% (13/23) of Latin American countries, and in most (62%, 8/13), there is only one center.[15] In addition, programs are usually in capital cities, and training in more modern technologies is not always available, 55% of programs offer training in SBRT, 70% in SRS, and 75% in Volumetric Modulated Arc Therapy (VMAT).[15] Although in countries like the US, Canada, Australia, and New Zealand, there is approximately one program per 0.57 to 3.7 million people, this proportion might be as high as one program per 50 million people (with two graduating residents per year).[15]

Currently, there are many initiatives to attract, engage, and assist trainees. The European societies annually offer a multidisciplinary course in oncology targeting medical students.[16] The American Society for Radiation Oncology grants a medical student fellowship award to promote radiation oncology as a career choice.[17] The IAEA also leads international cooperation initiatives that include fellowship programs and scientific visits.[18] Since 1985, American residents can count on the Association of Residents in Radiation Oncology, an independent organization created, to represent them,[19] along with the Global Health Subcommittee, created in 2009.[20] In addition to Medical Societies' lead initiatives, there are many online resources focused on radiation oncology education and research that can contribute to training.[21] Examples include contouring platforms,[22] key studies databases,[23] case vignettes,[24] anatomy platforms,[25,26] and platforms for discussing clinical situations with experts.[27] **Table 1** provides a list of some resources.

Those resources and initiatives have an undeniable value. However, they also illustrate the pattern of gaps in cancer care. Although most of these resources are free, some have associated costs, and trainees may be unaware of some of these resources. In addition, most of those resources are in English and are usually led in HICs. According to the Common European Framework of Reference for Languages (CEFR), the ability to "understand the main ideas of complex text on both concrete and abstract topics, including technical discussions in his/her field of specialization"

Table 1
List of available resources focused on radiation oncology education and research[a]

Resources List[a]			Costs
ROECSG—Radiation Oncology Collaborative Study Group	List of Web Resources Related to Radiation Oncology	https://roecsg.org/web-resources/	Free
International Societies, Associations, and Organizations			
ESO—European School of Oncology	Promotes continuing education initiatives, including online and offline learning opportunities, conferences and events, individualized career development programs, and fellowships.	https://www.eso.net/en/en/who-we-are/1-4986-1-	Some programs have associated costs. Some programs might have funding's resources.
ASTRO—American Society for Radiation Oncology	Guidelines, continuing education programs, funding opportunities, research resources, professional growth resources	https://www.astro.org/	$705 for annual membership, $440 for international membership, free to residents
ARRO—Association of Residents in Radiation Oncology	Residents resources, content for medical students, global health initiatives	https://www.astro.org/Affiliate/ARRO	Free to residents
ESTRO—European Society for Radiotherapy and Oncology	Guidelines, continuing education programs, funding opportunities, research resources, professional growth resources	https://www.estro.org/	Ranges from €55–150 per year, not free for residents
IAEA—International Atomic Energy Agency	Educational resources, documents, fellowship programs, scientific visits programs	https://www.iaea.org/services/technical-cooperation-programme/fellowships	Some resources have associated costs. Some programs might have funding's resources.

Point of care useful resources

eContour	Interactive contouring guidelines	https://econtour.org/	Free
RadOncTables	Key radiation oncology studies	https://radonctables.com/	Free
theMednet	A physician-only Q&A platform for expert answers to real-world clinical situations	https://www.themednet.org/	Free
i.treatsafely	Peer-to-peer learning site dedicated with practical learning videos for radiation oncology professionals	https://i.treatsafely.org/	Free
Anatomy			
IMAIOS	Radiological anatomy resources	https://www.imaios.com/en/e-anatomy	$95 per year for E-anatomy, $350 per year with question bank, can get group/institutional discounts
ACR—The Anatomy and Radiology Contouring Bootcamp	Anatomy and radiology course with hands-on contouring practice for radiation oncology	https://arcbootcamp.teachable.com/	$99 for course can get group discount and possible discount in LMICs!

Prices were last updated in March 2023.
a The presented resource list is not an exhaustive list, but rather a representation of some of the resources available.

is achieved in CEFR level B2.[28] This means that those with a level below B2 (A1, A2, B1) do not have the necessary English proficiency to understand the technical content in those resources. The 2022 English Proficiency Index report showed that health care professionals worldwide have a very low English proficiency level (lower half of CEFR level B1 and A2).[29] In addition, average scores in Africa and Latin America are in the low proficiency bands (upper half of CEFR level B1), and in the Middle East, they fall in the very low bands (lower half of CEFR level B1 and A2),[29] making the utilization of such resources increasingly difficult. The National Comprehensive Cancer Network addresses some of those issues by providing translated and resource-stratified practice guidelines,[30] thus aiding in the decision-making process in low-resource scenarios. However, there is a paucity of translated resources focused on trainee education. In LMICs, trainee engagement initiates can benefit by increasing access to such translated resources and addressing regional problems.

As reported in the trainee survey conducted in Latin America, trainees in this setting experience isolation and the feeling of practicing suboptimal treatments.[11] Latin America and other LMIC regions frequently do not have the newest RT technologies available. Trainees and clinicians have reported that this situation can be highly challenging. For example, proton therapy is a newer radiation technique that has been shown to decrease treatment side effects in certain patient populations and potentially improve oncologic outcomes.[31,32] Access to proton therapy, however, is limited globally, particularly in LMIC settings.[33]

Furthermore, trainees in LMICs must develop analytical and quantitative skills to identify the most appropriate and cost-effective treatments in limited-resource settings. For example, IMRT has been shown to decrease treatment-related toxicity[32] and, in some situations, improve survival, though its availability is limited.[34] In 2014, 30% of European countries were not equipped for IMRT, and 50% were not equipped for IGRT.[35] There was a correlation between socioeconomic status and the availability of RT technologies, with middle-income European countries having less technology access than higher income countries.[35] Even though this scenario may have improved in the last decade, this analysis illustrates the pattern of decreased access to RT treatment in lower income countries.[35] In 2020, the proportion of RT centers that could deliver advanced RT technologies in the Brazilian public health care system (which cares for 70% of the country's population) was 21% for IMRT, 14% for VMAT and IGRT, 15% for SRS, and 12% for SBRT.[14] Therefore, clinicians may have to choose which patients will or will not be offered a more advanced treatment modality, and they may be responsible for triaging and making decisions regarding resource allocation.

Trainees in LMICs also require training in technologies no longer currently used in HICs. The IAEA recommends cobalt RT machines in low-resource settings because they have a lower cost, a high level of robustness, and can increase treatment access for underserved populations.[36] Still, these machines are used scarcely in HICs. Given this, training resources usually focus on modern RT machines and techniques. One resource available, the i.treatsafely platform provides peer-to-peer practical learning videos for users across 50 countries from different specialties in RT.[20,37] Most users (61%) come from North America and the European Union, and it is important to increase awareness of the existence of such resources for health care professionals in other countries, especially considering that they provide videos with multilingual narration in English, Spanish, French, Portuguese, Mandarin, and Thai.[20] The content in i.treatsafely covers a wide range of RT platforms[37] and can serve to provide resources for training for older equipment and technologies.[20] However, expanding access to training in more modern RT technologies is also necessary. As discussed above, in Latin America, a 2022 analysis showed that training in IMRT, SRS, and SBRT is unavailable respectively in 25%, 30%, and 45% of programs in Latin America.[15] Even if treatment advances take longer to reach LMICs, the personnel must be trained to be able to deliver those treatments when they arrive.

Trainees in LMIC settings have reported another challenging aspect to be providing guideline-discordant care due the existing resource limitations. Patients can present with an advanced disease without proper staging and with guideline-discordant previous treatment pathways. For example, long wait times to start RT can lead to patients' first undergoing induction chemotherapy, even when this does not represent the standard of care. Clinical trials typically do not address the scenarios created by treatment access barriers. Therefore, trainees may feel like they are performing suboptimal care, leading to frustration and demotivation and hampering the implementation of evidence-based practices in real-world scenarios.

Last, collaborations between academic institutions in HICs and LMICs can also improve training and patient outcomes. Botswana has successfully implemented a collaboration including regular tumor boards and on-site visits that resulted in the introduction of new approaches to treatment and perceived improvements in care (BOTSOGO Collaborative Partnership).[38] Developing more partnerships like this, in which technological access and education is at the forefront, could improve trainee engagement in global radiation oncology. In addition, online remote training is a potential strategy to improve training and exchange between different centers.[39] The outline below summarizes the key areas discussed above to improve trainee engagement internationally. See **Fig. 1**.

Solutions: Practical Guideline

1. Creation of a global registry of RT network and training: an appropriate assessment is the first step to allowing effective interventions.
2. Expand access to English learning tools.
3. Access to translated versions of the available training resources.
4. Expand evidence-based medicine training.
5. Creation of a network connecting professionals
   a. Interactive online tumor boards — special focus on low-resource particularities
   b. Mentorship
   c. Learning resources

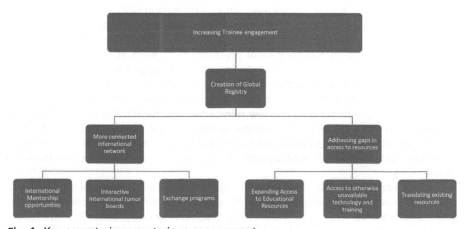

Fig. 1. Key areas to improve trainee engagement.

d. Exchange programs
6. Strengthening of professional support networks

PARTNERSHIPS WITH INDUSTRY

Despite potential conflicts of interest related to partnerships with industry, it should be recognized that these partnerships have contributed to major medical advances, especially in oncology.[40] Lately, there has been an increasing dependence on these partnerships.[41] In addition to enabling treatment advances, industry partnerships can improve grant support, the establishment of collaborative networks, facilities development, and health care management.[42] Therefore, industry partnerships should be considered when developing strategies to decrease gaps in cancer care.[39]

Radiation oncology has unique considerations that influence industry partnerships. Unlike medical and surgical oncology, RT requires significant capital investments to acquire machines and initiate treatment.[20] Because of that, policymakers may be hesitant to invest in RT, even if it may be more cost-effective in the long term.[20] To address this issue, vendors have already been reported to be working on novel funding approaches, developing more cost-conscious equipment, and engaging in private-public partnerships.[20] Despite the IAEA recommendation that less technologically advanced equipment might be more effective in low-resource settings,[36] lower-cost alternatives are often rejected because they are perceived as inferior equipment.[3] Finding cost-effective investments that are not considered outdated is a challenging task. Thus, it is important for the industry to consider the local context and regional preferences and beliefs to propose individualized solutions.

Public–private partnerships (PPPs) are "long-term contracts between a public and a private entity."[43] In these contracts, the public entity pays the private entity for health care delivery.[43] The PPPs are an emerging strategy to acquire and maintain RT equipment, overcoming government funding limitations and expanding access to treatment.[44] There are many examples of successful implementations of PPPs. In Nigeria, PPPs have increased the country's RT network, treating high patient volumes with minimal interruptions.[44] Government machines represented 80% of Nigeria's network; however, they were nonfunctional 35% of the year and treated 60% fewer patients than PPP machines.[44] In Botswana, RT development was led by a private initiative in the 1990s, and after a successful partnership with the government, public-sector patients represent more than 90% of patients undergoing RT.[45] The PPPs are considered responsible for enabling private-sector investments in Botswana.[45] Last, the My Child Matters program was a PPP that has improved survival outcomes for pediatric cancer patients in Latin America, Africa, and Eastern European countries by sponsoring different projects targeting local problems.[46] Despite such successes, such industry and PPP partnerships often rely on industry headquarters usually located in high-resource regions, without awareness of local challenges in LMICs.

One of the difficulties in accessing more advanced RT technologies in many countries is related to underfunding and low reimbursement for RT. Industry partnerships focused on developing cost-effectiveness analyses could help inform policymakers that modern RT techniques can support shorter overall treatment durations (hypofractionation) and increase treatment capacity. This could potentially contribute to fostering investments.

Artificial intelligence and machine learning (AI&ML) have an enormous potential to contribute toward decreasing the global RT gap. Those technologies can reduce the need for human intervention, contribute to the decision-making processes, and execute repetitive and time-consuming tasks.[47] Because of that, AI&ML can potentially increase efficiency and optimization in low-resource settings.[47] In many fields of medicine, AI&ML have already been integrated into health care operations. For example, the Laura Robot was the world's first risk management cognitive robot.[48] It now adds to other AI&ML initiatives that contribute to the decision-making process, helping target resources and improve outcomes.[49] Even though these initiatives were not directly related to RT, they are a model that could be adapted and applied in the RT workflow because such algorithms could help address staff shortages by monitoring patients during treatment and helping identify those who need urgent evaluations (eg, weight loss monitoring in head and neck treatments). Automatic contouring algorithms are another AI&ML application that can help overcome staff shortages, allowing health care professionals to focus on direct patient care and critical activities (such as target volume definitions). In a recent validation of a Python system, high contour accuracy scores were obtained in 98.5% of the images.[50] Partnerships with industry could foster technological advancements, provide solutions to local challenges, and help validate AI&ML models. To transform this potential into real improvements, it is fundamental to ground those partnerships on ethical principles.[20,41] Still, challenges remain in integrating such technologies into the landscape of LMICs, for example, the lack of electronic patient management and record systems might represent a barrier.

Solutions: Practical Guideline

1. Ethical committees focused on partnerships with industry to provide guidance and supervision.
2. Promotion and education of evidence-based innovation and how to assess innovation.
3. PPP networks are designed to allow centers to share their success and barriers and collaborate toward solutions.
4. Global opportunities with grants focusing on technological development in LMICs.
5. AI&ML initiatives that involve point-of-care, academic centers, and industry, enabling the development of solutions to real-life problems.

SUMMARY

Increasing trainee engagement and promoting industry partnerships are strategies to address the global gap in radiation oncology with the potential to decrease it and thus promote a meaningful impact in cancer care. Investments and the development of actions, such as expanding access to medical education tools, strengthening professional support networks, and increasing PPPS, are needed to create and expand such initiatives. Stakeholders in radiation oncology should work together with governments, academic institutions, and those in the point of care toward a more equitable and accessible future.

CLINICS CARE POINTS

- Establish mentorship programs to facilitate the transfer of knowledge and skills from experienced practitioners to trainees.
- Forge strategic partnerships with industry leaders in radiation oncology to leverage their expertise, resources, and technological advancements.
- Encourage the sharing of knowledge and best practices between clinics and industry partners to drive continuous improvement and optimize patient care.

DISCLOSURE

G.N. Marta is the Vice President of the Brazilian Society for Radiation Oncology (SBRT); leadership roles in those societies were pro bono. F.Y. Moraes received consulting fee from Cancer em foco (Elekta), and honoraria from AstraZeneca and IASLC; they are all unrelated to the present work. The other authors have nothing to disclose.

REFERENCES

1. Delaney G, Jacob S, Featherstone C, et al. The role of radiotherapy in cancer treatment: estimating optimal utilization from a review of evidence-based clinical guidelines. Cancer 2005;104(6):1129–37.
2. Khor R, Bressel M, Tai KH, et al. Patterns of retreatment with radiotherapy in a large academic centre. J Med Imaging Radiat Oncol 2013;57(5):610–6.
3. Atun R, Jaffray DA, Barton MB, et al. Expanding global access to radiotherapy. Lancet Oncol 2015;16(10):1153–86.
4. McDonald BA, Zachiu C, Christodouleas J, et al. Dose accumulation for MR-guided adaptive radiotherapy: From practical considerations to state-of-the-art clinical implementation. Front Oncol 2022;12:1086258.
5. Yan D. Adaptive radiotherapy: merging principle into clinical practice. Semin Radiat Oncol 2010;20(2):79–83.
6. Parkinson C, Matthams C, Foley K, et al. Artificial intelligence in radiation oncology: a review of its current status and potential application for the radiotherapy workforce. Radiogr Lond Engl 1995 2021;(27 Suppl 1):S63–8. https://doi.org/10.1016/j.radi.2021.07.012.
7. Bray F, Jemal A, Grey N, et al. Global cancer transitions according to the human development Index (2008-2030): a population-based study. Lancet Oncol 2012; 13(8):790–801.
8. Sung H, Ferlay J, Siegel RL, et al. Global cancer statistics 2020: GLOBOCAN estimates of incidence and mortality worldwide for 36 cancers in 185 countries. CA Cancer J Clin 2021;71(3):209–49.
9. Bishr MK, Zaghloul MS. Radiation therapy availability in Africa and Latin America: two models of low and middle income countries. Int J Radiat Oncol 2018;102(3): 490–8.
10. Barrios CH, Werutsky G, Mohar A, et al. Cancer control in latin America and the caribbean: recent advances and opportunities to move forward. Lancet Oncol 2021;22(11):e474–87.
11. Duma N, Moraes FY. Oncology training in latin America: are we ready for 2040? Lancet Oncol 2020;21(10):1267–8.
12. Slotman BJ, Cottier B, Bentzen SM, et al. Overview of national guidelines for infrastructure and staffing of radiotherapy. ESTRO-QUARTS: work package 1. Radiother Oncol J Eur Soc Ther Radiol Oncol 2005;75(3):349–54.
13. Norma CNEN NN 6.10 - Resolução CNEN 277/21 - Agosto/2021. Available at: https://www.gov.br/cnen/pt-br/acesso-rapido/normas/grupo-6/grupo6-nrm610.pdf. Accessed November 23, 2022.
14. Sociedade Brasileira de Radioterapia - RT2030 (2020).pdf. Available at: https://sbradioterapia.com.br/wp-content/uploads/2021/08/Relatorio_Projeto_RT2030.pdf. Accessed March 5, 2023.
15. Li B, Salazar JF, Rivera AF, et al. Radiation oncology residency training in Latin America: a call to attention. Adv Radiat Oncol 2022;7(3). https://doi.org/10.1016/j.adro.2022.100898.

16. www.evtel.com. ET. ESO-ESSO-ESTRO Multidisciplinary Course in Oncology for Medical Students - ESO - European School of Oncology. eso. Available at: https://www.eso.net/en/what-we-do/past-events/events2022/eso-esso-estro-multi disciplinary-course-in-oncology-for-medical-students/3-5611-0-. Accessed February 18, 2023.

17. Medical Student Fellowship Award - Funding Opportunities - American Society for Radiation Oncology (ASTRO) - American Society for Radiation Oncology (ASTRO). ASTRO. Available at: https://www.astro.org/Patient-Care-and-Research/Research/Funding-Opportunities/ASTRO-Medical-Student-Fellowship-Award Accessed February 18, 2023.

18. IAEA - Fellowship programme and Scientific visits. Published September 20, 2016. Available at: https://www.iaea.org/services/technical-cooperation-programme/fellowships. Accessed March 29, 2023.

19. Association of Residents in Radiation Oncology - American Society for Radiation Oncology (ASTRO) - American Society for Radiation Oncology (ASTRO). ASTRO. Available at: https://www.astro.org/Affiliate/ARRO. Accessed February 18, 2023.

20. Dad L, Royce TJ, Morris Z, et al. Bridging innovation and outreach to overcome global gaps in radiation oncology through information and communication tools, trainee advancement, engaging industry, attention to ethical challenges, and political advocacy. Semin Radiat Oncol 2017;27(2):98–108.

21. Web Resources. ROECSG. Published June 28, 2018. Available at: https://roecsg.org/web-resources/. Accessed February 18, 2023.

22. eContour. Available at: https://econtour.org/. Accessed February 18, 2023.

23. RadOncTables. RadOncTables. Published May 25, 2022. Available at: https://radonctables.com/. Accessed February 18, 2023.

24. ARROCase - American Society for Radiation Oncology (ASTRO) - American Society for Radiation Oncology (ASTRO). ASTRO. Available at: https://www.astro.org/Affiliate/ARRO/Resident-Resources/Educational-Resources/ARROCase. Accessed February 18, 2023.

25. Gray, Henry. 1918. Anatomy of the Human Body. Available at: https://www.bartleby.com/107/. Accessed February 18, 2023.

26. e-Anatomy, the Anatomy of Imaging. IMAIOS. Available at: https://www.imaios.com/en/e-anatomy. Accessed February 18, 2023.

27. theMednet. Available at: https://www.themednet.org/physicians. Accessed February 27, 2023.

28. Global scale - Table 1 (CEFR 3.3): Common Reference levels - Common European Framework of Reference for Languages (CEFR) - publi.coe.int. Common European Framework of Reference for Languages (CEFR). Available at: https://www.coe.int/en/web/common-european-framework-reference-languages/table-1-cefr-3.3-common-reference-levels-global-scale. Accessed February 19, 2023.

29. EF EPI 2022 – EF English Proficiency Index. Available at: https://www.ef.com/wwen/epi/. Accessed February 18, 2023.

30. National Comprehensive Cancer Network - Home. Available at: https://www.nccn.org/. Accessed February 18, 2023.

31. St Clair WH, Adams JA, Bues M, et al. Advantage of protons compared to conventional X-ray or IMRT in the treatment of a pediatric patient with medulloblastoma. Int J Radiat Oncol Biol Phys 2004;58(3):727–34.

32. Zhou J, Yang B, Wang X, et al. Comparison of the effectiveness of radiotherapy with photons and particles for chordoma after surgery: a meta-analysis. World Neurosurg 2018;117:46–53.

33. PTCOG - Facilities in Operation. Available at: https://www.ptcog.ch/index.php/facilities-in-operation-restricted. Accessed February 18, 2023.

34. Yeung AR, Deshmukh S, Klopp AH, et al. Intensity-modulated radiation therapy reduces patient-reported chronic toxicity compared with conventional pelvic radiation therapy: updated results of a phase III trial. J Clin Oncol Off J Am Soc Clin Oncol 2022;40(27):3115–9.

35. Grau C, Defourny N, Malicki J, et al. Radiotherapy equipment and departments in the European countries: final results from the ESTRO-HERO survey. Radiother Oncol 2014;112(2):155–64.

36. INTERNATIONAL ATOMIC ENERGY AGENCY, Setting Up a Radiotherapy Programme, Non-serial Publications , IAEA, Vienna. 2008. Available at: https://www.iaea.org/publications/7694/setting-up-a-radiotherapy-programme.

37. i.treatsafely – about us. Available at: https://i.treatsafely.org/about. Accessed February 18, 2023.

38. Efstathiou JA, Bvochora-Nsingo M, Gierga DP, et al. Addressing the growing cancer burden in the wake of the AIDS epidemic in Botswana: The BOTSOGO collaborative partnership. Int J Radiat Oncol Biol Phys 2014;89(3):468–75.

39. Laskar SG, Sinha S, Krishnatry R, et al. Access to radiation therapy: from local to global and equality to equity. JCO Glob Oncol 2022;(8):e2100358. https://doi.org/10.1200/GO.21.00358.

40. Royce TJ, Gupta GP, Chera BS. Increasing nonresearch-related industry funding in radiation oncology: cause for concern? Int J Radiat Oncol Biol Phys 2021;109(1):26–8.

41. Tringale KR, Hattangadi-Gluth JA. Are we for sale? Awareness of industry-related financial conflicts of interest in radiation oncology. Int J Radiat Oncol Biol Phys 2017;99(2):255–8.

42. Nwogu CE, Mahoney M, Okoye I, et al. Role of private enterprise in cancer control in low to middle income countries. J Cancer Epidemiol 2016;2016:7121527.

43. Hellowell M. Are public–private partnerships the future of healthcare delivery in sub-Saharan Africa? Lessons from Lesotho. BMJ Glob Health 2019;4(2):e001217.

44. Anakwenze Akinfenwa CP, Ibraheem A, Nwankwo K, et al. Emerging use of public-private partnerships in public radiotherapy facilities in Nigeria. JCO Glob Oncol 2021;7:1260–9.

45. Efstathiou JA, Heunis M, Karumekayi T, et al. Establishing and delivering quality radiation therapy in resource-constrained settings: the story of Botswana. J Clin Oncol 2016;34(1):27–35.

46. Howard SC, Zaidi A, Cao X, et al. The My Child Matters programme: effect of public-private partnerships on paediatric cancer care in low-income and middle-income countries. Lancet Oncol 2018;19(5):e252–66.

47. Krishnamurthy R, Mummudi N, Goda JS, et al. Using artificial intelligence for optimization of the processes and resource utilization in radiotherapy. JCO Glob Oncol 2022;8:e2100393.

48. LAURA ROBOT. Laura. Available at: https://laura-br.com/quem-somos/. Accessed February 18, 2023.

49. Hassan N, Slight R, Weiand D, et al. Preventing sepsis; how can artificial intelligence inform the clinical decision-making process? A systematic review. Int J Med Inf 2021;150:104457.

50. Pace E, Caruana CJ, Bosmans H, et al. CTContour: an open-source Python pipeline for automatic contouring and calculation of mean SSDE along the abdomino-pelvic region for CT images; validation on fifteen systems. Phys Medica PM Int J Devoted Appl Phys Med Biol 2022;103:190–8.

More Drugs Versus More Data: The Tug of War on Cancer in Low- and Middle-Income Countries

Mary Chamberlin, MD[a], Christopher Booth, MD[b],
Gabriel A. Brooks, MD[a], Achille Manirakiza, MD[c],
Fidel Rubagumya, MD[d], Verna Vanderpuye, MD[e],*

KEYWORDS

• Essential medicines • Clinical trials • LMICs • Prediction tools

KEY POINTS

- The New Public Health Order if applied to cancer will address key policies to advance the agenda for cancer control in Africa.
- There is an urgent need for global and country-level policy action to ensure patients with cancer globally have affordable access to high-priority medicines.
- There is a funding and publication bias against randomized clinical trials led by the investigators from LMICs. Building capacity and capability for randomized critical trials in variable resource settings is essential to determine the true risk versus benefit ratio for cancer treatments.
- Health services research is needed to understand the delivery of care and outcomes in these health systems.

INTRODUCTION

In June 2016, the chief executive office of a large pharmaceutical company stated "Giving out free cancer drugs will not help the poorest parts of Africa".[1] The investigator advocated that training more oncologists should be the focus, and the critics assessed that this stance was perpetuating the fallacy that cancer cannot be treated in Africa.[2] We would argue that all of the above are important but data are critical to best allocate the most essential medicines that make the biggest difference to those who will benefit the most.

[a] Dartmouth Cancer Center, 1 Medical Center Drive, Lebanon, NH 03765, USA; [b] Queen's University, Kingston, Canada; [c] Oncology Unit, Department of Medicine, King Faisal Hospital, Rwanda; [d] Department of Oncology, Rwanda Military Hospital, Kigali, Rwanda; [e] National Center for Radiotherapy, Oncology and Nuclear Medicine, Korlebu Teaching Hospital, PO Box KB 369, Accra
* Corresponding author.
E-mail address: vanaglat@yahoo.com

Hematol Oncol Clin N Am 38 (2024) 229–238
https://doi.org/10.1016/j.hoc.2023.06.010
0889-8588/24/© 2023 Elsevier Inc. All rights reserved.

BACKGROUND

Developing countries currently bear over 60% of the global cancer burden[3] and account for 70% of cancer deaths[4] with an estimated one million deaths per year predicted in Africa by 2030.[5] On September 29, 2022, the African Union Commission announced the New Public Health Order, calling on gov8ernments, multilateral organizations, philanthropic groups, the private sector, and civil society to support its full implementation. The Order includes elements essential for cancer control such as better access to vaccines, diagnostics and therapeutics, and an improved health workforce.[5] More than 800,000 new cases of cancer among 1.1 billion people were recorded in sub-Saharan African in 2020, according to data form the Global Cancer Observatory.[6] The New Public Health Order if applied to cancer would address the issues of workforce, infrastructure, and strong meaningful partnerships that are needed to advance the agenda for cancer control in Africa[3] with a set of innovative solutions regarding its funding and implementation.[5]

The narrative is not different for cancer control in Latin America and Caribbean recording an estimated 700,000 cancer deaths in 2020 and fraught with similar challenges. Latin America for many years has led the way to developing pragmatic and innovative strategies to overcoming the burden of high cost of cancer medicines; however, recent shortages of cancer drugs in Latin America fueled by inflationary prices as high as 54% in 2022 in countries such as Argentina are likely to compromise efforts at improving cancer outcomes control.

Drugmakers' attitudes toward helping Africa have changed since the late 1990s when Western companies were pilloried for refusing to lower prices on their acquired immune deficiency syndrome (AIDS) drugs as millions died. Now, nearly all companies offer a combination of donations and "tiered pricing" under which they charge poor countries a small fraction of what they charge rich ones, with safeguards to prevent smuggling of their products into wealthy markets.[4,7,8]

Companies compete to rise higher on the Access to Medicines Index which ranks them on how well they do at getting their products to the world's poor.[4]

In 2017, there was enthusiasm following the African Organization of Research and Training in Cancer annual meeting in Kigali, Rwanda, regarding a new program that was announced at the meeting and published shortly before in the New York Times[9]:

"In a deal similar to the one that turned the tide against AIDS, manufacturers and charities will make chemotherapy drugs available in six poor countries at steep discounts."[9]

Two major pharmaceutical companies working with the American Cancer Society were pledging steep discounts in the prices of cancer medicines in Africa. The recommended medicines for cancer are derived from the World Health Organization (WHO) essential medicine drug list. The WHO report indicates that only 32.0% to 57.7% of essential cancer medicines listed were available in resource constrained regions, additionally majority required full out-of-pocket payments.[1] Pfizer, based in New York and Cipla, based in Mumbai promised to charge rock bottom prices for 16 most commonly used chemotherapy drugs. The complicated deal was struck between the American Cancer Society, Clinton Health Access Initiative (CHAI), IBM, the US National Comprehensive Cancer Network, and the African Cancer Coalition (ACC), a network of 32 oncologists in 11 African countries. The ACC later evolved into an organization called Chemotherapy Access Partnership largely organized by African nations and then transformed again into Cancer Access Partnership in 2020 to increase the availability of high-quality affordable cancer medications, with participating companies Biocon biologics, Novartis, Pfizer, and Viatris. In 2021, Pfizer released an announcement to the press announcing a partnership with IDA Foundation, an independent social enterprise providing essential medicines to low- and middle-income countries including almost 70 developing countries across Latin America, Asia, Africa, and the Western Pacific region. This was announced as an agreement to build on the long-standing collaboration between Pfizer the American Cancer Society and CHAI that has provided access to oncology treatments in 11 sub-Saharan African countries to save an average of 56% on the cost of the medicines.[10] Complete chemotherapy protocols for breast, cervical, and prostate cancers, which make up most of the cancer burden on the continent, will be covered as well as drugs to cover 24 other cancer types under this agreement. Although these efforts are laudable, there are problems with this "drug first" approach without better understanding current models of care delivery, health system financing, workforce capacity, and patient needs.

Randomized clinical trials (RCTs) are largely considered the gold standard for determining effective treatment of cancer; however, recent work has identified some worrisome trends. Oncology trials are now predominantly funded by the pharmaceutical industry. Industry-funded trials are larger, more likely to be positive, predominantly test systemic therapies in the palliative setting and are published in higher impact journals than trials without industry support.[11] They are also almost always conducted in high-resource settings making their applicability to LMICs marginal at best due to competing comorbidities and vastly different disease patterns, biodiversity, and life expectancy.[12] RCTs from LMICs are more likely to identify effective therapies and have a larger effect size than RCTs from HICs.[10] The investigators have concluded that there is a funding and publication bias against RCTs led by investigators from LMICs. Policy makers, research funders, and journals need to address this issue with a range of measures including building capacity and capability in RCTs in variable resource settings to determine the true risk versus benefit ratio for cancer treatments.[12] An example of a high-impact clinical trial conducted in LMIC was the application of visual inspection of acetic acid and visual inspection of lugol's iodine for cervical cancer screening, a highly cost-effective method for low-resource regions without the capabilities for cytology-based papanicolaou testing, which is considered heavily resource-dependent.[2] There is a presumption that LMICs are incapable of hosting clinical trials; however, with increase in infrastructure, knowledge exchange, mentorship, international collaboration, and expanded use of information technology, there should be increased commitment to promote clinical investigations in LMIC.

Review of the Literature

As most oncologists are well aware, patients enrolled in clinical trials do not reflect "real-world" practice. This is even more so in LMICs and results cannot be ethically extrapolated to apply to globally diverse populations. For example, a prospective longitudinal study on patients with cancer in Southeast Asia determined the impact of a cancer diagnosis in Southeast Asia is potentially disastrous, with over 75% of patients experiencing death or financial catastrophe within 1 year.[13] These impacts are compounded by low socioeconomic status as participants in the low-income category within each country had significantly higher odds of financial catastrophe (odds ratio, 5.86; 95% confidence interval, 4.76–7.23) and death (5.52; 4.34–7.02) than participants with high income. Those without insurance were also more likely to experience financial catastrophe (1.27; 1.05–1.52) and die (1.51; 1.21–1.88) than participants with insurance. This study adds compelling evidence to the argument for policies that improve access to care and provide adequate financial protection from the costs of illness[13] but also points to the critical need for data-driven prediction tools for short-term mortality and side effects from treatment to spare these patients and families from potential catastrophic impacts of treatment. Drug regulation agencies and stakeholders including governments must be empowered with policies and incentives to halt the influx of substandard medicines so as to rebuild confidence in the pharmaceutical markets.[5]

This is not to say that access to appropriate medicine is not a priority. RCTs in HICs are clearly pointing to chemotherapy-sparing regimens with equal or better efficacy and less toxicity especially in the era of monoclonal antibodies, targeted therapies, and immunotherapies. However, these are the least likely drugs to be available in LMICs as a result of the associated high cost and need for expertise required to safely administer these drugs.

The WHO Essential Medicines List (EML) identifies priority medicines that are most important to public health. Over time, the EML has included an increasing number of cancer medicines.[14] Using an international cross-sectional survey, the investigators researching the use of cancer medicines determined that the most commonly selected medicines to make high priority were doxorubicin (by 499 [53%] of 948 respondents), cisplatin (by 470 [50%]), paclitaxel (by 423 [45%]), pembrolizumab (by 414 [44%]), trastuzumab (by 402 [42%]), carboplatin (by 390 [41%]), and 5-fluorouracil (by 386 [41%]). Of the 20 most frequently selected high-priority cancer medicines, 19 (95%) are currently on the WHO EML; 12 (60%) were cytotoxic agents, and 13 (65%) were granted US Food and Drug Administration regulatory approval before 2000. The proportion of respondents indicating universal availability of each top 20 medication was 9% to 54% in low-income and lower middle-income countries, 13% to 90% in upper middle-income countries, and 68% to 94% in high-income countries. The risk of catastrophic expenditure (spending >40% of total consumption net of spending on food) was more common in low-income and lower middle-income countries, with 13% to 68% of respondents indicating a substantial risk of catastrophic expenditures for each of the top 20 medications in lower middle-income countries versus 2% to 41% of respondents in upper middle-income countries and 0% to 9% in high-income countries. The investigators concluded that these data demonstrate major barriers in access to core cancer medicines worldwide. These findings challenge the feasibility of adding additional expensive cancer medicines to the EML. There is an urgent need for global and country-level policy action to ensure patients with cancer globally have access to high-priority medicines.[14] This difference in access to cancer care accounts for the variation in cancer mortality rates among LMIC even within the same continent. For example, 3-year crude breast cancer mortality is 45% in Zambia versus 36% in Nigeria, with increased access to early breast cancer diagnosis and treatments, one-third of these deaths could be averted[6] been articulated this way. At its core, the art of oncology involves guiding patients through complex treatment decisions to ensure that the care they receive aligns with their values and preferences. Although oncologists routinely discuss how treatments may (or may not) help patients live longer and how side effects may affect quality of life (QOL), we have not done a good job of helping patients understand the time required for cancer care and the inevitable trade-offs. With proper training, clinicians can do a better job of acknowledging this issue in care delivery, and the research community needs to generate data to guide these important discussions. Finally, although current value frameworks and economic models have allowed us to better quantify the net benefit associated with cancer therapy, holistic cancer care must consider patient time, which, for many, is the most important variable of all.[15] Trials completed in HICs cannot address the context, values, and health care delivery systems of low to middle income countries (LMICs). For example, in

Africa, fertility preservation is a cultural demand for women of childbearing age; therefore, cancer treatments that require ovarian suppression or hysterectomy are considered unacceptable resulting in high default rates. The way forward can follow the path started in high income countries (HICs) where biomarkers and predictive models have become a standard tool to assist with shared decision-making regarding the pros and cons of different systemic regimens for advanced cancer. Implementation science approaches can provide this context and lead to better models for LMICs.

Biomarker and Predictive Models in HICs

The role of chemotherapy in the curative treatment of breast cancer, for example, has been declining due to molecular tests validated to identify early-stage cancers that benefit most from chemotherapy versus those that do not. As such, the use of chemotherapy in early-stage breast cancer has been rapidly declining in high-income countries due to the predictive value of molecular sequencing that was validated in the prospective setting to show the mortality benefit of systemic chemotherapy was much smaller than that of hormone-based therapy in many cases of Estrogen receptor-positive breast cancer. It has become clear that the biology of the cancer was critically important in determining the benefit from chemotherapy, and without that information, nearly 20% to 30% of women with breast cancer are likely being overtreated at a high cost to society. With breast cancer being one of the most commonly treated cancers in LMICs, it is critically important to know which ones will benefit from chemotherapy and which ones are being treated with largely ineffective treatment with a high cost in quality of life. A study from 2014 reports a 14.5% difference in survival rates for patients with breast cancer living in Denmark compared with Lithuania (high income versus upper middle income).[16]

If one steps further back to include all cancers, of 277 cancer drug therapies for which clinical trials were published in 2011 to 2015, only 15% identified treatments that led to meaningful improvements in patient survival or quality of life.[12] In Asia, the proportion of patients who died in 1 year after being diagnosed with solid tumors such as breast or colorectal cancer, ranged from 12% in Malaysia to 45% in Myanmar according to a report published in 2012.

In the United States, 90% of women with breast cancer survive 5 years, in Uganda only 46% do, and in Gambia only 12%. The causes of this discrepancy is multifactorial, including access to care, sociocultural practices, low literacy and cannot be blamed solely on strength of the health system strengths.[17] If survival is that poor, the likelihood that systemic therapy is going to impact this is highly unlikely unless the confounding barriers to early health-seeking behaviors such as long distance to health care facilities, prolific use of complementary, and traditional medicines, financial toxicity, health illiteracy, and fractured health systems are addressed. In addition, the toxicity to the patient with very advanced disease in terms of time away from work and family, cost of transportation, lodging and food to receive treatment, and not to mention potential for serious side effects from the treatment mean that the benefit versus risk is considerably small.

Research priorities led by LMICs should focus on strategies for earlier diagnosis of cancer such as training of primary care workers and decentralizing aspects of early detection and diagnosis, artificial intelligence-assisted clinical breast and gynecological examination, self/health worker administered instant fecal occult blood test, be focused on cost-effective[4] predictive markers for response to therapy and mortality to individually estimate life expectancy, and a realistic discussion regarding expectations and reality of treatment effects.

The International Prognostic Index for hematologic malignancies and subsequent revisions is an example of a clinical biomarker rating scale that is well-validated and used for treatment stratification assigning one point each for age greater than 60, elevated lactate dehydrogenase (LDH), poor performance status, Stages III–IV, and one or more extra nodal sites for non-Hodgkin's lymphoma.[14]

Others have been developed for metastatic renal cell[18] and for toxicity in the elderly[19,20] but often require molecular testing and other data that are not readily available in low- or middle-income country health care facilities. For patients with advanced disease, basic laboratories and vital signs at the start of chemotherapy may be able to predict short-term mortality and less benefit from chemotherapy in resource-constrained settings. Two simple risk stratification models validated in HIC populations[21] to identify patients at risk for hospitalization during chemotherapy are an excellent example of how data can be used to risk stratify patients with cancer before treatment and similar models for toxicity and short-term mortality are needed in LMIC settings to clarify who will benefit most from chemotherapy. An example of data-driven prediction models is in the geriatric oncology literature where a risk stratification schema can establish the risk of chemotherapy toxicity in older adults.[22] Geriatric assessment variables have repeatedly been shown to independently predict the risk of toxicity.

In LMICs, the same geriatric principles could be used with the concept of vulnerability with the development of a vulnerable patient assessment (VPA). Chronological age alone cannot adequately predict the relative benefits of treatment. Vulnerability is common in patients with cancer everywhere but especially in LMICs where better assessments are critical. Social retributions may manifest in myriad ways such as increased domestic abuse, social isolation, and financial distress due to the loss of income that impacts access to cancer care facilities and these are topics not routinely captured in surveys developed in HICs.[23] It is imperative therefore that cancer research conducted in LMIC must be coled by local experts to assess pertinent contextual components of the social structure that hinder uptake of evidence-based recommendations. By 2030, it is expected that nearly 22 million people will be affected by cancer worldwide and the economic impact is estimated at nearly $460 billion US dollars, with worse impact in LMICs. Unfortunately, there are huge differences in mortality and morbidity depending on where someone lives and therefore differences in the benefit from treatment. The nuances of this discrepancy should be realistically integrated into global health frameworks for improving cancer outcomes in LMIC.

DISCUSSION

As the number of people diagnosed with cancer in LMICs increases, interventions such as surgery, radiation, targeted therapies, and chemotherapy will likely become increasingly available but the infrastructure varies widely sometimes even on a monthly basis. As a result, drug shortages, delays in treatment, and suboptimal optimal care delivery are a frequent occurrence. This means that the relative benefits of cancer treatments drawn from RCTs conducted in high-income settings likely do not apply in weaker health systems. Comorbidities from noncommunicable diseases are increasingly impacting people at younger ages and life expectancy is shorter. For example, it is often reported in the literature that breast cancer is more deadly in LMICs due to younger age at diagnosis and more aggressive biology compared with HICs but this must be put in the context of comparing to countries with screening mammogram programs which drives the age at diagnosis and the percentage of breast cancers with less aggressive biological phenotypes. This emphasizing the need for accurate cancer data in LMICs lest it continue to perpetuate the fallacy that it is impossible to treat cancer in LMICs. Furthermore, because LMICs are underrepresented in international clinical trials, the treatment algorithms may not be applicable either. As a result, shared decision-making approaches to cancer care management are not straight forward and must be applied in context. It could be a disregard for a patient and family financial and social circumstances especially in the absence of public or private health insurance when management decisions are discussed and often skewed to the treating physician's preferences. Multiple externally validated prognostic models estimating remaining life expectancy have been published and are widely used in high-income settings but are not applicable to other settings where they are most needed.[24,25] More research is needed to interject country-specific social determinants and demographic data in estimating the cost-effectiveness and disability/quality-adjusted life year measurements for cancer interventions in resource-constrained regions.

Life expectancy at 5 and 10 years is particularly relevant in the curative or adjuvant setting where competing risks of mortality from other causes such as human immunodeficiency virus (HIV), heart disease, diabetes, or malnutrition are common. At the same time, there is tremendous heterogeneity in health care delivery and resources. For example, a 55-year-old woman in a high-income country would have a life expectancy of 30+ years versus 10 year for a 55-year-old woman in a LMIC based on current data. Without reliable life expectancy estimates in LMICs, there is a serious risk of over- or undertreatment of people with cancer.[20,22,26–32] Treatment decisions for vulnerable patients with cancer is difficult for all involved and risks need to be carefully weighed against benefits within the context of the individual patient, each with their own priorities, goals, resources, and vulnerabilities.

De-intensified treatment options for early-stage hormone-positive breast cancer may include a lumpectomy plus endocrine therapy rather than additional radiotherapy if overall survival is likely to be the same.[33] This has clearly been proven in the population of women who are 65 years and older in high-income settings due to competing comorbidities, without the burden of travel for a vulnerable patient who lives far from the radiotherapy center which is often the case. Implementation of this guideline may be hampered by a lack of data to determine if the age cutoff may be different in LMICs or compliance issues with oral chemotherapy intake.[8,9]

Data from geriatric oncology literature support the development of the concept of the VPA to achieve a higher rate of treatment completion and less toxicity with similar oncology outcomes in the control arm. Other studies have shown higher rates of upfront dose reductions with better treatment tolerance and better outcomes.[17,34]

A VPA could assist in allocating treatments optimally to tailor care and prevent both over- and undertreatment while maintaining similar overall survival by incorporating non-oncologic interventions to address comorbidities, medication optimization, nutrition, and psychosocial issues. With the growing population of patients with geriatric cancer in LMICs and the paucity of geriatric clinicians,[10] the role of multidisciplinary care is key to improving outcomes and an impetus to generate data to support resource appropriate treatment choices for this group of patients.

SUMMARY

As LMICs improve their cancer management, infrastructure pharmaceutical companies are expanding the distribution of chemotherapy that will improve access to essential medicines. Data to better define those who benefit given the complexity and variability of resources in individual countries and communities are critically needed. Training programs for medical oncologists in LMICs are expanding and need to train oncologists to be skilled in data collection and analysis, research, international collaborations, and leading careful shared decision-making conversations.

CLINICS CARE POINTS

- Cancer treatments are increasingly available but must be put in the context of the patients' values, social structure, risk of financial and social toxicity, and overall life expectancy.
- A global data base of cancer treatment-related data will help create a universally applicable prediction tool for use to define risks and benefits of cancer treatments on an individualized level.

DISCLOSURE

The authors have nothing to disclose.

REFERENCES

1. "There's no point giving free cancer drugs to Africa" - BBC News. Available at: https://www.bbc.com/news/health-36482367. Accessed May 26, 2023.
2. Lifesaving treatment for cancer: a necessity from Australia to Zambia | HuffPost Contributor. Available at: https://www.huffpost.com/entry/lifesaving-treatment-for-cancer-a-necessity-from-australia_b_57619fc8e4b02081542fa3ab. Accessed May 26, 2023.
3. Makoni M. Hope for africa's new public health order to fight cancer. Lancet Oncol 2022;23(11):1362.
4. As Cancer Tears Through Africa, Drug Makers Draw Up a Battle Plan - The New York Times. Available at: https://www.nytimes.com/2017/10/07/health/africa-cancer-drugs.html. Accessed May 26, 2023.
5. The Lancet Oncology. Strengthening cancer control in Africa gathers momentum. Lancet Oncol 2022;23(11):1343.
6. Bray F, Parkin DM, Gnangnon F, et al. Cancer in sub-Saharan Africa in 2020: a review of current estimates of the national burden, data gaps, and future needs. Lancet Oncol 2022;23(6):719–28.
7. 2016 Access to Medicines Index published | SpringerLink. Available at: https://link.springer.com/article/10.1007/s40274-016-3522-2. Accessed May 26, 2023.
8. Hogerzeil H, Bleimund E, Gitahl G, et al. Available at: https://accesstomedicine foundation.org/medialibrary/2022-access-to-medicine-index-1668514375.pdf.
9. Haskell DG. Opinion | The Seasons Aren't What They Used to Be. *The New York Times*. Available at: https://www.nytimes.com/2017/03/17/opinion/sunday/the-seasons-arent-what-they-used-to-be.html. Published March 17, 2017. Accessed May 26, 2023.
10. "Skyrocketing" Launch Prices for New Cancer Drug Need Reform. Available at: https://www.medscape.com/viewarticle/983765. Accessed May 26, 2023.
11. Fundytus A, Wells JC, Sharma S, et al. Industry funding of oncology randomised controlled trials: implications for design, results and interpretation. Clin Oncol 2022;34(1):28–35.
12. Wells JC, Sharma S, Del Paggio JC, et al. An analysis of contemporary oncology randomized clinical trials from low/middle-income vs high-income countries. JAMA Oncol 2021;7(3):379.

13. The ACTION Study Group. Catastrophic health expenditure and 12-month mortality associated with cancer in Southeast Asia: results from a longitudinal study in eight countries. BMC Med 2015;13(1):190.

14. Fundytus A, Sengar M, Lombe D, et al. Access to cancer medicines deemed essential by oncologists in 82 countries: an international, cross-sectional survey. Lancet Oncol 2021;22(10):1367–77.

15. Fundytus A, Prasad V, Booth CM. Has the current oncology value paradigm forgotten patients' time?: too little of a good thing. JAMA Oncol 2021;7(12):1757.

16. Sullivan R, Pramesh CS, Booth CM. Cancer patients need better care, not just more technology. Nature 2017;549(7672):325–8.

17. Hamaker ME, Te Molder M, Thielen N, et al. The effect of a geriatric evaluation on treatment decisions and outcome for older cancer patients – A systematic review. J Geriatr Oncol 2018;9(5):430–40.

18. Heng DY, Xie W, Regan MM, et al. External validation and comparison with other models of the International Metastatic Renal-Cell Carcinoma Database Consortium prognostic model: a population-based study. Lancet Oncol 2013;14(2): 141–8.

19. Owusu C, Cohen HJ, Feng T, et al. Anemia and functional disability in older adults with cancer. J Natl Compr Cancer Netw 2015;13(10):1233–9.

20. Hurria A, Cirrincione CT, Muss HB, et al. Implementing a geriatric assessment in cooperative group clinical cancer trials: CALGB 360401. J Clin Oncol 2011; 29(10):1290–6.

21. Brooks GA, Uno H, Aiello Bowles EJ, et al. Hospitalization risk during chemotherapy for advanced cancer: development and validation of risk stratification models using real-world data. JCO Clin Cancer Inform 2019;(3):1–10. https://doi.org/10.1200/CCI.18.00147.

22. Hurria A, Togawa K, Mohile SG, et al. Predicting chemotherapy toxicity in older adults with cancer: a prospective multicenter study. J Clin Oncol 2011;29(25): 3457–65.

23. Mohile SG, Epstein RM, Hurria A, et al. Communication with older patients with cancer using geriatric assessment: a cluster-randomized clinical trial from the national cancer institute community oncology research program. JAMA Oncol 2020; 6(2):196.

24. Lee SJ. Development and Validation of a Prognostic Index for 4-Year Mortality in Older Adults. JAMA 2006;295(7):801.

25. Schonberg MA, Davis RB, McCarthy EP, et al. External validation of an index to predict up to 9-year mortality of community-dwelling adults aged 65 and older: external validation of mortality index. J Am Geriatr Soc 2011;59(8):1444–51.

26. Walter LC. Development and validation of a prognostic index for 1-year mortality in older adults after hospitalization. JAMA 2001;285(23):2987.

27. Walter LC, Covinsky KE. Cancer screening in elderly patients: a framework for individualized decision making. JAMA 2001;285(21):2750.

28. DuMontier C, Loh KP, Bain PA, et al. Defining undertreatment and overtreatment in older adults with cancer: a scoping literature review. J Clin Oncol 2020;38(22): 2558–69.

29. Krishnan M, Temel J, Wright A, et al. Predicting life expectancy in patients with advanced incurable cancer: a review. J Support Oncol 2013;11(2):68–74.

30. Krishnan MS, Epstein-Peterson Z, Chen YH, et al. Predicting life expectancy in patients with metastatic cancer receiving palliative radiotherapy: the TEACHH model: life expectancy in metastatic cancer. Cancer 2014;120(1):134–41.

31. Hurria A. Embracing the complexity of comorbidity. J Clin Oncol 2011;29(32): 4217–8.
32. Extermann M, Boler I, Reich RR, et al. Predicting the risk of chemotherapy toxicity in older patients: the chemotherapy risk assessment scale for high-age patients (CRASH) score: CRASH score. Cancer 2012;118(13):3377–86.
33. Hoxha I, Islami DA, Uwizeye G, et al. Forty-five years of research and progress in breast cancer: progress for some, disparities for most. JCO Glob Oncol 2022;(8): e2100424. https://doi.org/10.1200/GO.21.00424.
34. Kalsi T, Babic-Illman G, Ross PJ, et al. The impact of comprehensive geriatric assessment interventions on tolerance to chemotherapy in older people. Br J Cancer 2015;112(9):1435–44.

Subspecialty Breast Imaging Education in Tanzania; Clinical, Infrastructure, and Logistical Paradigms for Best Practices in the Low- and Middle-Income Settings

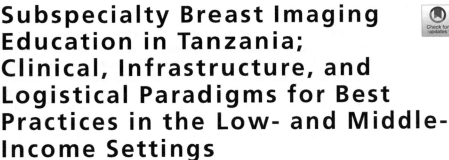

Toma S. Omofoye, MD[a], Anganile Kalinga, MD[b],
Ramapriya Ganti, MD, PhD[c], Frank J. Minja, MD[d],
Timothy B. Rooney, MD[e],*

KEYWORDS

- Breast imaging • Low and middle income countries • Breast imaging fellowship
- Breast ultrasound • Image-guided breast biopsy

KEY POINTS

- Subspecialty breast radiology training in the LMIC environment of sub-Saharan Africa (Tanzania) is presented as a paradigm for remote and in-person education.
- Tailoring BI-RADS in the resource-limited LMIC environment, emphasizing breast ultrasound for image-guided intervention and diagnosis.
- Presenting a scalable education program for adoption in the LMIC setting, with goals of improving interdisciplinary breast care through training, radiology/pathology correlation, and optimization of local resources.
- Providing bidirectional travel opportunities for global health care providers as an example of an alliance to care for underserved populations and acknowledging the global rise in breast malignancy.

[a] Department of Breast Imaging, The University of Texas MD Anderson Cancer Center, 1515 Holcombe Boulevard, Unit 1350, Houston, TX 77030, USA; [b] Department of Radiology and Medical Imaging, Muhimbili University of Health and Allied Sciences Main campus, United Nations Road, in Upanga West, Dar Es Salaam, Tanzania; [c] Department of Radiology and Medical Imaging, University of Virginia, 1215 Lee Street, Charlottesville, VA 22908, USA; [d] Department of Radiology and Imaging Sciences, Emory University School of Medicine, Atlanta, GA 30307, USA; [e] Department of Radiology and Medical Imaging, UVA Health, 1215 Lee Street, Charlottesville VA 22908, USA
* Corresponding author.
E-mail address: CWM4JW@UVAHealth.org

Hematol Oncol Clin N Am 38 (2024) 239–249
https://doi.org/10.1016/j.hoc.2023.05.016
hemonc.theclinics.com

INTRODUCTION

Only 18 of the 54 countries in Africa have well-established radiology residency training programs, and only five countries have documented radiology subspecialty training programs.[1] This severely limited access to formal diagnostic radiology and radiology subspecialty training programs is one of the key drivers for global radiology disparities. On average, there is less than one radiologist per million population in Africa.[2,3] With reports of the increasing incidence and mortality of breast cancer in Africa,[4] our subspecialty training paradigm directly addresses the need for a trained health care workforce to improve detection, diagnosis, and treatment of breast cancer in Africa, with a specific focus on Tanzania.

Breast cancer is the second leading cause of cancer mortality, after cervical cancer, among women in Tanzania based on the 2017 Tanzania Ministry of Health (MoH) commissioned report on breast cancer in the country.[5] The lifetime risk for developing breast cancer in Tanzania is approximately 1 in 20.[6] Approximately 80% of women diagnosed with breast cancer in Tanzania are diagnosed at advanced stages (III or IV), when treatment is less effective, and outcomes are poor.[5–9] Currently in Tanzania, in the absence of any screening program, breast disease is generally discovered as a palpable lesion by the patient and/or provider, and biopsy is accomplished surgically, without the benefit of image guidance. Recommendations from this assessment emphasized a resource-stratified, phased implementation approach to breast cancer detection, diagnosis, and treatment. Prerequisites to implementation included standardized guidelines, protocols, and a trained health care workforce. The phased recommendations start with the systematic triage and diagnosis of palpable breast disease (phase 1) and culminate in systematic upgrading of technology and training necessary for the management of nonpalpable breast disease using screening mammography (phase 4).[5] Our training paradigm directly addresses the need for a trained health care workforce, who will lead these phased implementation efforts.

We describe efforts to establish a 2-year Women's Imaging (WI) Fellowship program which includes breast and body imaging subspecialty training at Muhimbili University of Health and Allied Sciences and its main teaching hospital Muhimbili National Hospital (MUHAS/MNH) in Dar es Salaam, Tanzania. MUHAS/MNH is the main tertiary referral center in the country receiving patients from the entire nation. These training efforts are organized and supported by the Radiological Society of North America (RSNA) Global Learning Center (GLC) program in Tanzania. RSNA-GLC programs aim to create regional centers of excellence in radiology education around the world.[10] In 2020, MUHAS/MNH was selected as the second GLC site (2021–2024) after Stellenbosch University, Cape Town, South Africa. Recognizing the need for radiology subspecialty training, MUHAS/MNH chose to focus on establishing 2-year radiology subspecialty training programs to build on its well-established 3-year diagnostic radiology residency training program. Interventional radiology (IR), neuroradiology (NR), and WI were identified as high-priority subspecialty areas and addressed sequentially as opportunities for additional subspecialty training. Our WI Fellowship program is primarily hosted at the MUHAS/MNH complex, with an inaugural cohort of 3 Tanzanian fellows enrolled in 2022.

The few available radiology subspecialty training opportunities in Africa consist of unstructured clinical apprenticeships or short-term observer-based models, with limited published details available.[1] To our knowledge, our WI fellowship program represents the first documented 2-year curriculum-based formal WI training program in Africa and has evolved alongside subspecialty training programs in IR and NR at MUHAS in Dar es Salaam, Tanzania.

EDUCATIONAL PARADIGM
Background and Perceived Need

Tanzania, a member of the East African community (EAC), with a population of approximately 61 million, contains a tiered national medical system encompassing increasing levels of care, culminating in the MNH complex, in Dar Es Salaam, providing the highest specialization/tertiary care.

In Tanzania, medical education is structured differently from what it is in the United States. The Doctor of Medicine (MD) degree is a 5-year program and directly follows secondary school.[11,12] Subsequent provider specialization is available as a 3-year degree program, known as a masters in medicine (MMed), which qualifies the graduate to practice in a specific specialty, that is, diagnostic radiology. An additional 2-year degree for subspecialty training is currently available for the radiologist in IR, NR, and now in WI, as a masters in Science (MSc).

Specialty care in diagnostic radiology is relatively new, with the first trained radiologists in Tanzania receiving training in Kenya, Uganda, and Cuba, beginning in approximately the 1990s. MUHAS started a 3-year diagnostic radiology residency training program in 2005 and only embarked on the 2-year radiology subspecialty training programs in IR in 2019 and NR in 2021.

Diagnostic radiology training has grown to 2 sites in the country, with the largest training site at MNH/MUHAS in Dar Es Salaam, currently including 68 residents, 18 fellows, and 18 faculty/staff radiologists. Most radiologists are now trained in Tanzania, rather than at sites in India or China. As radiology is a relatively new specialty in Tanzania, as recently as 5 to 10 years ago, many radiologists were trained in other countries. As the number of trained radiologists has increased, and equipment has improved, almost all radiologists are now able to complete their training in Tanzania. The MNH diagnostic radiology program is currently the largest radiologist training cohort in the EAC. While the number of radiologists per capita remains small (approximately 1 radiologist per million people),[3] a need for subspecialty image-based diagnosis and intervention has been emphasized. Examples include the need for temporizing care for advanced cervical cancer patients by IR and the need for image-guided breast biopsy to guide breast cancer therapy, among many other gaps in medical care for benign and malignant disease.

Secondary to this perceived need, and over the last approximately 7 years, intermittent teaching efforts have coalesced into formal curriculum-driven degree courses. The MSc in IR has now graduated 10 fellows, who are practicing in Tanzania (8), Rwanda (1), and Nigeria (1). The NR MSc program graduated two inaugural fellows in 2022, one of whom has joined MUHAS as faculty; and an additional four NR fellows are currently enrolled. With the success of subspecialty radiology care in NR and IR, leaders at MNH/MUHAS turned attention to the state of breast health in the country.

Tanzania, like many developed and low- to middle-income country (LMIC) environments around the globe, experiences significant morbidity secondary to breast malignancy. In Tanzania, the 5-year survival rate of breast cancer patients is 45%, compared to 90% in the United States.[6,13] These mortality statistics in Tanzania are representative of those seen in similar LMIC settings. Tanzania suffers from high mortality rates as the disease is often discovered in a more advanced/symptomatic phase; 78% of cases in Tanzania are diagnosed at stages III-IV, compared to 35% in the United States.[13] In Tanzania, once diagnosed, the management of breast cancer is largely limited to mastectomy and axillary dissection.[7-9] Receptor status until recently has been unavailable, and chemotherapy regimens are therefore nontargeted and limited.

CURRICULUM

The 2-year WI fellowship includes both breast and body imaging training. We will only discuss the breast imaging portion of the WI fellowship.

The overarching design of the curriculum is to address the challenges of this population while optimizing and leveraging the available resources currently available in Tanzania. Specifically, in the LMIC environment, ultrasound equipment, training, and expertise are relatively advanced in comparison to the more-resource-heavy modalities of mammography and magnetic resonance imaging (MRI). In addition, the historical purview of the radiologist in Tanzania is in imaging-based diagnosis, rather than in image-guided intervention.[14]

Adhering to the principles of postgraduate medical education design, the creation of customized WI curriculum addressed the recommended components by experts: goals and objectives, content, learners, faculty, resources and methods, assessment and evaluation, governance, and continuous improvement.[15,16]

Goals and Objectives

The stakeholders (MNH/MUHAS hospital leadership, practicing radiologists and leaders in the department of radiology, interested trainees, and prospective faculty) engaged the government in the creation of the MSc course. The necessary regulatory guidelines were identified and met to ensure incorporation of the program (and eventually, acceptance of certification) into the national training model.

Content

Using the American College of Radiology (ACR)/Society of Breast Imaging breast imaging fellowship training recommendations as a guide,[17] we collaboratively developed a comprehensive breast imaging curriculum for the WI fellowship aligned with phased implementation recommendations from the 2017 Tanzania Breast Health Care Assessment.[5] Our WI fellowship curriculum for breast imaging emphasizes the diagnosis and management of palpable breast disease using breast ultrasound during the first year; then the diagnosis and management of nonpalpable breast disease using mammography and breast MRI during the second year. The four-semester breast imaging curriculum includes the following courses: Introduction to Breast Imaging (semester 1), Breast Ultrasound (semester 2), Mammography (semester 3), and Breast MRI and Other Modalities (semester 4).

Learners

For the first training cohort, interested applicants were solicited and evaluated. Based on the program guidelines, admission policy had been drafted with selection criteria including the need for qualified applicants to have completed diagnostic radiology residency (MMed) training and demonstrate sustained interest in WI. Three promising applicants were selected for the first training cohort; two were practicing radiologists at MNH, and the third practiced at Ocean Road Cancer Institute (ORCI). All three had completed their diagnostic radiology residency (MMed) training at MUHAS within the preceding 5 years. The WI MSc program provides the fellows with protected time for didactic activities and case discussions, in addition to the fellows taking on increasing responsibility for challenging WI cases in their daily practices. Each of the fellows are supported financially by their respective employers MNH and OCRI, as employees in training.

Faculty

RSNA is the largest professional organization of radiologists worldwide with more than 50,000 members in 145 countries. Leveraging this large membership base, the

RSNA-GLC program solicited volunteer academic faculty for the WI fellowship. We sought academic faculty with experience in teaching and mentorship, a willingness to participate in virtual and in-person education, and a commitment to participate for the 2-year training timeline. Experience with global radiology was encouraged, but not mandatory. A total of five USA-based academic faculty were selected to participate in the breast imaging portion of the WI MSc program. An onboarding process was created whereby selected volunteer faculty met with the lead faculty to learn about their specific roles and goals of the training program.

RESOURCES AND METHODS

A mix of on-demand web-based and live virtual lectures (synchronous and asynchronous) methods are used.

Synchronous Teaching

Didactics are provided remotely and in person. A cadre of 5 U.S. academic radiologists schedule one- to two-week travel for in-person teaching/training at the fellows' institutions. These on-site interventions include case presentations, formal lectures in breast disease topics, image-guided biopsy workshops and consultation, radiology/pathology correlation, and multidisciplinary consultation with referring providers in Tanzania. While all five academic radiologists travel to teach in person, schedules and situations are variable, and each radiologist travels to teach on-site for 1 to 4 weeks during each academic year.

Remote teaching is accomplished by weekly virtual meetings which predominantly consist of case presentations by the fellows for the participating U.S. faculty member.

Asynchronous Teaching via Web-Based Lectures

Recognizing the advantages of remote teaching, we incorporated customized web-based learning materials into the course.[18] Remote lecture materials are provided as a recorded lecture series with pretests and posttests, and topics are assigned as appropriate for the curriculum. Future interventions include recurring multidisciplinary tumor conferences, using the U.S. paradigm as an example of best practice.

Observerships

The fellows will travel to the U.S. to participate in 2-month observer experiences at one of our academic centers. The fellows will participate in a research project, observe screening and diagnostic imaging and technologist and radiologist workflows, and observe multidisciplinary and radiology/pathology correlation conferences.

Assessment and Evaluation

Learning assessments

Trainees undergo two midterm examinations and a final examination each semester, consisting of written, practical, and oral evaluations. The faculty create a variety of learning assessments: multiple-choice image-rich exams and oral exams. The learning assessments follow recommendations for constructing high-quality questions.[19,20]

Research project

Each fellow will be expected to participate in design and implementation of a research project with mentorship by the US-based faculty.

Governance

The curriculum for the WI MSc program was vetted by MUHAS, then accredited by the Tanzania Commission of Universities over a 2-year period (2021–2022). The training program adheres to the MUHAS academic calendar, which consists of two semesters: October-February and March-August. Following the MUHAS academic calendar ensures structure and accountability for the training program.

Continuous Improvement

Faculty

The faculty provide continuous feedback on the program to stakeholders through routine meetings, after in-person trips, after assessments/semesters, and on an ad hoc basis. Feedback includes assessment of trainee progress, ongoing challenges, and by participating in virtual and in-person teaching assignments.

Trainees

The trainees, as adult learners, are encouraged to provide feedback to all stakeholders (faculty, MNH/MUHAS, and RSNA leadership). Their feedback is used to make improvements to the program.

Other stakeholders

The overseeing bodies National MoH and MNH/MUHAS, leaders of the successful NR and IR fellowship programs, provide suggestions to improve the training program.

BREAST IMAGING SERVICE

In addition to the curriculum-based didactics, the fellows will simultaneously begin a breast imaging service at two sites in Dar Es Salaam: at the MNH complex and at the ORCI.

The goals of breast imaging in the low-resource environment of LMICs are different from high-resource countries. Screening mammography is virtually nonexistent. In the United States, the current guidelines by the ACR/SBI are for asymptomatic women at average risk of breast cancer to receive screening starting at the age of 40 years.[21] Breast cancer mortality has decreased 40% since the 1990s due to screening mammography and early detection.[22] However, screening in the United States is achieved with yearly mammograms, which in LMIC is challenging for many reasons. These include markedly limited access to mammography, which is only available in urban areas with a high examination cost.[23] In addition, with few trained personnel for mammography installation, maintenance, and interpretation, widespread mammography use is not feasible for most of sub-Saharan Africa, particularly in a high-volume screening context. In addition, routine breast MRI is not currently feasible in most LMICs.

According to the WHO, the goal in low-resource settings is for earlier detection of breast cancer.[24,25] This occurs through community education of breast health, education of community health workers, and increasing capacity at national referral centers.[26]

Thus, in our program, we are developing breast imaging, focusing on earlier detection of breast cancer, while utilizing technologies currently locally available, such as high-frequency ultrasound and ultrasound-guided biopsy. Patients who are symptomatic, and who present to their primary care provider, are subsequently scheduled for diagnostic image-based evaluation beginning with breast ultrasound.[14] At the fellowship training sites (MNH/ORCI), the breast fellow trainees perform diagnostic ultrasound for the symptomatic patient. At each site, a 2D digital mammography full field digital mammography (FFDM) unit is available for diagnostic use and additional imaging/confirmation. However, secondary to challenges with mammography maintenance and quality, and little to no mammography technologist training, there are significant limitations to the use of this modality. Additional barriers include a lack of reading room lighting standards, poor reading monitor quality, and limited picture archiving and communication system (PACS) storage capability for large mammography files. Breast MRI, while the most sensitive examination, also has limited utility in this low-resource setting.

Ultrasound technology is generally available in low-resource settings. Hand-held ultrasound is widely used as point-of-care and for formal diagnosis and is used by physicians, allied health providers, and sonographers as an inexpensive, accurate, and efficient tool. In the LMIC breast imaging setting, ultrasound technology is comparable to more developed countries, and high-frequency linear probes are available and widely used. With the introduction of this curriculum, we are providing trainees with the breast-imaging-approved data-driven lexicon, Breast Imaging Reporting and Data System Atlas, 5th Edition (BI-RADS), to align their interpretation, assessment, and recommendations of abnormalities.[27] The trainees are required to obtain feedback on case interpretation and recommendations for management from our USA-based teaching faculty.

Image-guided biopsy intervention for breast lesions is a novel concept for Tanzanian radiologists, and few faculty or trainees have prior experience.[13] Therefore, patient data, consent, time-out procedures, interventional competence, and radiology/pathology concordance are all new concepts for the fellows. In-person visits by our faculty emphasize these skills in the context of a day-to-day workflow.

Reporting

To address uniformity and to standardize reporting in mammography, the BI-RADS was instituted by the ACR.[27] The lexicon of imaging features is one of the most important aspects of BI-RADS. While directly implementing BI-RADS in its current form in LMIC may be a challenge, modified versions can be made available to enable structured and uniform reporting.[28] Structured reporting is currently not available in Tanzania and will be one of the major areas of focus of this training program where templates will be provided and adapted to suit the needs and challenges of this area. Specific use of BI-RADS lexicon and image-guided recommendations are specific areas where the Tanzanian fellows can improve their reporting acumen and begin to train and assimilate both their radiologist colleagues and their referring providers.

Interprofessional Considerations

Breast cancer diagnosis and treatment involves a multidisciplinary team of professionals including those from primary care, radiology, pathology, breast surgery, medical oncology, radiation oncology, and often, plastic surgery. Typically, in high-resource contexts, the breast imager detects the lesion on imaging (mammogram, ultrasound, and/or MRI), samples the lesion using image guidance, and sends the tissue to the pathologist for diagnosis. After diagnosis, the patient is seen by medical or surgical oncology, to discuss further management. The current paradigm at MUHAS/MNH does not include this multidisciplinary team, and one of the major areas of work for the training program is to streamline this approach. This is most feasible if the radiologist is the central access point in the care of the patient until a cancer diagnosis has been established. This approach is also helpful since biopsies/tissue sampling can be performed under percutaneous image guidance without the need for more invasive procedures, thereby reducing morbidity compared with open surgical biopsy.

The expectation of the Tanzanian fellow is to image the patient, perform a percutaneous biopsy using the appropriate modality, send the tissue sample to pathology, follow up on the results of the biopsy, and notify the patient of the results. Following the diagnosis, the patient will be seen by medical or surgical oncology, facilitated by the radiologist. Subsequently, the case will be discussed at a multidisciplinary case conference to discuss optimal care for the patient. The goal of the training program, in addition to developing expertise in breast imaging and performing image-guided procedures, is to also develop a multidisciplinary breast cancer program that will continue to educate all members of the care team on the importance of earlier detection and multidisciplinary treatment to increase rates of breast conservation as well as improve survival.

INFRASTRUCTURE

As with most radiology-based training, specific technology/equipment is essential. Breast imaging is particularly technology-intensive, secondary to the large file sizes of mammography, specialized linear high-frequency ultrasound transducers, image-guided biopsy devices, quality control of mammography modalities, the complexity of the reading station/environment, PACS challenges, and multidisciplinary meetings, among other issues. We use as many locally available processes and equipment as possible, while continuing to emphasize quality and sustainable practices. Reports indicate that up to 80% of medical equipment in LMICs is donated, and up to 40% is nonfunctioning.[29] Biomedical engineers and medical physicists, necessary for optimization of quality, safety, and efficiency of breast imaging equipment, are rare in LMICs.[29] While the specifics of our acquisition of new and additional equipment are beyond this discussion, we continue to leverage expertise in medical physicists involved in global health and vendors established in sub-Saharan Africa. In addition, breast imaging training in the USA includes necessary quality metrics, audits, and inspections. We integrate this essential training into the curriculum with the goal of creating a sustainable cadre of imaging professionals in Tanzania. This approach necessitates inclusion of breast imaging technologists and physicists, as well as vendor maintenance contracts to emphasize continued quality. While early in the implementation phase currently, as radiologists begin to play a central role in the diagnosis and management of breast disease, we anticipate scaling up of quality image-based care, enabling training and technology advances as demand and sophistication increases.

FUTURE DIRECTIONS

Creating a sustainable breast imaging and intervention team in the LMIC setting will remain a significant challenge in the short and medium term. Fortunately, our current program benefits from a vibrant group of Tanzanian trainees, faculty, allied providers, and technologists who remain motivated allies in providing and improving the care of their patients. While our immediate goals to provide a breast service and trained subspecialists, the longer-term goals of interdisciplinary care teams are not yet realized. Constant improvement, novel uses of BI-RADS in the LMIC setting, and continued commitment to global health are mandatory if we are to continue this work and scale up throughout sub-Saharan Africa and beyond.

Because ultrasound remains widespread and inexpensive in most settings, it may be the most effective way to improve the currently poor morbidity and mortality statistics in LMICs. As we are training breast imaging professionals, next steps may include creating training opportunities for allied health providers/sonographers who can serve as an expanding referral base for this underserved patient population.

SUMMARY

Breast cancer is the most frequent cancer affecting women in sub-Saharan Africa. Similar to developed countries, the LMIC setting is experiencing increasing breast cancer incidence with attendant morbidity and mortality. Partnerships in research and education are needed to address this critical issue. Our model, in creating the first WI fellowship in Tanzania, is an opportunity for capacity building to address women's health goals in sub-Saharan Africa. To date, our trainee Tanzanian colleagues have performed very well, expanding their knowledge of breast imaging, documented in oral and written examinations, interdisciplinary tumor board presentations, and on-going research projects.

REFERENCES

1. Iyawe E, Idowu B, Radiology OOSJ of, 2021 undefined. Corrigendum. Radiology subspecialisation in Africa: A review of the current status. SA J Radiol 2022;1921–2009. https://doi.org/10.4102/sajr. Available at: http://www.scielo.org.za/scielo.php?script=sci_arttext&pid=S2078-67782021000100025. Accessed March 29, 2023.
2. Kawooya MG, Kisembo HN, Remedios D, et al. An Africa point of view on quality and safety in imaging. Insights Imaging 2022;13(1):1–10. https://doi.org/10.1186/S13244-022-01203-W/FIGURES/1.
3. Gaupp F, Solomon N, Rukundo I, ANJ of V and, 2019 undefined. Tanzania IR initiative: training the first generation of interventional radiologists. Elsevier. Available at: https://www.sciencedirect.com/science/article/pii/S1051044319306876. Accessed March 29, 2023.
4. Sung H, Ferlay J, Siegel RL, et al. Global Cancer Statistics 2020: GLOBOCAN Estimates of Incidence and Mortality Worldwide for 36 Cancers in 185 Countries. CA Cancer J Clin 2021;71(3):209–49.
5. TANZANIA BREAST HEALTH CARE ASSESSMENT 2017 An Assessment of Breast Cancer Early Detection, Diagnosis and Treatment in Tanzania.
6. Yang K, Msami K, Calixte R, et al. Educational Opportunities for Down-Staging Breast Cancer in Low-Income Countries: an Example from Tanzania. J Cancer Educ 2019;34(6):1225–30.
7. Oncology SMTL, Service review: improving breast cancer care in Tanzania. Lancet. Available at: https://www.thelancet.com/journals/lanonc/article/PIIS1470-2045(17)30160-2/fulltext. Accessed March 29, 2023.
8. Sood R, Masalu N, Connolly RM, et al. Invasive breast Cancer treatment in Tanzania: landscape assessment to prepare for implementation of standardized treatment guidelines. BMC Cancer 2021;21(1). https://doi.org/10.1186/S12885-021-08252-2.
9. Sakafu LL, Philipo GS, Malichewe CV, et al. Delayed diagnostic evaluation of symptomatic breast cancer in sub-Saharan Africa: A qualitative study of Tanzanian women. PLoS One 2022;17(10 October). https://doi.org/10.1371/JOURNAL.PONE.0275639.
10. Global Learning Centers | RSNA. Available at: https://www.rsna.org/education/global-learning-centers. Accessed March 30, 2023.
11. Rehani B, Brown I, Dandekar S, et al. Radiology education in Africa: analysis of results from 13 African countries. Elsevier; 2017 undefined. Available at: https://www.sciencedirect.com/science/article/pii/S1546144016307554. Accessed March 29, 2023.

12. Lugossy A-M. Tanzania country profile; 2020. - Google Scholar. Accessed March 29, 2023. Available at: https://scholar.google.com/scholar?hl=en&as_sdt=0%2C44&q=Lugossy+A-M.+Tanzania+country+profile%3B+2020.+&btnG=.
13. Breast Cancer Statistics | CDC. Accessed March 30, 2023. Available at: https://www.cdc.gov/cancer/breast/statistics/index.htm.
14. Okello R, Rooney T, Jumbe M, ... LSJ of B, 2020 undefined. Breast Imaging and Image-guided Intervention in Tanzania: Initial Experience. academic.oup.com. https://academic.oup.com/jbi/article-abstract/2/3/269/5820901. Accessed March 29, 2023.
15. Grant J. Principles of curriculum design. Understanding Medical Education: Evidence, Theory, and Practice 2018;71–88. https://doi.org/10.1002/9781119373780.CH5. Published online October 5.
16. Radiology JCA, 2000 undefined. Curriculum in radiology for residents: what, why, how, when, and where. Elsevier. https://www.sciencedirect.com/science/article/pii/S1076633200804584. Accessed March 29, 2023.
17. Katzen J, Grimm L, Imaging RBJ of B, 2021 undefined. The American College of Radiology/Society of Breast Imaging updated fellowship training curriculum for breast imaging. academic.oup.com Available at: https://academic.oup.com/jbi/article-abstract/3/4/498/6067554. Accessed March 29, 2023.
18. Omofoye T, Leong L, Kalambo M, et al. Responsive web-based breast imaging core curriculum for international radiology residents with self-assessment: a pilot study. Elsevier; 2022. https://www.sciencedirect.com/science/article/pii/S1076633221003123. Accessed March 29, 2023.
19. Catanzano T, Jordan S, of PLJ of the AC, 2022 undefined. Great question! The art and science of crafting high-quality multiple-choice questions. Elsevier. https://www.sciencedirect.com/science/article/pii/S1546144022001715. Accessed March 29, 2023.
20. Radiological JCR a review publication of the, 2006 undefined. Education techniques for lifelong learning: writing multiple-choice questions for continuing medical education activities and self-assessment modules. *europepmc.org*. https://europepmc.org/article/med/16549616. Accessed March 29, 2023.
21. Lee C, Dershaw D, Kopans D, PEJ of the A, 2010 undefined. Breast cancer screening with imaging: recommendations from the Society of Breast Imaging and the ACR on the use of mammography, breast MRI, breast. Elsevier. https://www.sciencedirect.com/science/article/pii/S1546144009004803. Accessed March 29, 2023.
22. Siegel R, Miller K, clinicians AJ. A cancer journal for, 2018 undefined. Cancer statistics 2018;68(1):7–30. Wiley Online Library.
23. Black E, Richmond R. Improving early detection of breast cancer in sub-Saharan Africa: Why mammography may not be the way forward. Global Health 2019;15(1). https://doi.org/10.1186/S12992-018-0446-6.
24. Organization WH. WHO report on cancer: setting priorities, investing wisely and providing care for all. Published online 2020. https://apps.who.int/iris/bitstream/handle/10665/330745/9789240001299-eng.pdf. Accessed March 29, 2023.
25. Newman L, & MPBP& RCO, 2022 undefined. Breast cancer screening in low and middle-income countries. Elsevier. Available at: https://www.sciencedirect.com/science/article/pii/S1521693422000578. Accessed March 29, 2023.
26. New global breast cancer initiative highlights renewed commitment to improve survival. https://www.who.int/news/item/08-03-2021-new-global-breast-cancer-initiative-highlights-renewed-commitment-to-improve-survival. Accessed March 29, 2023.

27. ACR BI-RADS® Atlas, Breast Imaging Reporting and - Google Scholar. https:// scholar.google.com/scholar?hl=en&as_sdt=0%2C44&q=ACR+BI-RADS%C2% AE+Atlas%2C+Breast+Imaging+Reporting+and+Data+System.+Reston% 2C+VA%2C+American+College+of+Radiology%3B+2013&btnG=. Accessed March 29, 2023.

28. Scheel J, Peacock S, Orem J, et al, 2016 undefined. Improving breast ultrasound interpretation in Uganda using a condensed breast imaging reporting and data system. Elsevier. https://www.sciencedirect.com/science/article/pii/S1076633216 300976. Accessed March 29, 2023.

29. Perry L, Malkin R. Effectiveness of medical equipment donations to improve health systems: How much medical equipment is broken in the developing world? Med Biol Eng Comput 2011;49(7):719–22.

Diagnostic Accuracy of Biomarkers and International Ovarian Tumor Analysis Simple Rules in Diagnosis of Ovarian Cancer

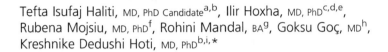

Tefta Isufaj Haliti, MD, PhD Candidate[a,b], Ilir Hoxha, MD, PhD[c,d,e],
Rubena Mojsiu, MD, PhD[f], Rohini Mandal, BA[g], Goksu Goç, MD[h],
Kreshnike Dedushi Hoti, MD, PhD[b,i],*

KEYWORDS

- Kosovo • Ovarian cancer • ROC analysis • Tumor biomarkers • IOTA Simple Rules

KEY POINTS

- This study investigates whether combining IOTA Simple Rules with tumor biomarkers would improve the diagnostic accuracy for the early detection of adnexal malignancies.
- We performed a ROC curve analysis of suspected adnexal tumors in 226 women admitted for surgery at the University Clinical Center of Kosovo.
- IOTA Simple Rules combined with biomarker indications increased the diagnostic accuracy of classifying adnexal masses.

INTRODUCTION

Ovarian cancer is the 8th most common cancer in women worldwide and is the second most common and fatal cancer in gynecology.[1] Malignancy rates of ovarian cancer continue to be high and late-stage diagnosis is the main factor in the mortality in this category of malignant gynecologic tumors.[2] Early detection of ovarian malignancy

[a] Clinic of Obstetrics and Gynecology, University Clinical Centre of Kosovo, Prishtina, Kosovo; [b] Faculty of Medicine, University of Hasan Prishtina, Prishtina, Kosovo; [c] The Dartmouth Institute for Health Policy and Clinical Practice, Geisel School of Medicine at Dartmouth, Lebanon, NH, USA; [d] Evidence Synthesis Group, Prishtina, Kosovo; [e] Research Unit, Heimerer College, Prishtina, Kosovo; [f] Obstetric Gynecologic University Hospital "Koco Gliozheni", Tirana, Albania; [g] Dartmouth College, Hanover, NH, USA; [h] Department of Obstetrics and Gynecology, American Hospital, Prishtina, Kosovo; [i] Clinic of Radiology, University Clinical Centre of Kosovo, Prishtina, Kosovo
* Corresponding author. Clinic of Radiology, University Clinical Centre of Kosovo, Prishtina, Kosovo.
E-mail address: kreshnike.dedushi@uni-pr.edu

Hematol Oncol Clin N Am 38 (2024) 251–265
https://doi.org/10.1016/j.hoc.2023.06.011

is challenging for the entire medical community due to the clinical variability and non-specific symptoms, even in the advanced stages of the disease.[3] Many studies have been focused on the development of more sensitive imaging and detection methods that could lead to the early detection of adnexal masses and improve the differentiation between benign and malignant ovarian tumors.[4–10] Serum biomarkers can be useful in the diagnosis of ovarian cancer together with clinical and ultrasonography examination.[10] Therefore the research for novel biomarkers and the application of ultrasound features, in particular, International Ovarian Tumor Analysis Simple Rules (IOTA SR) is of the utmost importance in the early detection of ovarian cancer.[6]

Ovarian cancer in low-to-middle-income countries (LMICs) is difficult to detect due to structural barriers (ie, lack of funding, lack of resources, capacity of staff) preventing this way effective diagnosis. Women often cannot access follow-up visits, and health systems lack the infrastructure to support several rounds of diagnostic testing.[11] Hence, the need for accurate diagnostic tests in these countries is particularly urgent. Kosovo, which only recently has moved from being an LMIC to upper-middle-income country, faces similar barriers.[12] In 2021, the incidence of ovarian cancer was 2.75%, and the incidence of fallopian tube and parametrium cancer was 0.06%.[13–15]

The most-used diagnostic tests for the detection of ovarian cancer in medical practice are tumor markers and imaging methods. However, none of them are reliable in their diagnostic accuracy. Therefore there is a need for a more dependable method or combination of methods that could lead to an early and timely diagnosis.[7] There is no specific biomarker to date for the early detection of ovarian cancer, but the most common serum marker for the differentiation of pelvic adnexal masses with prognostic value in clinical settings is cancer antigen 125 (CA125). However, CA125 is nonspecific for cancer as it can be elevated in other benign gynecologic conditions such as myomas, endometriomas, and menstrual cycle.[6] Some ovarian cancers in the early stages do not generate sufficient CA125, and CA125 used alone can have a worse performance than ultrasonography methods. Hence the need for a novel biomarkers or their use in combination with ultrasonography is vital for the detection of ovarian cancer.[6,8]

Ferritin is a cytosol protein that serves for the storage of intracellular iron, and its serum values are changed when there is an alteration in the metabolism of iron, such as in the neoplastic process.[6,16] An abnormal distribution of ferritin and a reduction of serum iron is found in patients with ovarian cancer.[17] However, ferritin has a low specificity and may be released from several types of malignancies. Therefore, its diagnostic accuracy alone is not useful for the early detection of ovarian cancer, and only in combination with other biomarkers (ie, carcinoembryonic antigen, neuron-specific enolase, cytokeratin 19, α-fetoprotein, carbohydrate antigen-125, and carbohydrate antigen-19.9) may prove valuable for the improvement of diagnosis.[16]

The American College of Obstetrics and Gynecology (ACOG) recommends a multivariable approach for the pre-operative diagnosis of women with suspicious adnexal masses by combining demographic, laboratory, and imaging parameters, as it improves diagnostic accuracy.[6,18] The most common and first-line tool for the diagnosis of pelvic pathology is the abdominal and transvaginal ultrasound. Kosovo clinicians try to stick to these guidelines and approaches given their resources and abilities. Furthermore, various classification systems for the categorization of adnexal masses have been designed, combining ultrasonography with other parameters to differentiate the nature of adnexal masses.[7] However, the most common and easy-to-use predictive model for the assessment of the adnexal masses is the IOTA SR, with a sensitivity of 91% and specificity of 93% for the model.[7,19,20] This technique is easily applicable and can be used by practitioners as well as non-expert examiners trained to use it.[20]

This research article examines whether the combination of tumor markers in preoperative settings with IOTA SR will improve the accurate detection of adnexal masses, particularly ovarian cancer. We predict that this combination will significantly improve diagnostic accuracy in the early detection of ovarian cancer. Therefore, the main objective of this study was to determine the diagnostic accuracy of biochemical and ultrasonography parameters in the early detection of ovarian cancer by comparison with histopathologic diagnosis of adnexal masses after the surgical intervention utilizing data from the University Clinical Center of Kosovo (UCCK). A study of this kind has never been conducted using Kosovo data, and the analysis is crucial in assessing the efficacy of clinical work in the diagnosis of ovarian cancer.

METHODS
Design and Setting

A prospective cross-sectional analysis of a cohort of women with adnexal masses scheduled for surgery was conducted to evaluate the early detection of ovarian cancer by comparing biochemical and ultrasonography parameters with histopathologic diagnosis after the surgical intervention. The data were collected from June 2020 to June 2022 in the Clinic of Obstetrics and Gynecology (COG), Institute of Pathology, and Institute of Biochemistry within the University Clinical Center of Kosovo (UCCK), which is a tertiary health care center affiliated with the University of Prishtina.

A total of 226 female patients participated in this research, all with suspicious adnexal masses. Women selected for this study were evaluated by referring practitioners for elective surgery when conservative treatment failed or was inappropriate. Women were admitted to the surgery and oncology ward after being evaluated by the clinic's panel, comprised of three physician consultants of COG, to establish indications for surgery. The authors of this study were not included in the panel. Following their admission, a history of the disease was taken from the subjects with all the necessary data for our research using a questionnaire. We provided to each study subject information about the aim of the study and methods to be employed, and finally, study subjects were offered and signed an informed consent document. The questionnaire consisted of questions on patients' demographic data, family, lifestyle, and socio-epidemiologic anamnesis. The study was approved by the Ethical Committee of the Faculty of Medicine at the University of Prishtina.

Study Population and Data Collection

The study population included women aged 13 to 84 years with suspicious adnexal masses that were referred to UCCK for surgery. Women with metastatic cancer, subserosal myomas, endometriotic cysts, ectopic pregnancy, tubo-ovarian abscesses, and ruptured or twisted cysts were ineligible for the study. Surgical intervention for the removal of adnexal masses was carried out in COG. Techniques and surgical procedures were selected and conducted based on medical indications. Treatment involved laparotomic cystectomy, oophorectomy, hysterectomy, and debulking surgery. Specimens were taken during the surgery and put in formaldehyde 10% for fixation and then taken to the Institute of Pathology for further preparation. Samples were then processed and stained with hematoxylin and eosin (H&E), covered with Canada Balsam, and were prepared for microscopic analysis by a pathologist who was blinded in regard to IOTA SR assessment by referring gynecologist.

Pre-surgical assessment and surgical staging were based in International Federation of Gynecology and Obstetrics (FIGO) system for ovarian, fallopian tube, and peritoneal cancer. Histopathologic (HP) diagnosis was assessed based on World Health Organization (WHO) guidelines. Only patients with HP diagnoses were included in the final analysis. Women whose HP reports were not ready or had failed to determine ovarian or tubal tumor were excluded from the study.

Eligible women were examined via ultrasound following hospital admission by assessing the morphology of the adnexal masses with a 2D real-time and color doppler. The assessment included a detailed examination using initially a transabdominal approach and then a transvaginal probe. This was performed before the surgery and histopathologic analysis. Sonographic assessment of the given adnexal masses was performed using a 2 to 5 MHz curved transducer for transabdominal sonography and a transducer with a frequency of 5 to 12 MHz for transvaginal sonography. A power Doppler with a setting of Pulse Repetition Frequency (PRF) 0.3 and a velocity scale of 3 to 6 cm/s was used to score the color flow.

The ultrasound assessment was performed by an expert examiner in a supine position by applying a transabdominal ultrasound probe with a full urinary bladder. After requesting the patient to empty the bladder, an additional vaginal examination was conducted. The examiner was blinded in relation to the clinical presentation and laboratory workup. IOTA SR were used for all tumor types, and in cases of undetermined origin of tumors, MRI was performed to assist in the selection of the surgical method approach for the removal of the tumor. The IOTA group is a multicentric collaboration with the aim of designing models for pre-operative diagnosis of ovarian cancer, which can be used by non-expert ultrasound examiners.[21] IOTA SR, a preoperative classification system for ovarian tumors, consists of five features that categorize tumors as benign, malignant, or inconclusive. Approximately 80% of adnexal masses classified using IOTA SR are found to be benign (B) or malignant (M), with the remaining 20% classified as inconclusive.[19]

B features include unilocular cyst, presence of solid components less than 7 mm in diameter, presence of acoustic shadow, smooth multilocular tumor with the tumor measuring less than 100 mm, and no blood flow on color doppler. M features include irregular solid tumors, the presence of ascites, at least four papillary structures, irregular multilocular solid tumor with the largest diameter greater than 100 mm, and very strong blood flow.[7] If one or more M features were present in the absence of the B features, the tumor was classified as malignant. If one or more B features were present in the absence of M features, the tumor was classified as benign. When both B features and M features were present, or none of the features was present, the mass was considered inconclusive.[8] Tumor size was measured in three dimensions, including the volume, which was calculated in cubic centimeters (cm^3). We also assessed the unilaterality or bilaterally of the tumor.

The following day, peripheral blood was drawn for the measurement of tumor markers. The average time to acquire the blood sample was two days prior to the surgical intervention.

Measurement and Measures Used for Analysis

Blood samples collected from patients were drawn in 10 mL serum tubes and were left to clot at room temperature for at least 30 minutes, then centrifuged at 3000 RPM for 10 minutes. Any sample above the normal range (for ferritin 13–150 ng/mL and for CA125 0–35 U/mL) was considered elevated. Serum ferritin was detected with ElectroChemiLuminescence (ECLIA) Cobas e411 (Roche Diagnostics GmbH) and the correspondent kit (Roche Diagnostics GmbH). Values were expressed in ng/mL. Serum CA125 was detected with Cobas e411 analyzers, using the electrochemiluminescence technique in the Cobas e411 analyzers (Roche Diagnostics GmbH) and correspondent kit (Roche Diagnostics GmbH). Values were expressed in U/mL.

Statistical Analysis

For analytical purposes, tumors in our sample were grouped into five categories (benign, malignant and borderline, only malignant, malignant early stage, that is, stages I and II, and malignant advanced stage, that is, stages II and IV).

To express the distribution of continuous data with normal distribution, we calculated the mean and standard deviation. Normal distribution was determined using a histogram, QQ plot, and Shapiro-Wilk test. For continuous data without normal distribution, we calculated the median and interquartile range. A Welch t-test or a Mann-Whitney U test was used to compare the differences in continuous data as appropriate. Frequencies and percentages were used to describe categorical data. A Chi-square test was used to compare the differences in categorical data between groups, that is, benign versus different categories of malign cancers (malign or borderline, malign only, early stage malign, advanced stage malign). We then calculated malignancy rates comparing IOTA SR with histopathological findings. We calculated the malignancy rate for borderline tumors and malignant tumors, and the malignancy rate for malignant only tumors.

Next, we calculated the Receiver Operating Characteristic (ROC) and Areas Under the Curves (AUC) for CA125, ferritin, IOTA SR, and their combinations which assess and describe the performance of biomarkers and screening tests. The ROC curve is a graphical representation that illustrates the trade-off between sensitivity and specificity for different cut-off values of a test and allows us to determine the ability of the score to classify tumors via biomarkers and IOTA SR classification. In this study, we use ROC and AUC analysis to determine the optimal cut-off value for decision-making thresholds of IOTA SR and biomarkers in determining the malignancy of adnexal masses. By using the AUC, we can compare different biomarkers or other diagnostic tests and assess their ability to distinguish between patients with the disease and those without the disease.

The AUC, which ranges from 0 to 1, quantifies the overall discriminative ability of a test. A higher AUC indicates better discrimination and suggests that the test has a higher ability to correctly classify patients as either having the disease or not having the disease. An AUC value over 0.9 indicates a high clinical diagnostic value. We performed this calculation for each set of group comparisons, that is, benign versus malignant and borderline, benign versus only malignant, benign versus malignant early stage, and benign versus malignant advanced stage. We used histopathological results as a reference for all ROC analyses. Statistical analyses were performed with STATA 17BE (Stata Corp).

RESULTS
Pathologic Diagnosis of Adnexal Masses and Ultrasound Classification

The final pathologic diagnosis of adnexal masses, final ultrasound classification, and clinical characteristics of the tumors are described in **Table 1**. Out of a total of 226 women included in our analysis, 52 women (23%) had malignant early and advanced stage ovarian tumors, 160 women (70.8%) had benign tumors, and 14 women (6.2%) were designated as borderline.

In total, 201, or 88.9% of women in the cohort, were correctly classified. 92.5% of women with suspected benign tumors were correctly classified, 50% of women with borderline tumors were correctly classified. Out of 52 malignant tumors, based on final pathologic diagnosis, 30 were at the early malignant stage, out of which 26 (86.7%) were correctly classified, and 22 were at the malignant advanced stage, out of which 20 (90.9%) were correctly classified. The most common histologic type among 52 malignant tumors was serous adenocarcinoma which was observed in 28 (53.8%) cases.

Table 1
Final pathologic diagnosis of adnexal masses and their final ultrasound classification

Histologic Type	Total		Correctly Classified	
	n	%	n	%
Benign	*160*	*100.0*	*148*	*92.5*
Brenner tumor	1	0.6	1	100.0
Cystadenofibroma	13	8.1	12	92.3
Fibroma	8	5.0	5	62.5
Fibrothecoma	8	5.0	1	12.5
Functional cysts	40	25.0	40	100.0
Mucinous cystadenoma	25	15.6	24	96.0
Myolipoma	1	0.6	1	100.0
Serous cystadenoma	43	26.9	43	100.0
Struma ovarii	2	1.3	2	100.0
Teratoma	19	11.9	19	100.0
Borderline	*14*	*100.0*	*7*	*50.0*
Mucinous borderline tumor	9	64.3	5	55.6
Mucinous cystadenoma	1	7.1	0	0.0
Serous borderline tumor	4	28.6	2	50.0
Malign early stage	*30*	*100.0*	*26*	*86.7*
Clear cell carcinoma	1	3.3	0	0.0
Endometrioid adenocarcinoma	3	10.0	3	100.0
Fibrosarcoma	1	3.3	1	100.0
Granulosa cell tumor	6	20.0	3	50.0
Immature teratoma	1	3.3	1	100.0
Malignant Brenner tumor	1	3.3	1	100.0
Mucinous adenocarcinoma	3	10.0	3	100.0
Serous adenocarcinoma	12	40.0	12	100.0
Sertoli-Leydig cell tumor	1	3.3	1	100.0
Squamos cell carcinoma	1	3.3	1	100.0
Malign advanced stage	*22*	*100.0*	*20*	*90.9*
Endometrioid adenocarcinoma	3	13.6	3	100.0
Malignant Mullerian tube mixed tumor	1	4.5	0	0.0
Mucinous adenocarcinoma	2	9.1	2	100.0
Serous adenocarcinoma	16	72.7	15	93.8
Total	*226*	*100.0*	*201*	*88.9*

Sample Characteristics

Table 2 shows clinical characteristics, biomarkers, and features of the IOTA SR among the cohort of women. The rates of tumor categorization between IOTA SR classifications were significant in all comparison groups. In the benign group, 86 (53.8%) of tumors were epithelial, 16 (10.0%) were stromal, 21 (13.1%) were germ cell, and 37 (23.1%) were tumor-like lesions. In the malign cancer group, 42 (80.8%) of cancers were epithelial, 8 (15.4%) were stromal, and 2 (3.8%) were germ cell. Bilateral location of tumors was found in 5 (3.1%) out of 160 benign tumors and 22 (42.3%) out of 52 malignant tumors.

Malignancy Rates

Table 3 compares malignancy rates according to IOTA SR with findings based on histopathology for a subset of women in the original cohort. Of 160 women diagnosed with benign tumors according to histopathological results, IOTA SR classified 145 of them (90.6%) as benign. Of 52 women diagnosed with malign tumors according to histopathological results, IOTA SR classified 46 (88.5%) them as malign. Malignancy rates found by IOTA SR overall were similar to histopathological-concluded malignant cases.

Diagnostic Performance of Biomarkers and International Ovarian Tumor Analysis Simple Rules

ROC analysis for each set of group comparisons, that is, benign versus malignant and borderline, benign versus only malignant, benign versus malignant early stage, and benign versus malignant advanced stage, is presented in **Table 4**, **Fig. 1**, and Online Appendix.

The ROC curve showed that the best cutoff value for CA125 in distinguishing benign from malignant or borderline adnexal masses was ≥ 40.8 and ≥ 75.0 for ferritin. The AUCs for the CA125, ferritin, and IOTA SR in discriminating benign from malignant or borderline adnexal masses were 0.881 (95% CI, 0.823–0.938), 0.710 (95% CI, 0.638–0.782) and 0.929 (95% CI, 0.888–0.971), respectively (see **Table 4**). In addition, the sensitivity of CA125, ferritin, and IOTA SR was 83.33%, 65.08% and 75.76%, respectively, and their specificity was 84.38%, 63.46% and 97.50%, respectively, while their accuracy was 84.07%, 63.93% and 91.15%, respectively (see **Table 4**). Moreover, ROC analysis showed that a combination of CA125 and IOTA SR had a larger AUC than the combination of CA125 and ferritin or the combination of CA125, ferritin, and IOTA SR (0.962 vs 0.892 and 0.957, respectively, see **Fig. 1**).

The best cutoff value for CA125 in distinguishing benign from malignant only adnexal masses was ≥ 63.4 and ≥ 119.9 for ferritin. The AUCs for the CA125, ferritin, and IOTA SR in discriminating benign from malignant only adnexal masses were 0.895 (95% CI, 0.831–0.959), 0.775 (95% CI, 0.707–0.843) and 0.942 (95% CI, 0.899–0.985), respectively (see **Table 4**). In addition, the sensitivity of CA125, ferritin, and IOTA SR was 84.62%, 67.35% and 88.46%, respectively, and their specificity was 88.13%, 75.00% and 97.50%, respectively, while their accuracy was 87.26%, 73.17% and 95.28%, respectively (see **Table 4**). Moreover, ROC analysis showed that a combination of CA125 and IOTA SR had a larger AUC than the combination of CA125 and ferritin or the combination of CA125, ferritin, and IOTA SR (0.969 vs 0.915 and 0.964, respectively, Online Appendix). Results follow similar trends for early stage and advanced stage cancers versus benign comparisons, with advanced stage AUC being the highest (Online Appendix).

Table 2
Sample characteristics

	Benign (n = 160)		Malign or Borderline (n = 66)			Malign (n = 52)			Early Stage (n = 30)			Advanced Stage (n = 22)		
	n	%	n	%	P value	n	%	P value	n	%	P value	n	%	P value
Age (years)[a]	42.14	17.60	53.95	13.27	<0.001	55.79	10.57	<0.001	54.40	11.42	<0.001	57.68	9.19	<0.001
Urban residence	92	57.5	30	45.5	0.099	25	48.1	0.235	16	53.3	0.672	9	40.9	0.142
Married	110	68.8	57	86.4	0.006	46	88.5	0.005	27	90.0	0.017	19	86.4	0.088
Body-Mass Index					0.046			0.050			0.413			0.070
Underweight	5	3.1	1	1.5		1	1.9		1	3.3		0	0.0	
Normal	63	39.4	14	21.2		10	19.2		7	23.3		3	13.6	
Overweight	44	27.5	26	39.4		21	40.4		11	36.7		10	45.5	
Obese	48	30.0	25	37.9		20	38.5		11	36.7		9	40.9	
Age at menarch (years)[a]	13.58	1.58	14.05	1.55	0.044	14.04	1.61	0.077	14.07	1.82	0.179	14.00	1.31	0.181
Nulliparae	62	38.8	10	15.2	0.001	6	11.5	<0.001	3	10.0	0.002	3	13.6	0.021
Premenopause	104	65.0	25	37.9	<0.001	17	32.7	<0.001	10	33.3	0.001	7	31.8	0.003
Oral contraceptives intake	13	8.1	4	6.1	0.920	4	7.7	0.593	3	10.0	0.734	1	4.5	0.555
Previous history of ovarian cancer	6	3.8	11	16.7	0.001	9	17.3	0.001	5	16.7	0.005	4	18.2	0.005
Previous history of breast cancer	11	6.9	11	16.7	0.024	9	17.3	0.025	3	10.0	0.548	6	27.3	0.002
Existing conditions	46	28.8	35	53.0	0.001	30	57.7	<0.001	16	53.3	0.008	14	63.6	0.001
Tubal ligation	7	4.4	0	0.0	0.125	0	0.0	0.084	0	0.0	0.243	0	0.0	0.317
CA125[b]	19.1	12.3 (28.4)	209.3	63.4 (539.0)	<0.001	335.7	84.9 (943.8)	<0.001	193.2	34.9 (389.0)	<0.001	540.2	390.1 (2934.0)	<0.001
Ferritin[b]	52.8	29.8 (119.6)	126.0	58.2 (229.0)	<0.001	163.6	78.7 (238.1)	<0.001	151.0	69.7 (217.4)	<0.001	181.1	78.7 (245.5)	<0.001
Bilateral location of tumor	5	3.1	24	36.4	<0.001	22	42.3	<0.001	9	30.0	<0.001	13	59.1	<0.001

	Total	Group 1	p	Group 2	p	Group 3	p	Group 4	p
Volume of tumor (cm3)[b]	215.8 116.0 474.8	437.0 160.8 962.8	0.001	370.6 153.1 702.2	0.024	344.3 130.4 742.2	0.101	406.8 178.2 591.4	0.073
IOTA Simple Rules classification			<0.001		<0.001		<0.001		<0.001
Benign	145 90.6	6 9.1		4 7.7		3 10.0		1 4.5	
Inconclusive	11 6.9	10 15.2		2 3.8		1 3.3		1 4.5	
Malign	4 2.5	50 75.8		46 88.5		26 86.7		20 90.9	
Histologic type			<0.001		<0.001		0.003		0.001
Epithelial	86 53.8	56 84.8		42 80.8		20 66.7		22 100.0	
Stromal	16 10.0	8 12.1		8 15.4		8 26.7		0 0.0	
Germ cell	21 13.1	2 3.0		2 3.8		2 6.7		0 0.0	
Tumor-like lesion	37 23.1	0 0.0		0 0.0		0 0.0		0 0.0	

Abbreviations: CA125, carbohydrate antigen; IOTA, the international ovarian tumor analysis.
[a] Mean and Standard Deviation.
[b] Median and Inter Quartile Range.

Table 3
Malignancy rates in comparison of IOTA Simple Rules with histopathological findings

Histopathology →	Benign (n = 160)		Malign or Borderline (n = 66)		Malign (n = 52)		Malignancy rate[a]	Malignancy Rate
	n	%	n	%	n	%	%	%
IOTA Simple Rules classification								
Benign	145	90.6	6	9.1	4	7.7	4.0	2.7
Inconclusive	11	6.9	10	15.2	2	3.8	47.6	15.4
Malign	4	2.5	50	75.8	46	88.5	92.6	92.0

[a] Inclusive of border line tumors.

Table 4
Efficacy of CA125, ferritin and IOTA Simple Rules

	AUC	95% CI		Sensitivity (%)	Specificity (%)	PPV	NPV	Accuracy (%)
Malign or borderline vs benign								
CA125	0.881	0.823	0.938	83.33	84.38	68.75	92.47	84.07
Ferritin	0.710	0.638	0.782	65.08	63.46	41.84	81.82	63.93
IOTA	0.929	0.888	0.971	75.76	97.50	92.59	90.70	91.15
Malign vs benign								
CA125	0.895	0.831	0.959	84.62	88.13	69.84	94.63	87.26
Ferritin	0.775	0.707	0.843	67.35	75.00	45.83	87.97	73.17
IOTA	0.942	0.899	0.985	88.46	97.50	92.00	96.30	95.28
Early stage vs benign								
CA125	0.820	0.712	0.927	73.33	88.13	53.66	94.63	85.79
Ferritin	0.756	0.671	0.841	74.07	66.03	27.40	93.64	67.21
IOTA	0.926	0.861	0.992	86.67	97.50	86.67	97.50	95.79
Advanced stage vs benign								
CA125	0.988	0.975	1.000	95.45	95.63	75.00	99.35	95.60
Ferritin	0.797	0.708	0.887	72.73	75.00	29.09	95.12	74.72
IOTA	0.961	0.912	1.000	90.91	97.50	83.33	98.73	96.70

Abbreviations: AUC, area under the curve; CA125, carbohydrate antigen; IOTA, the international ovarian tumor analysis; NPV, negative predictive value; PPV, positive predictive value.

DISCUSSION

This study demonstrates that using IOTA SR in combination with CA125 and ferritin can improve the accuracy of preoperative diagnosis in differentiating between malignant and benign tumors in women with adnexal masses who are scheduled for elective surgery. This combined approach is particularly useful in cases where there is no experienced sonographer available to provide a subjective evaluation of the masses, thereby ensuring a more accurate assessment.[5] IOTA SR combined with biomarker

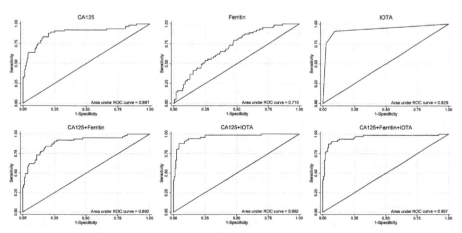

Fig. 1. ROC analysis of CA125, Ferritin, IOTA and their combinations for malign or borderline versus benign diagnosis.

indications increased the diagnostic accuracy of classifying adnexal masses. Data analysis of individual measures implicate ferritin with the lowest rate of sensitivity. The study results indicated that IOTA SR was more effective than CA125 and ferritin alone in diagnosing adnexal masses before surgery.

Strengths and Limitations

The strength of this study rests in analyzing the ROC curve for the combination of IOTA SR with tumor biomarkers, an approach that resulted in a higher discriminatory power than each diagnostic test individually. Such an approach could provide more clinical utility compared to using IOTA SR or biomarkers alone. Our ROC curve analysis allows for a comprehensive assessment of the diagnostic performance and helps identify the optimal diagnostic performance for the combined approach. Additionally, including almost every histologic type of ovarian tumor in our study enhances its generalizability and applicability to a wider range of patients. This comprehensive approach ensures that the findings can be relevant and informative for the diagnosis and management of various ovarian tumor subtypes. The use of both abdominal and vaginal ultrasonography for detecting ovarian masses is another strength of our study. This dual approach increases the chances of early detection and facilitates a more accurate assessment of ovarian masses. Vaginal ultrasonography, in particular, is known to provide better visualization and characterization of the ovaries, especially in cases where the masses are small or located deep within the pelvis. By leveraging these strengths, our study provides valuable insights into the combined approach of IOTA SR with tumor markers, offering a more comprehensive and accurate diagnostic strategy for the detection and characterization of ovarian masses. The main limitation of the study is the small sample size which limits the generalizability of the findings.

Context, Interpretation, and Implications

The prevalence of malignancy in similar studies, reporting IOTA Simple Rules for diagnosis of ovarian cancer, ranged from 10% to 44%.[22–26] Additionally, the study sizes varied considerably, with the number of women included ranging from 103 to 1938.[22] This diversity in study sizes reflects the varying sample populations and the inclusion of different cohorts of women with adnexal masses. It's worth noting that the wide range in prevalence and study sizes may be attributed to several factors, including differences in patient demographics, study designs, and geographic locations.[22] Considering these differences, it is important to interpret the results of individual studies within their specific context and consider the overall body of evidence when drawing conclusions or making clinical decisions. In our study, a sample of 226 women was included, with 52 having malignant tumors and 160 having benign tumors. The malignancy rate was 23% (see **Table 3**). When applying the IOTA SR criteria in ultrasound examinations, the sensitivity and specificity were found to be 88.4% and 97.5%, respectively, compared to 92% and 96% in the original IOTA study.[19] Other studies demonstrated similar results. For example, a prospective study conducted in the UK with a malignancy rate of 24.8% showed a sensitivity of 87% and specificity of 98% when applying the IOTA SR criteria.[27] Another prospective study conducted by Tantipalakorn and colleagues included 398 adnexal masses, with the IOTA SR applicable in 319 cases. The sensitivity and specificity were reported as 82.9% and 95.3%, respectively, with 19.9% of masses yielding inconclusive results.[28] A study in Spain reported a lower malignancy rate of 12.2% and demonstrated a sensitivity of 87.9% and specificity of 97.5%.[29] Fathallah and colleagues reported a malignancy rate of 11.5% in their study, with a sensitivity of 73% and specificity of 97% when applying the IOTA SR criteria.[30] This lower sensitivity may be attributed to the low malignancy rate in their sample. A study in Thailand involving 100 patients reported a sensitivity of 89.3% and specificity of 83.3% when using the IOTA Simple Rules.[28]

Overall, the findings from our study and other studies suggest that the IOTA SR criteria show promise in accurately diagnosing adnexal masses with generally high sensitivity and specificity. This will be important for low middle or upper middle income countries which can possess technology to use IOTA SR criteria as compared to other advanced tumor diagnostics technology which can be more expensive (ie, MRI). Provision of basic technology with proper capacity building to use IOTA SR may be the way forward. However, variations in malignancy rates and study populations can influence the performance of the criteria in different settings. It is indeed important to consider alternative options when the IOTA SR yield inconclusive results for adnexal tumors.[31] In our study, 6.9% of benign tumor cases and 3.8% of malignant tumor cases had inconclusive diagnoses using the IOTA SR criteria. This indicates that, in these cases, the criteria did not provide a clear distinction between benign and malignant tumors. When facing inconclusive results with the IOTA SR, it is necessary to consider alternative diagnostic approaches. In our case, we recommended referring patients for MRI examination to further clarify the nature of the adnexal masses. However, further research is needed before adopting this as a standardized protocol. By conducting additional studies, researchers can evaluate the effectiveness and reliability of MRI as an alternative diagnostic tool in cases where the IOTA SR criteria are inconclusive.[31] This ongoing research will help establish evidence-based protocols and guidelines for the management of adnexal masses, particularly in situations where the initial diagnostic criteria do not provide definitive results. It is important to note that the AUC values can vary across different studies due to variations in study populations, sample sizes, and other factors. Nonetheless, the consistent finding across these studies is that IOTA SR demonstrates good to strong discriminatory power in distinguishing between malignant and benign adnexal masses.

SUMMARY

The IOTA Simple Rules demonstrate high diagnostic performance in distinguishing between benign and malignant adnexal masses. They achieve a correct classification rate of approximately 95.28% for adnexal masses, which is superior to the performance of tumor biomarkers alone. However, when combined with CA125 and ferritin, the IOTA SR criteria further enhance the diagnostic accuracy in the early detection of ovarian cancer. The combination of these strategies leads to a significant improvement in the ability to differentiate between benign and malignant masses, providing clinicians with a more reliable tool for early diagnosis and appropriate management of ovarian cancer.

CLINICS CARE POINTS

- The IOTA Simple Rules demonstrate high diagnostic performance in distinguishing between benign and malignant adnexal masses.
- This is important for lower or upper middle income countries which possess technology to use IOTA Simple Rules criteria.
- IOTA Simple Rules in combination with CA125 and ferritin can improve the accuracy of preoperative diagnosis in differentiating between malignant and benign tumors in women with adnexal masses who are scheduled for elective surgery.

CONTRIBUTION STATEMENT

T.I. Haliti developed the idea for the study. T.I. Haliti and I. Hoxha designed the study. T.I. Haliti collected the data. I. Hoxha performed the data analysis. T.I. Haliti drafted the report with the support of I. Hoxha, R. Mandal. All authors critically reviewed the report.

DISCLOSURE

No external funding was received for this study. No potential conflicts of interest were reported.

SUPPLEMENTARY DATA

Supplementary data related to this article can be found online at https://doi.org/10.1016/j.hoc.2023.06.011.

REFERENCES

1. GLOBOCAN 2020: New Global Cancer Data. Available at: https://www.uicc.org/news/globocan-2020-new-global-cancer-data. Accsessed June 1, 2023.
2. Huang J, Chan WC, Ngai CH, et al. on behalf of NCD Global Health Research Group of Association of Pacific Rim Universities. Worldwide Burden, Risk Factors, and Temporal Trends of Ovarian Cancer: A Global Study. Cancers 2022;14(9):2230.
3. Rampes S, Choy SP. Early diagnosis of symptomatic ovarian cancer in primary care in the UK: opportunities and challenges. Prim Health Care Res Dev 2022; 23:e52.
4. Bast Robert C, Lu Zhen, Han Chae Young, et al. Biomarkers and Strategies for Early Detection of Ovarian Cancer. Cancer Epidemiol Biomarkers Prev 2020; 29(12):2504–12.
5. Phinyo P, Patumanond J, Saenrungmuaeng P, et al. Diagnostic Added-Value of Serum CA-125 on the IOTA Simple Rules and Derivation of Practical Combined Prediction Models (IOTA SR X CA-125). Diagnostics 2021;11(2):173.
6. Zhao J, Guo N, Zhang L, et al. Serum CA125 in combination with ferritin improves diagnostic accuracy for epithelial ovarian cancer. Br J Biomed Sci 2018;75(2):66–70.
7. Solanki V, Singh P, Sharma C, et al. Predicting malignancy in adnexal masses by the international ovarian tumor analysis-simple rules. J Mid-life Health 2020;11:217–23.
8. Hartman CA, Juliato CR, Sarian LO, et al. Ultrasound criteria and CA 125 as predictive variables of ovarian cancer in women with adnexal tumors. Ultrasound Obstet Gynecol 2012;40(3):360–6.
9. Terzic M, Dotlic J, Likic I, et al. Current diagnostic approach to patients with adnexal masses: Which tools are relevant in routine praxis? Chinese journal of cancer research = Chung-kuo yen cheng yen chiu 2013;25:55–62.
10. Yang D, Li H, Sun X, et al. Clinical usefulness of high levels of C-reactive protein for diagnosing epithelial ovarian cancer. Sci Rep 2020;10(1). 20056.
11. Mulisya O, Sikakulya FK, Mastaki M, et al. The Challenges of Managing Ovarian Cancer in the Developing World. Case Reports in Oncological Medicine 2020. https://doi.org/10.1155/2020/8379628. 8379628.
12. Hoxha I, Islami DA, Uwizeye G, et al. Forty-Five Years of Research and Progress in Breast Cancer: Progress for Some, Disparities for Most. JCO Glob Oncol 2022; 8:e2100424. https://doi.org/10.1200/GO.21.00424.
13. National Public Health Institute of Kosovo. Available at: https://niph-rks.org/. Accesed June 1, 2023.

14. Islami DA, Breast Cancer. Prishtina, Kosovo. October 2019;25:2019.
15. Oncology Clinic . Available at: www.shskuk.rks-gov.net. Accsessed June 1, 2023.
16. Li X, Lu J, Ren H, et al. Combining multiple serum biomarkers in tumor diagnosis: A clinical assessment. Mol Clin Oncol 2013;1(1):153–60.
17. Jiang J, Wang S, Zhang L, et al. Characteristics of the Distribution of Ferritin in Epithelial Ovarian Tumor Patients: Results of a Retrospective, Observational Study. Yangtze Medicine 2018;2:51–61.
18. American College of Obstetricians and Gynecologists' Committee on Practice Bulletins—Gynecology. Practice Bulletin No. 174: Evaluation and Management of Adnexal Masses. Obstet Gynecol 2016;128(5):e210–26.
19. Timmerman D, Planchamp F, Bourne T, et al. ESGO/ISUOG/IOTA/ESGE Consensus Statement on preoperative diagnosis of ovarian tumors. Ultrasound Obstet Gynecol 2021;58:148–68.
20. Abramowicz JS, Timmerman D. Ovarian mass–differentiating benign from malignant: the value of the International Ovarian Tumor Analysis ultrasound rules. Am J Obstet Gynecol 2017;217(6):652–60.
21. Xie WT, Wang YQ, Xiang ZS, et al. Efficacy of IOTA simple rules, O-RADS, and CA125 to distinguish benign and malignant adnexal masses. J Ovarian Res 2022;15(1):15.
22. Nunes N, Ambler G, Foo X, et al. Use of IOTA simple rules for diagnosis of ovarian cancer: meta-analysis. Ultrasound Obstet Gynecol 2014;44(5):503–14.
23. Van Calster B, Timmerman D, Bourne T, et al. Discrimination between benign and malignant adnexal masses by specialist ultrasound examination versus serum CA-125. J Natl Cancer Inst 2007;99(22):1706–14.
24. Crestani A, Theodore C, Levaillant JM, et al. Magnetic Resonance and Ultrasound Fusion Imaging to Characterise Ovarian Masses: A Feasibility Study. Anticancer Res 2020;40(7):4115–21.
25. Timmerman D, Ameye L, Fischerova D, et al. Simple ultrasound rules to distinguish between benign and malignant adnexal masses before surgery: prospective validation by IOTA group. BMJ 2010;341:c6839.
26. Shetty J, Saradha A, Pandey D, et al. IOTA Simple Ultrasound Rules for Triage of Adnexal Mass: Experience from South India. J Obstet Gynaecol India 2019;69(4): 356–62.
27. Sayasneh A, Kaijser J, Preisler J, et al. A multicenter prospective external validation of the diagnostic performance of IOTA simple descriptors and rules to characterize ovarian masses. Gynecol Oncol 2013;130(1):140–6.
28. Tantipalakorn C, Wanapirak C, Khunamornpong S, et al. IOTA simple rules in differentiating between benign and malignant ovarian tumors. Asian Pac J Cancer Prev 2014;15(13):5123–6.
29. Alcázar JL, Pascual MÁ, Olartecoechea B, et al. IOTA simple rules for discriminating between benign and malignant adnexal masses: prospective external validation. Ultrasound Obstet Gynecol 2013;42(4):467–71.
30. Fathallah K, Huchon C, Bats AS, et al. Validation externe des critères de Timmerman sur une série de 122 tumeurs ovariennes [External validation of simple ultrasound rules of Timmerman on 122 ovarian tumors]. Gynecol Obstet Fertil 2011; 39(9):477–81. French.
31. Bernardin L, Dilks P, Liyanage S, et al. Effectiveness of semi-quantitative multiphase dynamic contrast-enhanced MRI as a predictor of malignancy in complex adnexal masses: radiological and pathological correlation. Eur Radiol 2012;22: 880–90.

Moving?

Make sure your subscription moves with you!

To notify us of your new address, find your **Clinics Account Number** (located on your mailing label above your name), and contact customer service at:

Email: journalscustomerservice-usa@elsevier.com

800-654-2452 (subscribers in the U.S. & Canada)
314-447-8871 (subscribers outside of the U.S. & Canada)

Fax number: 314-447-8029

Elsevier Health Sciences Division
Subscription Customer Service
3251 Riverport Lane
Maryland Heights, MO 63043

*To ensure uninterrupted delivery of your subscription, please notify us at least 4 weeks in advance of move.